Psychosocial Interventions for Health and Well-Being

Girishwar Misra
Editor

Psychosocial Interventions for Health and Well-Being

Springer

Editor
Girishwar Misra
Mahatma Gandhi Antarrashtriya Hindi Vishwavidyalaya
Wardha
India

ISBN 978-81-322-3780-8 ISBN 978-81-322-3782-2 (eBook)
https://doi.org/10.1007/978-81-322-3782-2

Library of Congress Control Number: 2018930128

Printed on acid-free paper

This Springer imprint is published by the registered company Springer Nature India Private Limited
The registered company address is: 7th Floor, Vijaya Building, 17 Barakhamba Road, New Delhi 110 001, India

Foreword

The mass of men lead lives of quiet desperation. What is called resignation is confirmed desperation... A stereotyped but unconscious despair is concealed even under what are called games of amusement and amusements of mankind. But it is a characteristic of wisdom not to do desperate things.

Henry David Thoreau, *Walden* (August 9, 1854)

The Conditions for Human Health and Well-Being Reside in the Psycho-social Contexts of Life ©

Introduction

I call upon the timeless words of Henry David Thoreau, a nineteenth-century student of Ralph Waldo Emerson (1803–1882), to open this article on the critical consequences of the sociocultural context for human health and well-being. It is, perhaps, coincidental that this year is Thoreau's 200th year anniversary, a reminder of the enduring power of great thoughts and words. Guide me, Sir!

I offer only a few lines of Thoreau's words as an epigram, insufficient to honour the timelessness of his thoughts, but perhaps sufficient to acknowledge his special sensitivities to the human condition of his age and our age. Thoreau's entire works deserve reading. The unfolding industrial age in which he lived, was the source of problems paralleling the problems of our unfolding socio-technical age.

I can think of no better guide to justify the thoughts and words of this article. In so many ways, we have forgotten the tragic consequences of the psychosocial contexts of life for the human condition; we have become infatuated with 'reductionism', a wondrous gift of technological progress, but a distraction from the realities of human nature.

No one can deny the sheer wonder and glory of our growing knowledge of the central nervous system (CNS), brain, organs and genetics. Yet, the magnificence of our knowledge must not detract from our understanding the socioenvironmental determinants of our life milieu. Political powers, controlling funding have called for various national initiatives: 'Decade of the Brain'.

Similar initiatives, however, for increasing awareness of psychosocial topics have too hidden agendas (see TV documentary: *America's War on Drugs*, http://www.history.com/Shows/Americas-war-on-drugs). On the surface, they appear to be noble in their intent, a massive government effort to address the endemic drug problems, including enhanced criminal prosecution. However, hidden agendas supported arms deals, racial oppression and disguised foreign-relations policies.

Recall, proposals by President Nixon and President Reagan resulted in imprisonment of vast numbers of African-American offenders, even for minor offenses; Recall also, billions of dollars generated by illegal drugs funded government oppression of insurgents in Central America, and kept pro-USA governments in power. We reap the consequences of these corrupt efforts today in the epidemic opiate disorders and deaths.

Psychosocial Contexts

Kurt Lewin (1890–1947), one of psychology's great thinkers, contended behaviour is a function of the interaction of organism and environment ($B = O \times E$). It is the interaction of an organism and its milieu which generates behavior, and the problems of disease and disorder. Nothing exists apart from its inner and outer singular milieu. Although physicists may disagree, nothing exists in a vacuum! Life is connections.

As we become increasingly, and deservedly, awed by reductionist discoveries and revelations, and as we seek insights, answers, and solutions to major human problems within reductionist levels, we are failing to address and resolve the challenges of the psychosocial context of our lives. The psychosocial context is the life context in the behaviour equation. The psychosocial context has critical implications and consequences for health and well-being. It is a formative cause of problems, a precipitating, an exacerbating cause and a maintaining cause. The psychosocial context requires careful attention and understanding in all of the causal relations (Fig. 1).

The challenge of first grasping a causal pattern and then of disentangling its pattern for intervention is difficult, and serves as a deterrent even to well-intentioned social and political activists and officials. How much easier is it to simply turn to a pill to change a brain?

We may be excessively concerned and preoccupied with the physical aspects of our being, even to the extent of dividing solutions into medical specialties, sub-specialties, and sub-sub specialties. We journey across limb, organ, cell, gene, atom and molecular space; this journey has proven miraculous for many diseases and disorders. However, this journey alone cannot address nor resolve the tolls

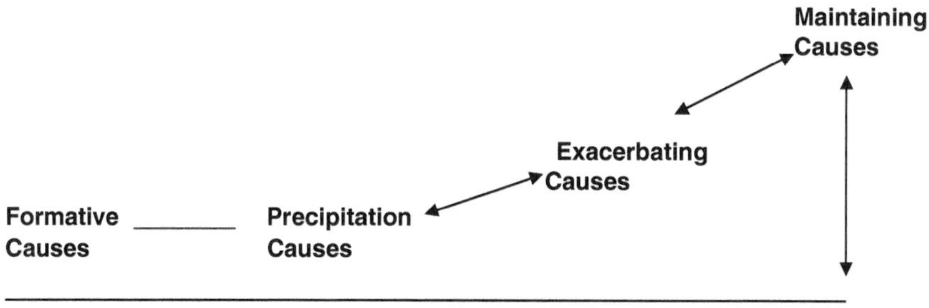

Fig. 1 Multi-dimensional causality: the complex ecology of causal relations

exacted on human health and well-being forged and sustained within the psychosocial contexts of our lives.

There are many empirical and theoretical reasons concluding many diseases, disorders, dysfunctions, deviancies, and distress arise from the psychosocial contexts of our life than from our body alone. Indeed, the experiences forged and sustained in the psychosocial contexts shape and generate many of these tragic 'D' words as the body and mind become war zones for survival struggles—lives of 'quiet desperation'.

Today, humans seek respite and relief from 'desperation' in prescription pills, illegal drugs and substances, and/or both. Pills and substances are often temporary palliatives, unable to treat and heal the broader destructive contexts of human life, located in the 'isms', poverty, violence, war and oppression.

There can be no doubt pills and substances alter behaviour via neurochemistry and anatomical structure. However, seeking solutions to the determinants of problems requires solutions appropriate to the level generating them and their consequences. Tragically, psychosocial contexts, though obvious, are too often ignored. These are big problems! Too often local, national and international leaders yield to the preferences of the wealthy, powerful and positioned. The result is the 'medicalization' of society and human existence. Abuse of power by those in power is history's story! It is said it is inevitable. The phrase 'Absolute power corrupts, absolutely is well known', and is now visibly apparent.

Many noble minds and hearts sought to awaken humanity to the psychosocial sources of their problems (e.g., Gandhi, Martin Luther King, Jr., Cesar Chavez, Nelson Mandela, President John Fitzgerald Kennedy), but those in power, continue to dominate, 'tossing bones of solace' to reaching hands. Today the world is gifted by many new heroic stalwarts, who are advancing peace and social justice (e.g., Mairead McGuire, Michael Knox, Antonio de Rosa, Glenn Paige and numerous others). The struggle, however, is endless, and requires a person become a social and political activist. As has been suggested by many, today's situation requires us to merge personal, occupational and civic lives; there must be a fusion or a

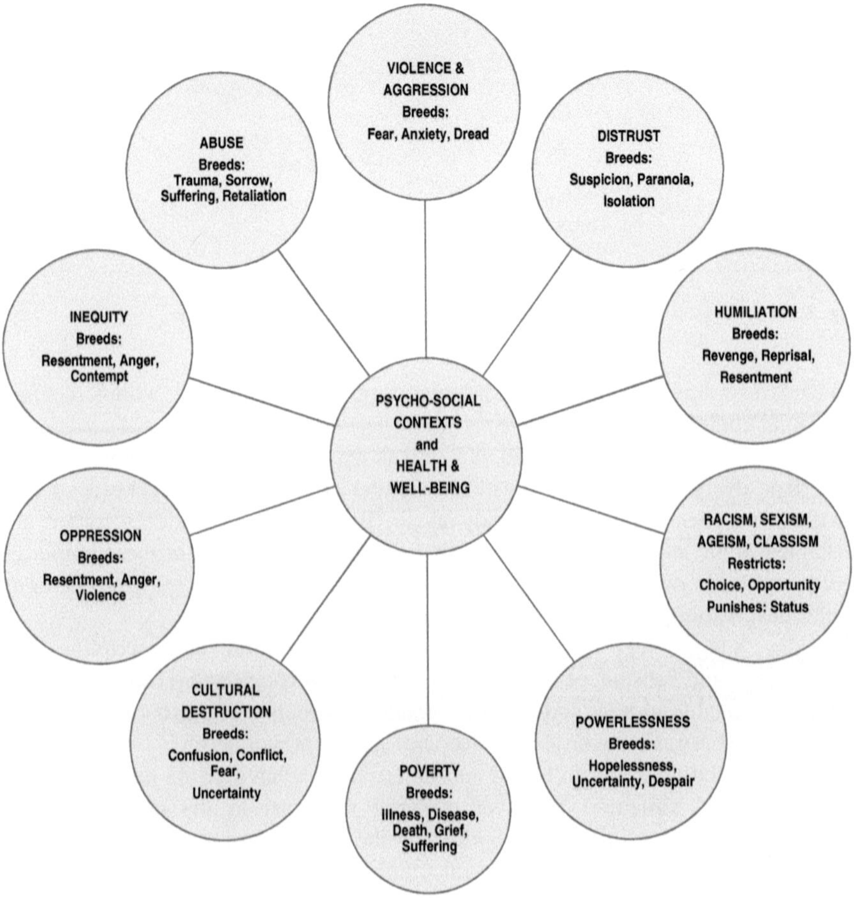

Fig. 2 Psychosocial contexts for health and well-being

gathering of 'self'. In two previous publications with the Transcend Media Service,[1] I suggested a number of psychosocial contexts determining health and well-being. These conditions and contexts, as well as others, are displayed in Fig. 2 and Table 1, along with suggestions of the human responses and conditions they breed and nurture.

The material in Fig. 2 is also offered in tabular form in Box 1. Readers may use either or both for purposes of teaching and other activities. Box 1 offers a few more assertions than Fig. 1 because of space limitations.

[1] See A.J. Marsella September 17, 2012: www.http://transcend.org/…/the-conditions-for-human-health-and-well-being-reside-in-the-psychosocial-contexts-of-life/; and A.J. Marsella, July 17, 2017: www.http://transcend.org/…/the conditions for human health and well-being reside in the psycho-social-contexts of life/.

Box 1: Psychosocial Contexts for Health and Wellbeing

We cannot have health and well-being where there is ***cultural destruction***, for this breeds **confusion, conflict, fear, and uncertainty**;

We cannot have health and well-being where there is ***oppression***, for this breeds **resentment, anger and violence**;

We cannot have health and well-being where there is ***powerlessness***, for this breeds **hopelessness, uncertainty and despair**;

We cannot have health and well-being where there is ***poverty***, for this breeds **illness, death, grief, suffering**;

We cannot have health and well-being where there is ***denigration, disdain, and contempt for others***, for this breeds **low self-esteem, worthlessness, identity confusion**;

We cannot have health and well-being where there is ***violence and aggression***, for this breeds **fear, anxiety and dread**;

We cannot have health and well-being where there is ***distrust***, for this breeds **paranoia, suspicion and isolation**;

We cannot have health and well-being where there is ***inequity and inequality***, for this breeds **resentment, anger, contempt**;

We cannot have health and well-being where there is ***humiliation***, for this breeds **revenge, resentment, and reprisal**;

We cannot have health and well-being where there are ***environmental toxins*** **(e.g., lead, mercury, radiation)**, for this breeds **disease, disorder and death**;

We cannot have health and well-being where there are ***tolerated and accepted power asymmetries and physical abuses (e.g., bulling, rape, familial violence)***, for this breeds **fear, injustice, hopelessness, and suicide**;

We cannot have health and well-being where there is ***asymmetric political partisanship***, for this corrupts **legal and moral local, regional and national governmental processes**.

We cannot have health and well-being where there is ***government corporate and military corruption, cronyism, favoritism, nepotism***, for this breeds **societal collapse, citizen and terrorism**.

Complexity, Interactions, Potentiation

There are many more items warranting inclusion, as 'interactions' foster new contexts and complexity. Amidst this challenging 'matrix', it is easy to become pessimistic, to give up on solutions, and to accept forces and fates as destiny. Do not!

As the struggles appear overwhelming, find inspiration and hope from those about you, especially at the local levels, making contributions to peace, justice and dignity. They are the new heroes of our times. Turn to them, model them; release your own heroic impulses, kept too often restrained, as Thoreau notes in the epigraph quoted above, by indifference, fear, and comfort.

There will only be one of you in this lifetime. Small contributions at local levels can escalate to larger contributions as institutions respond. While efforts to address social conditions and contexts are often met with resistance and delays by local officials, sometimes because of political graft and corruption, there are many options for activism.

Gandhi's life and its consequences offer a striking example of the determination of one person to address inequities and injustices of an imperial age. Gandhi's non-violence course was not easy, and many died in the struggle to free India from British domination. Today, there are many options for activism. There are letters to editors, petitions, peaceful protests, community organization, educational materials, newsletters, listservs, speaker bureaus, silent presence at community and government meetings, meetings with government officials, data collection of psychosocial consequences, involvement of teachers, doctors, lawyers and others in key positions. Move beyond 'quiet desperation'. Imagine it! Do it!

Honolulu, USA
2017

Anthony J. Marsella, Ph.D.
Member, TRANSCEND Network for Peace
Development and Environment
Past President Psychologists for Social Responsibility
Emeritus Professor of Psychology
University of Hawaii's Manoa Campus in Honolulu Hawaii; and
Past Director, World Health Organization
Psychiatric Research Center

Contents

Editor and Contributors

About the Editor

Girishwar Misra is Vice-Chancellor of Wardha University, Maharashtra, India. He was previously Professor of Psychology at the University of Delhi and Editor-in-chief of *Psychological Studies* (Springer).

Contributors

Manisha Agarwal Department of Psychology, Banaras Hindu University, Varanasi, India

Jayanti Basu Department of Applied Psychology, University of Calcutta, Kolkata, India

Sipra Basu Kolkata, India

Mahua Bhattacharya Department of Applied Psychology, University of Calcutta, Kolkata, India

Braj Bhushan Department of Humanities and Social Sciences, Indian Institute of Technology, Kanpur, India

Ajit K. Dalal Department of Psychology, Allahabad University, Allahabad, India

Amrita Deb Department of Liberal Arts, Indian Institute of Technology, Hyderabad, Telangana, India

Anubhuti Dubey Department of Psychology, DDU Gorakhpur University, Gorakhpur, India

Baiju Gopal Department of Psychology, CHRIST (Deemed to be University), Bangalore, India

Meena Hariharan Centre for Health Psychology, University of Hyderabad, Hyderabad, India

P. C. Joshi Department of Anthropology, University of Delhi, New Delhi, Delhi, India

S. Kapoor Assistant Professor, Jesus and Mary College, University of Delhi, New Delhi, India

Malavika Kapur National Institute of Advanced Studies, Indian Institute of Science Campus, Bangalore, India

Seema Mehrotra Department of Psychology, Bharathiar University, Coimbatore, India

M. Mehta Formerly Professor of Clinical Psychology Department of Psychiatry, AIIMS, New Delhi, India

Girishwar Misra Mahatma Gandhi Antarrashtriya Hindi Vishwavidyalaya, Wardha, India

Indiwar Misra Department of Psychology, B.R. Ambedkar College, University of Delhi, New Delhi, Delhi, India

Annalakshmi Narayanan Department of Psychology, Bharathiar University, Coimbatore, India

Gadiraju Padmaja Centre for Health Psychology, University of Hyderabad, Hyderabad, India

Nisha Mani Pandey Department of Geriatric Mental Health, King George's Medical University, Lucknow, Uttar Pradesh, India

Raghubir Singh Pirta Department of Psychology, Himachal Pradesh University, Shimla, India

Kumar Ravi Priya Department of Humanities and Social Sciences, Indian Institute of Technology Kanpur, Kanpur, Uttar Pradesh, India

Suvashisa Rana Centre for Health Psychology, University of Hyderabad, Hyderabad, India

Shubha Ranganathan Department of Liberal Arts, Indian Institute of Technology Hyderabad, Kandi, Sangareddy District, Telangana, India

Matangini Samanta Department of Applied Psychology, University of Calcutta, Kolkata, India

T. Sasidharan Department of Psychology, University of Calicut, Malappuram, Kerala, India

Prateeksha Sharma National Academy of Legal Studies and Research (NALSAR), Hyderabad, India

Sagar Sharma Department of Psychology, Panjab University, Chandigarh, India

Arun Pratap Singh Department of Psychology, Mahatma Gandhi Antarrashtriya Hindi Viswavidyalaya, Wardha, India

Shyodan Singh Department of Psychology, Zakir Husain College, University of Delhi, New Delhi, Delhi, India

Tissy Mariam Thomas Department of Psychology, University of Kerala, Thiruvananthapuram, Kerala, India

S. C. Tiwari Department of Geriatric Mental Health, King George's Medical University, Lucknow, Uttar Pradesh, India

Ravikesh Tripathi Institute of Behavioral Sciences, Gujarat Forensic Sciences University, Gandhinagar, Gujarat, India

Bal Krishna Upadhyay Faculty of Human Resource Management, Indian Institute of Forest Management, Bhopal, Madhya Pradesh, India

Nilisha Vashist Department of Anthropology, University of Delhi, New Delhi, Delhi, India

Chapter 1
Introduction: Perspectives on Interventions for Health and Well-Being

Girishwar Misra

The interventions for health promotion have twofold goals: preventing illness and enhancing wellness. Unfortunately, people address more to health breakdowns paying little attention to building resources for health and health maintenance. There is increasing realization among researchers that psychological factors like attitude and behaviour determine an individual's health and well-being; hence, attention to health maintenance including ways of coping with stress, preventing illness and promoting well-being have become crucial. In the wake of technological and socio-economic changes and increasing social mobility, stress factors have escalated. Prolonged or recurring stress causes cardio-vascular diseases, decreased immunity and other ailments; thus effective stress-management has become a necessity. Awareness about the benefits of exercise, biofeedback, yoga and relaxation, social support, spirituality and alternative medicine is gradually rising.

The phenomenon of health cannot be studied in a culture-free manner because its notions and contexts are culturally constructed and sustained. Concepts, theories and applications therefore need to be understood in specific cultural contexts. Also, with the rise in variety and complexity of health hazards there is a growing concern among health researchers about the medical, psychological and social factors that may improve and impair health and well-being of individuals. Their efforts often indicate that health and well-being is one of those few domains which reflect the inherent unity of mind and body; therefore the approach dealing with health problems need to be inclusive, broad in scope and cannot be confined to narrow disciplinary boundaries. Their analysis, therefore, draws from many social, as well as natural science disciplines and an interdisciplinary perspective becomes a must. Similarly it is widely felt that restoring and maintaining health and well-being and taking steps to prevent illness require deploying multipronged strategies.

G. Misra (✉)
Mahatma Gandhi Antarrashtriya Hindi Vishwavidyalaya, Wardha, Maharashtra, India
e-mail: misragirishwar@gmail.com

G. Misra (ed.), *Psychosocial Interventions for Health and Well-Being*,
https://doi.org/10.1007/978-81-322-3782-2_1

Interventions for Health Promotion

Psychosocial interventions in the domain of health and well-being are required as individual human rationality is limited and people's preferences are quite strong and deep seated. In order to prevent problems we need to use diverse modes of interventions. Health problems need to be attended to and treated and the negative labels attached to them should be removed through education. Attempts should also be made to make significant life contexts such as family, school and work more supportive and positive in their approach.

Health promotion involves interventions at many different levels. They range from individual level interventions focusing on health related cognitions, emotions and behaviour patterns through family and group interventions, organizational change interventions and whole community interventions and even to legislations. From the socio-ecological perspective, an integration of micro and macro level health-related intervention programmes offer a better option (Kok et al. 2008). The stakeholders at the higher level include community groups, health-related institutions, work organizations, and health providers. They may develop specific health promotion interventions. It may be noted that integrating interventions at different levels (e.g. individual, organization, community, and society) would prove more effective than organizing separate interventions at one or more levels.

The community-level interventions try to involve people in a geographically defined area in identifying local needs and assets and facilitating actions to create new resources, skills and health promoting behaviour patterns (Abraham et al. 2011). Empowerment and education of the masses is necessary to make them understand and offer health-related advice. In general combined environmental and institutional policy change with theory-based interventions and community involvement in designing community intervention are found most effective (Hingson and Howland 2002). Similarly, work-site interventions for health promotion are also required. The key imperatives of interventions in the area of health are outlined here.

The Cultural Context of Health and Well-Being

A person or community's health as well as abnormalities/pathologies/deviations are being challenged with multiple roots, which need holistic examination. Human lives in totality need to be understood and improved. This is important when we think of 'positive health'. At the same time we should also not forget that health issues are approached in the context of certain meta-theoretical conceptualizations endorsed by people as well as practitioners. They endorse certain views about the concepts of motivation, personality, self, identity, health, pathology and well-being employed in the discourse on health and well-being. Interestingly, these are context-bound concepts which operate within a conceptual network. They are primarily situated in our shared perspective about human nature (Marsella 2009; Marsella & White 1982; Sharma & Sharma 2010a).

Cultural Models of Self

A close perusal of the models of human beings prevalent in Euro-American psychological perspectives reveals that they often use 'animal', 'unique being' and 'machine' as metaphors of human functioning (Weiner 1992). A more inclusive view considers human beings as divine and spiritual (Rao and Paranjpe 2016). It situates self differently from its Western counterpart, which is often framed in terms of a 'bounded individual' (Kityama et al. 2007; Markus and Kitayama 1991). A relational orientation is prominent in the Asian context. The social presence of others is considered very important and the boundary between self and others is not sharply demarcated. It is the 'self in relationship with others' which is crucial since the self is relatively less differentiated. A person with relational self responds more to perceptions, social contingencies and obligations (Misra 2013).

The relational self is further supplemented by the quality of 'transcendence'. In the Indian tradition, a human being is conceived as a biopsychosocial-spiritual entity. It is a multilayered entity as reflected in the concept of *panchakosha*s or five sheaths (i.e., *annamaya* or bodily, *pranamaya* or vital, *vigyanamaya* or intellectual, *manomaya* or psychological and *anandamaya* or blissful), and the seven *chakra*s or centres located in the body. Ayurveda, the Indian science of health, also draws attention to the notion of *rashipurusha* or composite being (Misra 2005).

Going Beyond the Biomedical Model

Health/well-being is a complex and multidimensional concept. In this connection, it is pertinent to mention that in 1946 the World Health Organization (WHO) was established by the United Nations and the preamble of its constitution clearly stated that 'health is a state of complete physical, mental and social well-being, and not merely the absence of disease or infirmity'. It implies that health is not a 'default' concept, and is defined as a positive state that can be achieved through healthy behaviour and lifestyle. It is clear that biological mechanisms alone are insufficient to maintain or promote health (Anand 2009; Sunderrajan et al. 2013).

The Western system of medicine treats only the body, without considering mental, environmental or cultural factors. The underlying biomedical model is not enough; the search for alternative models is continuing. While present-day mainstream medicine has roots in alternative medicines of the past, modern medical schools generally do not teach alternative medicines. Various alternative medicines such as herbal medicine, manual healing, mind–body control, acupuncture, acupressure, massage therapy, Unani medicine, Siddha medicine, homeopathy and aroma therapy are gradually gaining attention and popularity. The Government of India has established a Ministry of Ayurveda, Yoga and Naturopathy, Unani, Siddha and Homoeopathy (AYUSH) to promote research in these areas. Also a Central Council of Indian Medicine (CCIM) has been established to promote research in these areas of traditional medicine. The US National Institute of Health has established the National Centre for Complementary and Alternative Medicine. Increasingly, a large number of modern hospitals are offering alternative therapies. In China, herbal therapies have a long tradition, as do acupressure and acupuncture therapies which claim to correct the imbalances of energy flow in the body causing the disease. In Germany, herbal remedies and homeopathy are quite popular. Contemporary healthcare systems are largely driven by the tradition of Western medicine. Most of its theories and concepts are borrowed from Western research though the conceptual richness of Indian and other Asian traditions has yet not been explored (see Sunderrajan et al. 2013).

Need for Plural Approach to Treatment and Intervention

Until recently, psychology did not show much interest in physical health, which was considered a specialty of medical science. Psychological research was primarily concerned with mental health problems. Clinical psychologists restricted themselves to investigate the classification of mental illnesses and determining its etiology, and to diagnose and treat the afflicted patients. They provided psychotherapeutic treatment to patients. However, their role was subsidiary to those of psychiatrists. This clear demarcation between mental and physical health was consistent with the notion of mind–body dualism.

In recent years, psychology's involvement with health has assumed many forms. In particular the emergence of sub disciplines of psychosomatic medicine, behavioural medicine, behavioural health and health psychology has paved several ways for the development of a variety of interventions for health promotion. The emerging discipline of health psychology got recognition only in the 1970s. Since then health psychology has been one of the rapidly growing fields of psychology. However, in India and other developing countries it is still in its infancy. Though there are many exciting possibilities of research and application, there is lack of appropriate teaching programmes and research agenda in this field. The scope of health psychology is now encompassing the strategies for health promotion and making preventive health measures more effective. Psychological rehabilitation of patients with chronic diseases and disabilities is another field that is gaining popularity.

In recent years, research regarding the role of cultural and social variables in health has substantially increased. It has led to changes in the study and practices related to the domain of health. It has been noted that cultural and ethnic contexts exert important influences on perceptions, attitudes and actions in the domain of health (Paniagua and Yamada 2013). As Angel and Williams (2013) have noted 'the subjective experience of illness, the help-seeking behaviour it elicits, as well as the response of society to an individual's symptoms and behaviour reflect more than purely scientific or clinical criteria. Cultural beliefs and practices, language, social norms, and even potential factors also come into play' (p. 51). While poverty is associated with poor health in developing countries, socio-economic hierarchies play an important part in affluent countries as well (Wilkinson 1996). Health and health-related behaviour patterns are embedded in legislative and social contexts. Government actions influence development of health infrastructure, economic policies, environmental policies and social policies. Sanctions against unhealthy behaviours like smoking and tobacco use are important. Formulation of national policies and adoption of legislative measures play primary role in public health promotion.

There is growing research evidence that psychological knowledge can make important contributions to a wide range of health-related domains. In Western behavioural science, spirituality now plays a central role. This is a radical departure from the secular and non-spiritual orientation of mainstream Western psychology, and has wide implications for the growth of health psychology (Susman 2004; Winkelman 2009). Several spiritual interventions such as meditation, prayer and *seva* (service) have been reported to be associated with different indicators of health/well-being (Sharma and Sharma 2007).

As human beings we are also located in the social and moral space, and spiritual living is a genuine part of our existence. Health thus refers to proper functioning of the body and the mind, as well as the capacity to participate in social activities, performing roles and abiding by moral principles. In fact, the idea of 'good health' is very close to the general well-being of a person. Health and well-being comprise people's evaluations, both affective and cognitive, of their lives. These are outcomes of a complex interplay of biological, socio-cultural, psychological, economic and spiritual factors.

An Indian Approach to Health and Well-Being

The Indian perspectives on health offer an ideal state of human functioning and constitute health and well-being as a state of mind which is peaceful, quiet, serene and free from conflicts and desires. The Indian notion of a *swastha* (healthy) individual who flourishes on the recognition of life force derived from material reality and, therefore, offers remedies for being healthy by opening a dialogue with its environment.

Going beyond the biomedical model of health, Ayurveda, the Indian science of life, offers a paradigm which articulates how body-mind-spirit interactions can be balanced and improved upon to enable people to live gracefully and harmoniously (Jaipal 2013). It focuses on one's relationship with the environment, seasons and events within which one is situated. There is emphasis on harmony/balance or equilibrium. The notion of *sama* (balance and moderation) is often emphasised.

Depending on the incongruence/congruence between the person and the environment anything can become health/disease promoting. *Ritusatmya*, for example, is the principle of adaptation that states that food should be consumed according to the season. The *Bhagavad Gita* considers this possibility and argues for a state of *sthitapragya* (steady intelligence) which allows equanimity. One's self, therefore, is a great friend as well as a great enemy. For one who has conquered the self it becomes a friend. Being healthy and experiencing the well-being is the natural or original state. The notion of *sat chit anand* (being, consciousness and bliss) is the true or the real nature. Instead, we identify ourselves with objects that are temporary attachments. *Swastha* means one who is located in one's own self. Contrarily, *aswastha* (illness or absence of health) denotes a condition of lack of self-control. Such a person is controlled by others or is externally controlled. One needs to realize one's true nature and live within its limitations. Birth and death are not within our control but the way we live is. Living a healthy, happy and empowered life is a choice that one can make (Salgame 2006, 2014).

Health policies, programmes and practices mirror the culture, society and political scenario. Ayurveda remained the basis of daily living and treatment of diseases for ages in the Indian subcontinent. In the Asian region, Siddha and Unani-Tibb, Japanese and Chinese traditions of medicine have also been practiced. They demonstrate that Western notion of health and illness has not been the only way of addressing medical care. From the late eighteenth and particularly the nineteenth century, Western medicine under British colonial rule became the official healthcare programme in the region. After political independence in 1947, India has witnessed a rapid expansion of healthcare infrastructure and medical institutions. The pressure of international agencies, like the WHO and World Bank, paved the way for shifts in policy. However, health and well-being are still emerging fields of study. Indian health sciences have not been able to build on the rich healing traditions and holistic curative practices of the region. There are intense efforts worldwide for the search of alternative healthcare systems, and India, along with other Asian countries, has much to offer in this respect.

Contemporary Challenges for Health

Today's life poses many issues which deserve the use of an interdisciplinary approach. The first set of issues deals with the world of work. To remain happy in a world which is in flux implicates that changes need to be brought about within the person too. Today, sources of psychological instability are increasing. Work–life balance is becoming a big issue. The professional career is also changing. Now it ceases to be a lifelong commitment and people change jobs and careers far more easily, adding to stress in daily life. In this context of lifestyle changes, the rich array of concepts, theories and practices available in Indian traditions of healing and meditation remain unexplored (Dalal and Misra 2012).

Enhancing the health status of people is another important issue. There is a realization among researchers, practitioners and policymakers that health status has complex linkages with poverty, deprivation, population growth and education (Sharma and Misra 2010). Health research needs to come out of the narrow disciplinary groves and has to accept the more challenging task of helping people to improve their physical and mental health.

Community-oriented health services are going to be a major research issue. Mapping the meaning of health and illness also needs interdisciplinary study. We need to know how people understand that they are sick and how cultural beliefs about health function to influence personal efficacy in everyday life (Dalal 2015, 2016; Dalal and Misra 2006). Well-being is undoubtedly one of the cherished goals of humanity. It involves the idea of good life or the state of optimal psychological functioning. Liberation (*moksha*) from suffering *(klesha)* was considered the highest goal of life as held by the ancient Indians. As Sen (1999) has argued freedom is a more rational goal for development. The idea of 'gross national product' is not enough. Sen (1999) has noted that in cultures where relative freedom has expanded both quality of life and economic growth have taken place.

The positive psychology movement has also drawn attention to human strengths and virtues (Peterson and Seligman 2004; Peterson et al. 2007). It has been established that material security and luxury alone do not guarantee well-being. In fact, it is lopsided to view well-being in terms of pleasure or happiness. The eudaimonic view of happiness invites societal engagement. Social well-being is a positive state associated with optimal functioning of a person within one's social network and community (Ryff 2014).

Broadening of Socio-cultural Concerns

The psychological perspective on health needs to attend to the cultural nuances of the contemporary world. Cross-cultural, cultural, psychological and anthropological works have demonstrated convincingly that many Western psychological assumptions about health and healing do not hold true in other parts of the world (Black 2013; Dwivedi 2005; Hopeworth 2006; Huey and Jones 2013; Kakar 1982; Klineman 1980; Rao 2005). Similarly, people do hold interdependent, relational and encompassing notions of self which go beyond the discrete and autonomous concepts of self-prevalence in Euro-American scholarship (Mascolo et al. 2004). At the same time, the processes of globalization, migration and communication revolution are restructuring the world of experience (Sharma and Sharma 2010b). This scenario is posing new challenges and offering opportunities for health researchers in the field of health. It is through innovative interdisciplinary research, teaching and training that emerging issues in the area of health psychology can be effectively dealt with. Such an approach will have multiple methods and will draw from various sources including literary works, folklore, life stories and ethnographic work.

Encompassing the Concerns of Well-Being

Until recently, the focus of work in the area of health has been predominantly on reducing death, disease and disability rather than promoting physical and mental well-being. It requires living in harmony with nature and pursuing wholeness, balance, wellness and bliss in life (Rao 2014). Heath involves enabling people to achieve their full health and well-being potential throughout the course of life.

Health for All

The key question is to maximize health as a fundamental right for all and not as a privilege for a few. Health is an asset for economic and social stability and for reducing poverty. Sustainable and equitable improvement in health and well-being or health equity is a must. The situation in India is alarming. The last national mental health survey by the National Institute of Mental Health and Neurosciences published in 2016 indicates that 15% Indian adults above 18 years are in need of active health intervention. We need the joint effort of health researchers from various areas and political will to achieve health and well-being of all.

The Layout of the Volume

In view of the overall organization of this volume, the chapters are sorted into four parts as outlined below.

Part I (*Conceptual Foundations*) consists of six chapters introducing the readers to an overview of the psychological factors in the management of health problems. The determinants of health and well-being and notions or resilience, post-traumatic growth and indigenous healing practices are discussed.

Part II (*Interventions across Life Span*) comprises eight chapters focusing on childhood, adolescence, mainstream and alternative interventions for the elderly. It also elaborates academic performance and lifestyle issues during adolescence, community-level behavioural intervention, religion-spiritual intervention, yoga.

Part III (*Cultural Perspectives on Intervention*) has three chapters offering anthropological perspectives on ethno-medicine, counselling and therapy, local institutions and practices.

Part IV (*Social Perspectives*) has five chapters focusing on disability, gender, perspective of the patient who has recovered, delivery of healthcare, and well-being and health in the aftermath of disaster.

The common goals across the four parts of the present volume are to enhance the understanding of interventions as complex undertakings situated in specific contexts. The multiple dimensions within and between developmental stages are examined to expand the discourse by relating to cultural contexts and to promote empirical understanding with culturally-based approaches.

Concluding Comments

In the contemporary era characterized by strong materialistic values and beliefs, people are increasingly engaged in cut-throat competition in the pursuit of ever-rising aspirations and lack tolerance for delays in gratification. These tendencies affect the social ethos. These are further complicated by diminishing levels of interpersonal trust and social support due to displacement, migration and concomitant changes in the traditional social institutions and networks like family, kinship and religion. At the same time, people are deeply engaged in pursuing self-interests which leads to anxiety, depression and other problems (Leary 2004). In such a scenario, people often indulge in various kinds of violence and are overpowered by the intense feelings of insecurity, loss, instability, and alienation (Sharma and Sharma 2010b). Also, there is lack of self-control and, therefore people frequently experience anxiety, pressure, frustration, conflict and mental imbalance. These factors put people at risk for mental health and well-being. Easy access to drugs and alcohol makes it possible for people to take recourse to addictive and intoxicating substances leading to various maladaptive behaviours. Hence, there is a serious need to formulate and launch interventions on a large scale for the promotion of health and well-being.

Health is a dynamic phenomenon and depends on a harmonious transaction with the surrounding environment and ecology within which human lives are embedded. Asian traditions favour the view that one's lifestyle has to be suitably adjusted and one's conduct has to be in accordance with the demands of time and place. In view of the fact that greed invites many problems, it is important to have correct assessment of needs, personal preferences, goals and pathways. People should be discouraged nurturing false self-conceptions and impressed upon to avoid overestimating their potential. Such moves often create problems in life. Nurturing mental peace through yoga and meditation in everyday life is important, as is self-control amidst a world of endless advertising and marketing.

References

Abraham, C., Kok, G., Schaalma, H. P., & Luszczynska, A. (2011). Health promotion. In P. R. Martin, F. M. Cheung, M. C. Knowles, M. Kyrios, L. Littlefield, & J. B. Overmeir (Eds.), *IAAP handbook of applied psychology* (pp. 83–111). West Sussex: Wiley-Blackwell.

Anand, J. (2009). Psychological healing and faith in the doctrine of Karma. *Mental Health, Religion & Culture, 12,* 817–832.

Angel, R. J., & Williams, K. (2013). Cultural models of health and illness. In F. A. Panuagua & A. M. Yamada (Eds.), *Handbook of multicultural health* (2nd Ed.) (pp. 49–68). Oxford: Academic Press, Elsevier.

Black, S. (2013). The mental health of culturally diverse older adults: Research and clinical issues. In F. A. Paniagua & A.-M. Yamada (Eds.), *Handbook of muticultual mental health* (pp. 411–426). Oxford: Academic Press, Elsevier.

Dalal, A. K. (2015). *Health beliefs and coping with chronic diseases*. New Delhi: Sage Publications.

Dalal, A. K. (2016). *Cultural psychology of health in India*. New Delhi: Sage Publications.

Dalal, A. K., & Misra, G. (2006). Psychology of health and wellbeing: Some emerging perspectives. *Psychological Studies, 51,* 91–104.

Dalal, A. K., & Misra, G. (Eds.). (2012). *New directions in health psychology*. New Delhi: Sage Publications.

Dwivedi, C. B. (2005). Swasthavrtta: The Ayurvedic model of health and wellbeing. In R. Singh, A. Yadav, & N. Sharma (Eds.), *Health psychology* (pp. 354–371). New Delhi: Global Vision.

Hingson, R. W., & Howland, J. (2002). Comprehensive community interventions to promote health: Implications for college-age drinking problems. *Journal of Studies on Alcohol. Supplement, 14,* 226–240.

Hopeworth, J. (2006). The emergence of critical health psychology: Can it contribute to promoting public health? *Journal of Health Psychology, 11,* 331–341.

Huey, S. J., & Jones, E. O. (2013). Improving treatment engagement and psychotherapy outcomes for culturally diverse youth and families. In F. A. Paniagua & A.-M. Yamada (Eds.), *Handbook of muticultural mental health* (pp. 427–444). Oxford: Academic Press, Elsevier.

Jaipal, R. (2013). Concepts of the person and health in Indian thought. In G. Misra (Ed.), *Psychology and psychoanalysis* (pp. 711–739). New Delhi: Centre for Studies in Civilizations.

Kakar, S. (1982). *Shamans, mystics and doctors*. Delhi: Oxford University Press.

Kityama, S., Duffy, S., & Uchida, Y. (2007). Self as cultural mode of being. In S. Kitayama & D. Cohen (Eds.), *Handbook of cultural psychology* (pp. 136–174). New York: Guilford Press.

Klineman, A. (1980). *Patients and healers in the contexts of culture*. Berkeley, CA: University of California Press.

Kok, G., Gottlieb, N. H., Commers, M., & Smerecnik, C. (2008). The ecological approach in health promotion programs: A decade later. *American Journal of Health Promotion, 23,* 437–442.

Leary, M. R. (2004). *The curse of self.* New York: Oxford University Press.

Markus, H. R., & Kitayama, S. (1991). Culture and self: Implications for cognition, emotion, and motivation. *Psychological Review, 98,* 224–253.

Marsella, A. J. (2009). Diversity in a global era: The context and consequences of differences. *Counselling Psychology Quarterly, 22,* 119–135.

Marsella, A. J., & White, G. M. (Eds.). (1982). *Cultural conceptions of mental health and therapy*. Boston: D. Reidel.

Mascolo, F. M., Misra, G., & Rapisardi, C. (2004). Individual and relational conceptions of self in India and the United States. *New Directions for Child and Adolescent Development, 104,* 9–26.

Misra, G. (2005). From disease to well-being perspectives from an indigenous tradition. In R. Singh, A. Yadav, & N. Sharma (Eds.), *Health psychology* (pp. 281–302). New Delhi: Global Vision.

Misra, G. (2013). Culture and self: Some emerging perspectives. In G. Misra (Ed.), *Psychology and psychoanalysis* (pp. 371–383). New Delhi: Centre for Studies in Civilizations.

Paniagua, F. A., & Yamada, A. M. (Ed.) (2013). *Handbook of multicultural health* (2nd Ed.) Oxford: Academic Press, Elsevier.

Peterson, C., Ruch, W., Beerman, U., Park, N., & Seligman, M. E. P. (2007). Strengths of character orientations to happiness and life satisfaction. *The Journal of Positive Psychology, 2,* 149–156.

Peterson, C., & Seligman, M. E. P. (2004). *Character strengths and virtues: A classification and handbook*. Washington, DC: American Psychological Association.

Rao, K. R. (2005). Psychology in the Indian tradition: A classical model with contemporary relevance. *Psychological Studies, 50,* 1–8.
Rao, K. R. (2014). Positive psychology and Indian psychology in need of mutual reinforcement. *Psychological Studies, 59,* 94–102.
Rao, K. R., & Paranjpe, A. C. (2016). *Psychology in the Indian tradition.* New Delhi: Springer.
Ryff, C. D. (2014). Psychological well-being revisited: Advances in science and practice. *Psychotherapy and Psychosomatic Medicine, 83,* 10–28.
Salgame, K. K. K. (2006). Happiness and well-being in Indian tradition. *Psychological Studies, 51,* 105–112.
Salgame, K. K. K. (2014). Positive psychology in the light of Indian tradition. In S. Saini (Ed.), *Positive psychology in the light of Indian traditions* (pp. 1–22). Hisar, India: Indian Association of Health Research and Welfare.
Sen, Amartya. (1999). *Development as freedom.* New York: Oxford University Press.
Sharma, S., & Misra, G. (2010). Health psychology: Progress and challenges. In G. Misra (Ed.), *Psychology in India Vol. 3 Clinical and health psychology* (pp. 265–316). New Delhi: Pearson.
Sharma, S., & Sharma, M. (2007). Preventing illness and promoting health and well-being: The stress perspective. *Psychological Studies, 52,* 70–76.
Sharma, S., & Sharma, M. (2010a). Self, social identity and psychological wellbeing. *Psychological Studies, 55,* 118–136.
Sharma, S., & Sharma, M. (2010b). Globalization, threatened identities, coping, and well-being. *Psychological Studies, 55,* 313–322.
Sunderrajan, L., Misra, G., & Marsella, A. J. (2013). Indigenous approaches to assessment, diagnosis, and treatment of mental disorders. In F. A. Paniagua & A.-M. Yamada (Eds.), *Handbook of muticultural mental health* (pp. 69–87). Oxford: Academic Press, Elsevier.
Susman, L. K. (2004). The role of culture in definition, interpretation and management of illness. In U. Gielen, J. Fish, & J. Draguns (Eds.), *Handbook of culture, therapy and healing* (pp. 37–65). New York: Lawrence Erlbaum Associates.
Weiner, B. (1992). *Human motivation: Metaphors, theories and research.* London: Sage Publications.
Wilkinson, R. (1996). *Unhealthy societies: The affliction of inequality.* New stork: Routledge.
Winkelman, M. (2009). *Culture and health: Applying medical anthropology.* San Francisco, CA: Jossey-Bass.

Part I
Conceptual Foundations

Chapter 2
Role of Psychosocial Factors in the Management of Health Problems

M. Mehta and S. Kapoor

Recent years have seen a rise in both chronic medical conditions as well as lifestyle disorders. Problems such as cancer, diabetes, sleep disorders, cardiovascular diseases, renal problems, as well as severe skin conditions are becoming increasingly prevalent. Though medicine has advanced by leaps and bounds in the management of these disorders, much work is left to be desired in the area of the psychological sequelae of these conditions. Importance of psychological factors involved in medical conditions, particularly chronic or terminal illnesses, has come to light in recent years, with much work focusing on the psychosocial aspects involved in initiation or exacerbation of symptoms. The role of psychosocial factors in management and therapy is now widely accepted and psychotherapy is increasingly beginning to serve as an adjunct to traditional forms of therapy where chronic, debilitating conditions are concerned. Medicine has, therefore, moved from a purely biological perspective of causation and management to a more biopsychosocial model of disease and treatment.

Biopsychosocial Model of Health and Illness

The biopsychosocial approach, proposed by Engel (1977), reduces emphasis on biological aspects while considering biological, psychological and social factors and their interactions in understanding health, illness and management.

M. Mehta (✉)
Formerly Professor of Clinical Psychology Department of Psychiatry, AIIMS, New Delhi, India
e-mail: drmanju.mehta@gmail.com

S. Kapoor
Assistant Professor, Jesus and Mary College, University of Delhi, New Delhi, India

G. Misra (ed.), *Psychosocial Interventions for Health and Well-Being*,
https://doi.org/10.1007/978-81-322-3782-2_2

The biological component of the biopsychosocial model focuses on physical functioning and genetic aspects as involved in causation. The psychological component looks for aspects of personality, cognitive functioning, emotional regulation, etc., while the social aspect investigates how different social factors such as socioeconomic status, culture, poverty, technology and religion influence health. In recent years, focus has moved beyond causation into looking at how the biopsychosocial model can be incorporated into healthcare—how it affects patients' understanding and acceptance of healthcare that is provided, as also the clinical course and outcome of the condition (Fig. 2.1).

Awareness and effective application of the model is, therefore, expected to result in improved healthcare practices. It is essential that the clinician follow certain basic principles for effective application of the model to clinical practice. Recognizing that relationships are central to providing healthcare and eliciting the patient's history in the context of life circumstances is crucial to be able to develop a comprehensive model of the patients' illness. Further, it is important to decide which aspects of biological, psychological and social domains are most important to understand and promote a patient's health.

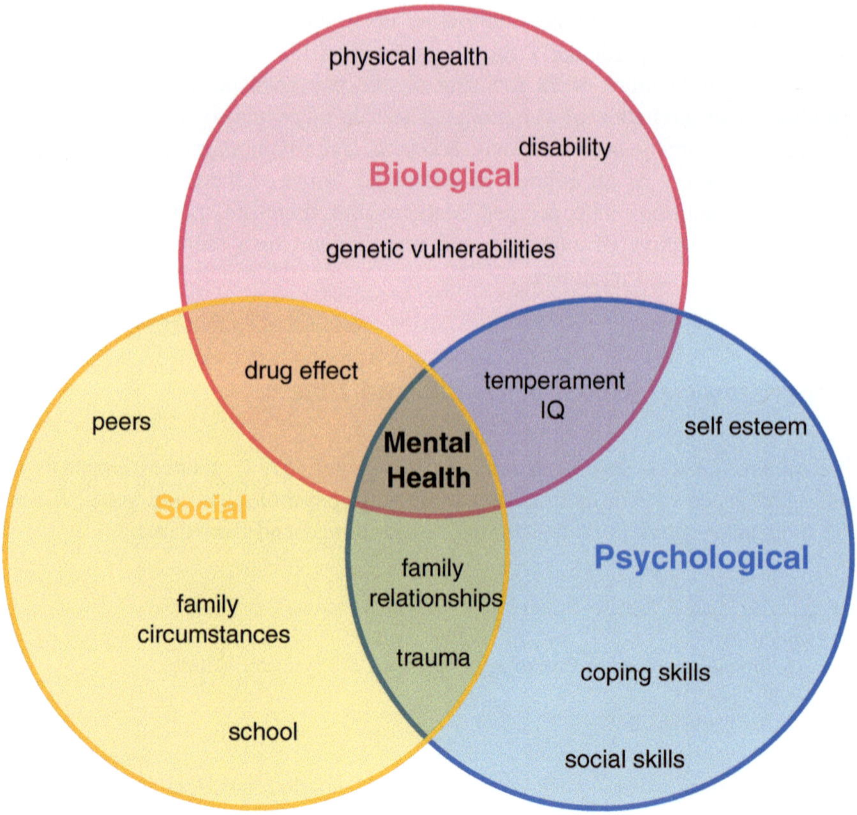

Fig. 2.1 Biopsychosocial model of health. *Source* http://chiro.org/wordpress/2017/06/the-biopsychosocial-model-and-chiropractic/

Following from this, DSM IV contains a category on psychological factors affecting mental health, which involves the 'occurrence of one or more emotional or behavioural factors that aggravate or adversely affect the physical health problem or condition' (American Psychiatric Association 2000). Subsumed under it are the following conditions:

Mental disorders affecting a medical condition
Psychological symptoms affecting a medical condition
Personality traits or coping style affecting a medical condition
Maladaptive health behaviours affecting medical condition
Stress-related physiological response affecting medical condition
Other or unspecified psychological factors affecting medical condition

As is evident from the categories, a number of conditions can be said to contribute to initiate or exacerbate of medical conditions or to interfere with treatment and outcome. For example, prolonged stress due to interpersonal difficulties or poor coping styles may result in physical problems, such as heart disease. Chronic anxiety or depression resulting from these interpersonal difficulties may then interfere with treatment or prolong recovery period even after the completion of treatment.

Psychosocial Factors as Risk and Protective Factors

Psychosocial factors that are often implicated in medical conditions are prolong or severe stress, anxiety, depression, ineffective coping, personality problems, interpersonal difficulties, maladaptive behaviours such as smoking, etc., among many others.

Enlisted in Table 2.1 are some of the prominent risk and protective factors implicated in poor psychological health complicating medical conditions.

Role of individual factors has been studied in populations widely varied in demographics. Among adolescents, it was found that searching for a coherent meaning in life served as a protective factor against poor psychological health (Brassai et al. 2011). Studies suggest that adolescents who are depressed and those who attempt suicide share many psychosocial risk factors. A few strong predictors of suicide attempt have been listed as—having a history of past attempt, current suicidal ideation and depression, recent attempt by a friend, low self-esteem and being born to a teenage mother (Lewinsohn et al. 1994).

Role of psychosocial variables in predicting mortality amongst old-age patients has also been extensively studied. Zuckerman et al. (1984) found three psychosocial variables as significant predictors: religiousness, happiness (as rated by the interviewers) and presence of a living offspring. The first two reduced the risk of mortality primarily among the elderly who were in poor health, while the third one did not interact with health status. Another study stressed on the importance of depressive symptoms as one determinant of recovery from hip fracture and indicates the need to attend to the affective status of hip fracture patients following surgery (Mossey et al. 1989).

Table 2.1 Psychosocial risk and protective factors

Domain	Risk factors	Protective factors
Individual	Difficult temperament	Easy-going temperament
	Chronic physical illness	Physical fitness
	High stress	High activity levels
		Social skills, self-efficacy
		Intelligence
Family	Severe interpersonal discord	Closeness, warmth, trust
	Overcrowded homes	Open communication
	Parental/familial psychopathology	Close extended family relationships
	Lack of significant relationships	High quality relationships, particularly with regard to parent and child
	Abuse and exposure to violence	Secured attachment pattern
	Authoritarian/indifferent parenting style	Authoritative parenting style
	Inconsistent parenting	Consistent parenting through established patterns of reinforcement and punishment
	High expressed emotion	
Social/community	Poverty	Age relevant resources
	Violence/sustained fear of crime in the neighbourhood	High quality health care and access to services
	Social isolation/discrimination	Community/social network and support
	Poor quality of schooling	Good quality schooling

In a study on clinical course of depression, it was found that better clinical course of depression was associated with patients who had high levels of social support, were more active and had less avoidant coping styles, who were physically active, and who had fewer co-morbid chronic conditions. Improvements in measures of functioning and well-being associated with patients who were employed, drank less alcohol, and had active coping styles (Sherbourne et al. 1995).

Understanding Health Related Behaviour

The **Health Belief Model** (Rosenstock 1974) attempts to explain and predict health behaviour by focusing on beliefs and attitudes of the individual. From a cost-benefit analysis, the model elaborates on perceived threats and benefits in terms of four constructs:

- *Perceived susceptibility* of being afflicted by a condition
- *Perceived severity* or seriousness of the condition and its consequences

- *Perceived benefits* of the advised action to reduce risk or severity
- *Perceived barriers* or costs to the advised action

The model proposed that an evaluation of these four constructs determines to what extent an individual will initiate and comply with a suggested treatment programme. Combined with these, two constructs were later included into the model to better explain health-related action undertaken by individuals—'*cues to action*' which include strategies designed to activate readiness in the patient, and '*perceived self-efficacy*' or the individuals' belief in their ability to carry out the required health action (Fig. 2.2).

The health belief model has been applied to a range of health behaviours. Conner and Norman (1996) identified three broad areas where the model has found great applicability: (a) preventive health behaviour, including health-promoting and health-risk behaviours; (b) compliance with recommended medical action; (c) regular follow-up.

Much research has found evidence for the four constructs in predicting health behaviours. In the area of smoking cessation, it has been found that providing information about the effects of smoking and the extent of consequences is effective in initiating cessation (e.g., Sutton 1982). Studies in the area of breast self-examination have found that perceived barriers and perceived susceptibility (Wyper 1990) were the best predictors of healthy behaviours. Rimer et al. (1991) found that knowledge about breast cancer was related to having regular mammograms.

Protection Motivation Theory (Rogers 1983) examines two appraisal processes as being involved in adaptive or maladaptive coping with a health threat. The model posits that health-related behaviours are a product of five components:

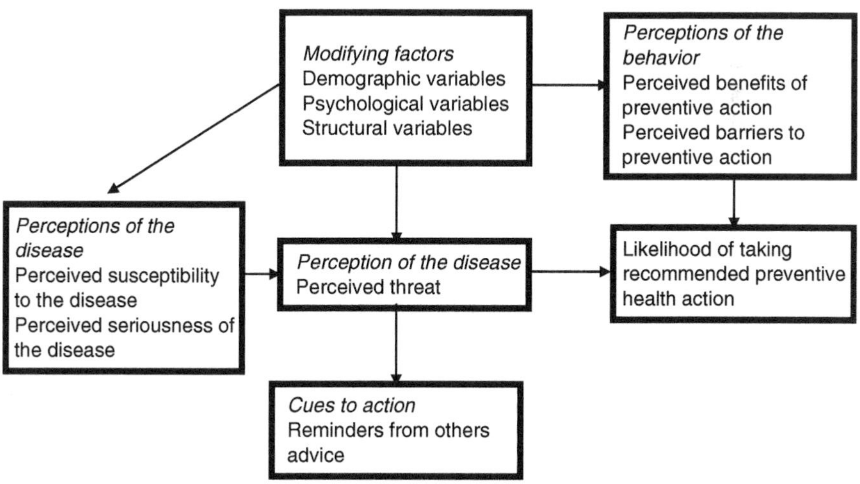

Fig. 2.2 Conceptual model: health belief model. *Source* Author's representation

- Coping Appraisal
  - *Self-efficacy (e.g. 'I am confident that I can quit smoking');*
  - *Response effectiveness (e.g. 'Quitting smoking would improve my health');*
- Threat Appraisal
  - *Severity (e.g. 'Lung cancer is a serious illness');*
  - *Vulnerability (e.g. 'My chances of getting lung cancer are high');*
  - *Fear.*

According to the Protection Motivation Theory, there are two sources of information—Environmental (e.g., verbal persuasion, observational learning) and Intrapersonal (e.g., prior direct or indirect experience). This information elicits either an 'adaptive' coping response (i.e., the intention to improve one's health) or a 'maladaptive' coping response (e.g., avoidance, denial). Protection motivation is a mediating variable whose function is to arouse, sustain and direct protective health behaviour (Boer and Seydel 1996) (Fig. 2.3).

The above example of smoking cessation illustrates the principles of the model.

Health Locus of Control (LOC), given by Wallston and Wallston, evaluates the degree to which individuals believe that their health is controlled by internal or external factors. Those with an external health LOC are likely to believe that their health is controlled by powerful others, such as medical professionals, or by chance or luck; while those with an internal health LOC are likely to view health as controllable and a consequence of their own actions.

Internal LOC has been linked to positive health beliefs and behaviours. Individuals with internal LOC have ability to stop smoking (Coan 1973), adherence to a medical regimen (Lewis et al. 1978), getting preventive inoculations (Dabbs and Kirscht 1971) etc. Developing an understanding of the origin and nature of LOC is essential to understand individual health-related behaviour and devising individualized treatment programmes and interventions to modify maladaptive

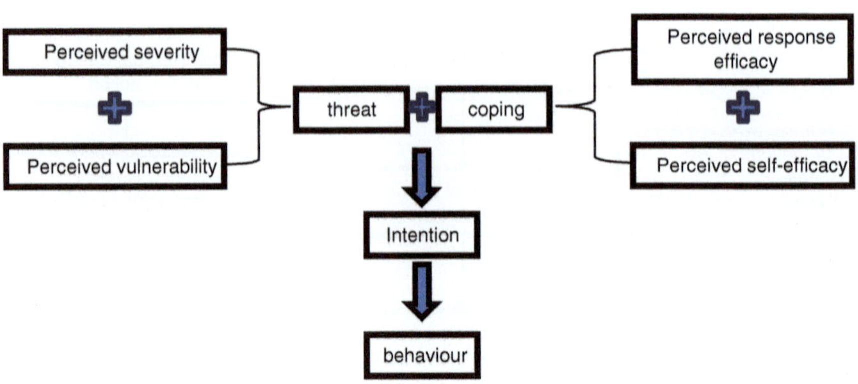

Fig. 2.3 Conceptual model: protection motivation theory. *Source* https://www.researchgate.net/figure/6341971_fig1_Flow-chart-of-Protection-Motivation-Theory

LOC. It is believed that development of LOC is affected by parenting style (where a nurturant, consistent style of parenting is correlated with an internal LOC), consistent reinforcement, socioeconomic status and prior experience with sickness and health. Those belonging to a lower socioeconomic status are more likely to have an external LOC due to fewer reinforcements; their general circumstances make them more reliant on external sources of reinforcement. Prior experiences with disease are also important determinants of LOC, wherein an individual who may have continued to suffer through an illness despite all health-related behaviours may start to develop an external LOC. Such knowledge about development of health LOC is important at the individual and social level in developing healthcare practices; and is also related to how individuals change their behaviour and to the kind of communications style they require from health professionals.

Social cognition models such as **Theory of Planned Behaviour** (TPB) and **Theory of Reasoned Action** (TRA), proposed by Ajzen and Fishbein (1980), seek to explain health-related behaviour intentions and actions as a combination of beliefs. Theory of Reasoned Action suggests that a person's *attitude* towards a particular action along with his/her *subjective norm* regarding that action determine an individual's intention to perform that action or behaviour. Behaviour is most likely to be predicted by *intention*, which is the cognitive representation of a person's readiness to perform a given behaviour. TRA was related to voluntary behaviour. Theory of planned behaviour is an extension of the TRA, and includes a component of '*Perceived behavioural control*'. Perceived behavioural control refers to people's perceptions of their ability to perform a given behaviour. These predictors lead to intention, in addition to the previously mentioned attitudes and subjective norms. As a general rule, the more favourable the attitude and the subjective norm, the greater is the perceived control and stronger the person's intention to perform the behaviour in question (Figs. 2.4 and 2.5).

The **Health Action Process Approach**, developed by Schwarzer in 1992, posits two stages of change—motivation stage and action maintenance stage.

According to this approach, the *motivation* stage involves a combination of *self-efficacy* (e.g., 'I believe I can cut down on unhealthy foods'); *outcome expectancies*

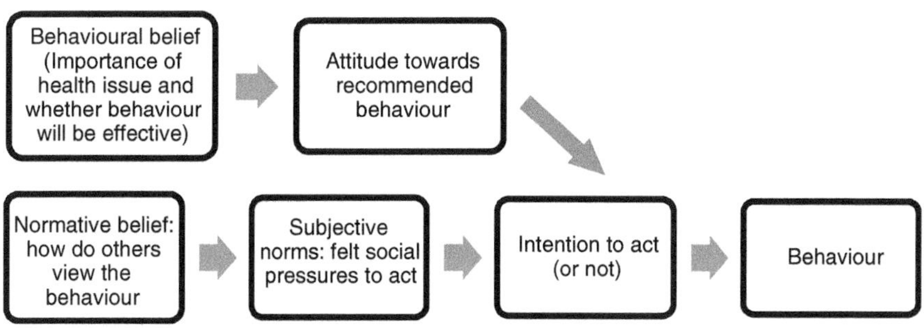

Fig. 2.4 Conceptual model: theory of reasoned action. *Source* Adapted from: https://www.med.uottawa.ca/sim/data/BehaviorChange_e.htm

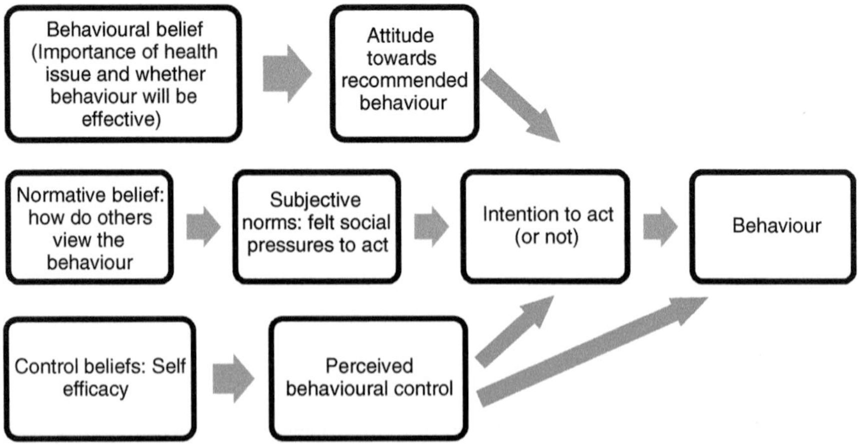

Fig. 2.5 Conceptual model: theory of planned behaviour. *Source* Adapted from: https://www.med.uottawa.ca/sim/data/BehaviorChange_e.htm

(e.g., 'Cutting down on unhealthy food will improve my health'), *social outcome expectancies* (e.g., 'Other people want me to cut down on bad eating and doing so will be favourable to them') as well as *threat appraisal*, which involves beliefs about perceived susceptibility and severity. The *action* stage comprises *action plans* (e.g., 'When tempted with unhealthy food I can think of healthier options') and *action control* (e.g., 'I can resist temptation by thinking of my resolve to be healthier'). Presence of social support and absence of social barriers are mediating factors in the process (Fig. 2.6).

The **Transtheoretical Model of Change** emphasizes on the dynamic nature of beliefs, time, and costs and benefits, and proposes the following stages of change:

Precontemplation: not intending to make any changes
Contemplation: considering a change
Preparation: making small changes
Action: actively engaging in a new behaviour
Maintenance: sustaining change over time

People in the later stages, e.g., maintenance, would tend to focus on the benefits (I feel healthier after giving up smoking), whereas people in the earlier stages tend to focus on the costs (I will be at a social disadvantage if I give up smoking). Strategies such as motivation enhancement, and supportive therapy are primarily used in the precontemplation stage while more structured cognitive behavioural methods are applied in the later stages, such as problem-focused CBT for the contemplation stage and self-management CBT and coping effectiveness are used in the action stage (Fig. 2.7).

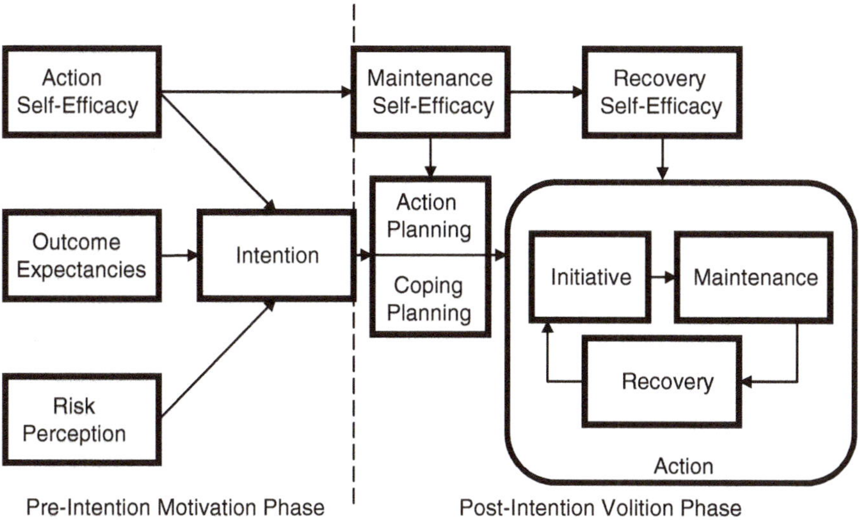

Fig. 2.6 Conceptual model: health action process approach. *Source* Adapted from Schwarzer (2008)

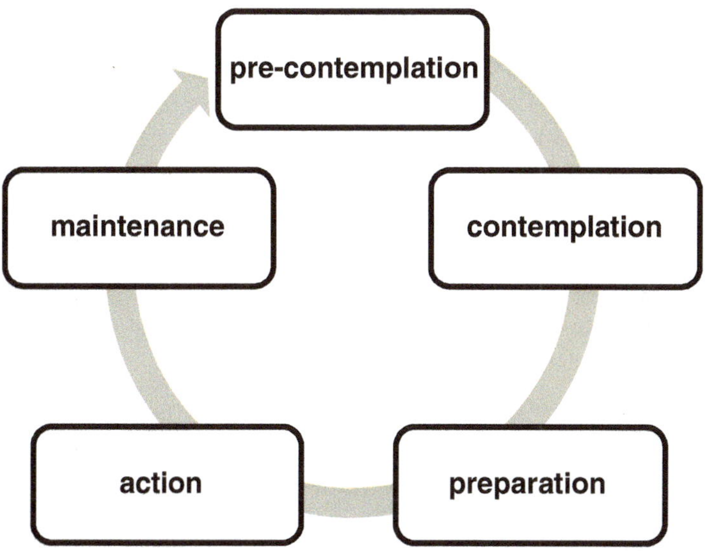

Fig. 2.7 Conceptual model: transtheoretical model of change. *Source* Authors' representation

Psychosocial Intervention for Health Problems

Chronic illness is a pervasive, often distressing condition that may cause significant psychological changes and impact one's psychological adjustment. According to a report by the Institute of Medicine (2008), people with a chronic illness need help to learn how to:

- Cope with the intense, sometimes debilitating, emotions related to their illness.
- Change behaviours in order to minimize the impact of their disease and maximize treatment protocol.
- Manage the disruptions their illness may cause to their work, school and family life.

A large number of psychological interventions for general health conditions have been developed and researched over the years. A brief overview of the main approaches is provided in this section.

- Psychoeducation

The models of health behaviour suggest that an essential predictor of health-related action is the set of beliefs and attitudes that an individual holds about the illness, particularly pertaining to the likelihood of their getting the illness and the severity of its consequences. Research has found that information in the form of fear-arousing warnings may change attitudes and health behaviour in such areas as dental health, safe driving and smoking (Sutton 1982). Several studies have also indicated a positive correlation between knowledge about Breast Self-examination (BSE) and breast cancer and performing BSE (Alagna et al. 1987; Champion 1984).

- Stress management training
  - Relaxation
  - Guided Imagery
  - Stress Inoculation Training
  - Coping Effectiveness Training: Helping to evaluate and develop a regimen between problem and coping style

- Cognitive Behaviour Therapy
  A large body of work has focused on using Cognitive Behaviour Therapy (CBT) for a range of conditions such as skin conditions, insomnia, pain management (particularly in cases where pain is chronic, such as cancer, fibromyalgia), cardiovascular diseases, etc. Management techniques have been developed using a combination of the following techniques:

- Problem-focused counselling
- Cognitive restructuring
- Enhancing self-efficacy
- Behavioural activation
- Activity scheduling
- Operant conditioning techniques

• Emotional disclosure and supportive counselling
• Family intervention

- Consistent and nurturant parenting styles
- Decreasing discord
- Facilitating open and warm communication
- Managing Expressed Emotion

• Self-management approach
This approach involves transferring the responsibility of treatment to patient by teaching the relevant skills and expecting application of the same in own settings. It has found great applicability in lifestyle disorders such as diabetes, where insulin treatments, compliance and dietary and lifestyle modifications are established as targets. It has also found useful in the treatment of alcohol and drug abuse.

Fekete et al. (2007) reviewed recent studies that have used behavioural or psychosocial interventions aimed at preventing type 2 diabetes mellitus, cardiovascular disease and HIV/AIDS as well as the psychosocial management of cardiovascular disease, HIV and cancer. Behavioural (lifestyle) interventions can decrease risk of type 2 diabetes mellitus and cardiovascular disease. Psychosocial interventions have proven efficacy for alleviating distress in patients medically treated for cancer, cardiovascular disease and HIV/AIDS. Behavioural and psychosocial interventions are useful in preventing some chronic diseases and for alleviating distress in patients who have been medically treated for diseases such as cancer, cardiovascular disease and HIV/AIDS. Barton et al. (2003) carried out interventions to improve coping strategies in patients with asthma and found them effective in reducing symptoms and psychological distress.

Use of psychosocial management as an adjunct to pharmacological treatment in cancer has been extensively studied. Certain modalities of treatment have been shown to be more efficacious at different stages of cancer treatment. Though psychoeducation may be the primary mode of patient interaction in the earlier stage and during diagnosis, group therapy may be more advantageous post diagnosis and to facilitate coping and adjustment (Blake-Mortimer et al. 1999). During extended treatments and chemotherapy, cognitive-behaviour techniques such as relaxation, stress management and cognitive coping may be the modality of choice (e.g., Fawzy et al. 1995; Bottomley 1996). Cunningham has identified a hierarchy of different types of therapy beginning with providing information, emotional support, behavioural training in coping skills, psychotherapy, leading up to spiritual/ existential therapy (Cunningham 1995).

Edelman et al. (1999) conducted 12 sessions of CBT for cancer patients, comprising cognitive behaviour therapy, behavioural strategies focusing on communication and coping, and self-expression. At the end of the therapy, depression and low mood states were reported lesser while a significant increase was seen in self-esteem scores. Menzies et al. (2004) used guided imagery of self-efficacy in patients with fibromyalgia and found reportedly decreased stress, fatigue, pain and depression.

It has also been found that behavioural intervention in patients with diabetes helped in increasing treatment compliance, decreasing anxiety and depression and shown positive changes in health LOC. In a conceptual review, Peyrot and Rubin (2007) proposed five Cs to effective psychosocial management in diabetes:

- Constructing problem definition
- Collaborative goal setting
- Collaborative problem solving
- Contracting for change
- Continuing support

The working alliance (patient–physician relationship) is important in medical treatment, as it is associated with patient adherence and satisfaction. Patients' self-efficacy ought to be assessed and promoted as it is also associated with treatment adherence (Fuertes et al. 2007).

Conclusion

The role of psychosocial factors is being increasingly recognized as a critical factor in maintenance as well as management of medical conditions. Understanding of health models, and effective application of psychotherapeutic techniques by experts can go a long way in speedy and effective management of such conditions and their psychological sequelae. Although a majority of the physicians seem to recognize the importance of addressing psychosocial issues, approximately one-third believe that addressing such factors would lead to minimal or no improvements in outcomes. A minority reports that their training regarding the role of psychosocial factors was effective, while relatively a few indicate interest in receiving further training in these areas (Astin et al. 2006). Adequate training of health professionals and appropriate referral systems are required to bridge the gap between medical and psychosocial work in current medical practice.

References

Ajzen, I., & Fishbein, M. (1980). *Understanding attitudes and predicting social behaviour*. Englewood Cliffs, NJ: Prentice Hall.

Alagna, S. W., Morokoff, P. J., Bevett, J. M., & Reddy, D. M. (1987). Performance of breast self-examination by women at high risk for breast cancer. *Women and Health, 12*, 29–46.

American Psychiatric Association. (2000). *Diagnostic and statistical manual of mental disorders* (4th ed., text revision). Washington, DC. American Psychiatric Association.

Astin, J. A., Soeken, K., Sierpina, V. S., & Clarridge, B. R. (2006). Barriers to the integration of psychosocial factors in medicine: Results of a national survey of physicians. *Journal of the American Board of Family Medicine, 19*, 557–565.

Barton, C., Clarke, D., Sulaimanc, N., & Abramson, M. (2003). Coping as a mediator of psychosocial impediments to optimal management and control of asthma. *Respiratory Medicine, 97*, 747–761.

Blake-Mortimer, J., Gore-Felton, C., Kimerling, R., Turner-Cobb, J. M., & Spiegel, D. (1999). Improving the quality and quantity of life among patients with cancer: A review of the effectiveness of group psychotherapy. *European Journal of Cancer, 35*, 1581–1586.

Boer, H., & Seydel, E. R. (1996). Protection motivation theory. In M. Connor & P. Norman (Eds.), *Predicting health behavior*. Buckingham: Open University Press.

Bottomley, A. (1996). Group cognitive behavioural therapy interventions with cancer patients: A review of the literature. *European Journal of Cancer Care (English Language Edition), 5*, 143–146.

Brassai, L., Piko, B. F., & Steger, M. F. (2011). Meaning in life: Is it a protective factor for adolescents' psychological health? *International Journal of Behavioural Medicine, 18*, 44–51.

Champion, V. L. (1984). Instrument development for health belief model constructs. *Advances in Nursing Science, 6*, 73–85.

Coan, R. W. (1973). Personality variables associated with cigarette smoking. *Journal of Personality and Social Psychology, 26*, 86–104.

Conner, M., & Norman, P. (1996). *Predicting health behavior: Search and practice with social cognition models*. Buckingham: Open University Press.

Cunningham, A. J. (1995). Group psychological therapy for cancer patients: A brief discussion of indications for its use, and the range of interventions available. *Supportive Care in Cancer, 3*, 244–247.

Dabbs, J. M., & Kirscht, J. P. (1971). Internal control and the taking of influenza shots. *Psychological Reports, 28*, 959–962.

Edelman, S., Bell, D. R., & Kidman, A. D. (1999). A group cognitive behaviour therapy programme with metastatic breast cancer patients. *Psychooncology, 8*, 295–305.

Engel, G. L. (1977). The need for a new medical model: A challenge for biomedicine. *Science, 196*, 129–136.

Fawzy, F. I., Fawzy, N. W., Arndt, L. A., & Pasnau, R. O. (1995). Critical review of psychosocial interventions in cancer care. *Archives of General Psychiatry, 52*, 100–113.

Fekete, E. M., Antoni, M. L., Schneiderman, N. (2007). Psycho-social and behavioural intervention for chronic medical condition. *Current Opinions in Psychiatry, 20*, 152–157.

Fuertes, J. N., Mislowack, A., Bennett, J., Paul, L., Gilbert, T. C., Fontan, G., et al. (2007). The physician-patient working alliance. *Patient Education and Counseling, 66*, 29–36.

Lewinsohn, P. M., Rohde, P., & Seeley, J. R. (1994). Psychosocial risk factors for future adolescent suicide attempts. *Journal of Consulting and Clinical Psychology, 62*, 297–305.

Lewis, F. M., Morisky, D. E., & Flynn, B. S. (1978). A test of construct validity of health locus of control: Effects of self-reported compliance for hypertensive patients. *Health Education Monographs, 6*, 138–148.

Menzies, V., Taylor, A. G., & Bourguignon, C. (2004). Effects of guided imagery on outcomes of pain, functional status, and self-efficacy in persons diagnosed with fibromyalgia. *Journal of Alternative and Complementary Medicine, 12*, 23–30.

Mossey, J. M., Mutran, E., Knott, K., & Craik, R. (1989). Determinants of recovery 12 months after hip fracture: The importance of psychosocial factors. *American Journal of PublicHealth, 79,* 279–286.

Peyrot, M., & Rubin, R. R. (2007). Behavioral and psychosocial interventions in Diabetes: A conceptual review. *Diabetes Care, 30*(10), 2433–2440.

Rimer, B. K., Trock, B., Engtorn, V. F., Lerman, C., & King, E. (1991). Why do some women get regular mammography? *American Journal of Preventive Medicine, 7,* 69–74

Rogers, R. W. (1983). Cognitive and physiological processes in fear appeals and attitude change: A revised theory of protection motivation. In J. Cacioppo & R. Petty (Eds.), *Social psychophysiology* (pp. 153–176). New York: Guilford Press.

Rosenstock, I. (1974). Historical origins of the health belief model. *Health Education Monographs, 2,* 328–335.

Schwarzer, R. (1992). Self-efficacy in the adoption and maintenance of health behaviors: Theoretical approaches and a new model. In R. Schwarzer (Ed.), *Self-efficacy: Thought control of action* (pp. 217–242). Washington, DC: Hemisphere.

Schwarzer, R. (2008). Modeling health behavior change: How to predict and modify the adoption and maintenance of health behaviors. *Applied Psychology: An International Review, 57*(1), 1–29.

Sherbourne, C. D., Hays, R. D., & Wells, K. B. (1995). Personal and psychosocial risk factors for physical and mental health outcomes and course of depression among depressed patients. *Journal of Consulting and Clinical Psychology, 63,* 345–355.

Sutton, S. R. (1982). Fear-arousing communications: a critical examination of theory and research. In J. R. Eiser (Ed.), *Social psychology and behavioral medicine* (pp. 303–337). London: Wiley.

Wyper, M. A. (1990). Breast self-examination and the health belief model: Variations on the theme. *Research in Nursing & Health, 13,* 421–428.

Zuckerman, D. M., Kasl, S. V., & Ostfeld, A. M. (1984). Psychosocial predictors of mortality among the elderly poor. The role of religion, well-being and social contacts. *American Journal of Epidemiology, 119,* 410–423.

Chapter 3
Determinants of Health and Well-Being: Empirical Analysis with Different Groups of Eastern Uttar Pradesh

Anubhuti Dubey

Concepts of Health and Well-Being

World Health Organization (WHO) (1948) has defined health, as a 'state of complete physical, mental and social well-being and not merely the absence of disease or infirmity'. Such a definition is very close to the definition enshrined in ancient treatises of Ayurveda, the Indian science of life. Shushrat defined health as 'a state of delight" or a feeling of spiritual, physical and mental well-being (Raina 1990; Rao 1983; Sharma 1981). The Sanskrit and Hindi equivalents for health is *swastha*; a person who possesses health is called *swasth*. It essentially involves a state of being located inside one's existential condition. It is being defined as 'being in one's self; being in one's natural state; relying upon one's self and self-sufficient' (Moneire-Williams Dictionary 2008; revised).

Thus the concept of health cannot be understood only as a medical, psychological and scientific concern but also needs to be placed in the larger societal context. Even one's perception of health is influenced by economic and political conditions, fashion trends, environmental support, cultural background and norms, standard of healthcare and so on. Therefore, the determinants of health are multiple and interactive.

Determinants of Well-Being

Health behaviour theories acknowledge that health behaviours may be influenced by numerous biological, psychological and social factors (Sutton 2004). In particular, residence, income, education, environment, genetic make-up, relationship

A. Dubey (✉)
Department of Psychology, DDU Gorakhpur University, Gorakhpur 273009, India
e-mail: anubhutiddu@rediffmail.com

G. Misra (ed.), *Psychosocial Interventions for Health and Well-Being*,
https://doi.org/10.1007/978-81-322-3782-2_3

with family and friends and also individual characteristics together determine the status of well-being. Based on the criteria used, Sumner (1996) has provided two categories of definitions—subjective and objective. Objective definition assumes that the criteria can be labelled without preferences, interests, ideals, values and attitude. The subjective definition acknowledges the individual's preferences, interests, ideals, values and attention. Diener and Suh (1997) asserted that health and well-being include people's evaluation (both affective and cognitive) of their lives. Biological, socio-cultural, psychological, economic and spiritual factors play a significant role.

Well-being is closer to the concept of mental health and happiness, life satisfaction and realization of one's full potential. General well-being is the subjective feeling of contentment, happiness and satisfaction with life's experiences and of one's role in one's field of work, thereby providing a sense of achievement, utility and belongingness without experiencing distress, dissatisfaction or worry (Verma and Verma 1989). Health and well-being both are linked with various domains of life including personal as well as social relationships (Diener 1984, 2000; Diener et al. 2003). The desire for the well-being of everyone (*Kamaye duhktanam praninamartinshanam*) has been a core Indian concern (Sharma and Misra 2010).

Education, Health and Well-Being

Education and literacy are graded as the key determinants of health, along with employment, income distribution, working conditions and social environment. The India Literacy Project (ILP 2000) mentions that India's literacy level is around 60%, and is particularly low with regard to women.

The education of women in rural India in general is still not satisfactory even though education has been endorsed as being the fundamental right and as an explicit goal for development. In a large part of the developing countries, women's access to schooling remains inadequate. Tripathi (2013) conducted a study on women of Sabia village of Kushinagar district of Eastern Uttar Pradesh and reported that educated women of all ages perceived their health status in a better way than women with no formal education. ANOVA findings indicated that educated women were engaged in health-enhancing practices more than those with no formal education. Content analyses of the interview data also confirmed these findings that educated women were taking healthy diet and precautions, providing their children with vaccinations, maintaining cleanliness at home and neighbouring areas and following a regular routine more than those who had no formal education. In case of a health-related problem, the educated women were more active in coping with it than any formal education group. Dubey (2013) also found that educated women access reproductive health services like regular checkups during pregnancy, institutional delivery, other prenatal and antenatal services, use of contraceptives etc. provided by the government more than the lesser educated or uneducated women.

Education provides skills and information to facilitate people to deal with the stresses of life. Moreover, education develops one's ability to gather and interpret information and solve problems at many levels; it increases one's potential to cope up with problems (Tripathi 2013). Other studies also show that educated people engage in a range of health-enhancing and self-maintenance activities (Lynch et al. 1997; Ross and Wu 1995). Tripathi and Dubey (2013) reported that high health literacy in women positively affect health practices and preventive health behaviours. Limited health literacy acts as independent risk factors for poor health (Baker et al. 1998) because of medication errors and inadequate understanding of diseases and treatment (Williams et al. 1998).

Education improves health directly as well as indirectly through work, economic conditions, social-psychological resources and healthy lifestyle (Ross and Wu 1995; Grossmann 2006). Educational attainment is associated with a broad array of psychosocial and biological conditions among the elderly (Dubey 2013).

Psychological Resources, Health and Well-Being

Psychological resources enable an individual to bounce back more quickly from life's setbacks. In this Sect. 1 will first look at the three psychological resources, i.e. optimism, future orientation and perceived control in health and well-being, which had been examined with diverse groups like cancer, diabetic and heart patients, healthcare professionals, homemakers, working and rural women, the elderly and students.

The diagnosis of a chronic disease like cancer, diabetes or cardiovascular diseases which are associated with life-threatening conditions poses manifold challenges before the person afflicted with the disease as well as his/her family. Dubey and Agarwal (2008, 2004) examined the predictive power of internal resources like future orientation, optimism and perceived control in maintaining quality of life as well as satisfaction with life in patients afflicted with chronic diseases. The findings of the multiple regression analysis showed that perception of control, optimism and future orientation explained 2–35% variance in predicting quality of life and satisfaction of life.

Dispositional Optimism is an individual difference variable that reflects the extent to which people hold generalized favourable expectancies for their future. In times of adversity or difficulty the higher levels of optimism have been related prospectively to better subjective well-being (Carver et al. 2010). Optimism is also related to indicators of better physical health and well-being (Carver et al. 2010; Dubey 2003; Peterson and Bossio 2001).

Optimism is not just a cognitive characteristic but it has inherent emotional and motivational components. Researchers have suggested links between pessimism, hopelessness and risk of heart disease (Dykema et al. 1995; Everson et al. 1996; Kubzansky et al. 2005) among the elderly (Giltay et al. 2006). However, extreme optimism can be damaging as it can put forward an underestimation of possible threats and an inadequate preparation for the same (Lovallo and Kahneman 2003). A pessimistic outlook is correlated with symptoms of depression and hopelessness (Koivumaa-Honkanen et al. 2000, 2001). Nevertheless, a moderate optimistic illusion can motivate adaptive behaviour in the present towards a future goal, and has been related to mental (Scheier and Carver 1987) and physical (Taylor and Brown 1988) health. Dispositional optimism was found to be positively associated with approach-coping strategies aiming to eliminate, reduce or manage stressors or emotions and negatively associated with avoidance-coping strategies seeking to ignore, avoid or withdraw from stressors or emotions (Nes and Segerstrom 2006; Dubey 2003, 2012a, b). Optimism negatively explained 9% variance in maladaptive coping for chronically ill patients (Dubey 2003).

The concept of future orientation, an aspect of time perspective is linked with individual hopes, expectations, aspirations, plans and strivings for goals, and has both motivational and cognitive components. People with high dispositional future orientation are prone to view a task as an open task (Agarwal 1993). This tendency leads dispositional future orientation to facilitate temporal coding. Dispositional future orientation mediated the perception of the utility of a material in the future, to affect its temporal coding (Agarwal and Tiwari 1988). High future-oriented persons had developed favourable attitude towards those whose names were associated with future-oriented cue statements (Tiwari and Agarwal 1989). This tendency was significantly more evident in high as compared to low future-oriented subjects. This showed the role of future orientation for the formation of other unrelated attitudes. Misra and Agarwal (2003) found that future orientation had significant positive association with women's possession of social skills and better psychological well-being. Women who have more structured future time perspective were more satisfied and happy with their lives.

Agarwal and Pandey (1998) observed that since future-oriented chronically ill patients are able to visualize hurdles in their path of achieving their goals, they also think and plan about ways and means of overcoming these hurdles and maintaining an optimistic outlook in spite of health problems. It was also noted by Agarwal and Tripathi (2000) that if the mothers of chronically ill children had future expectations about their children and had beliefs that health problems could be overcome in future by following present regimens, their children displayed better academic behaviour. Furthermore, mother's future expectations significantly predicted academic behaviour of children with chronic illness. As a protective factor, positive future orientation provides a measure of resilience against negative biopsychosocial outcomes through the utilization of active and adaptive coping strategies (Hirsh 2005). Individuals who are more future-oriented tend to be less involved in risk behaviour (Wills et al. 2001). Rothspan and Reed (1996) examined the present versus future time perspective among college students. They hypothesized that safer sex behaviours might reduce the exposure to HIV, positively correlating with future orientation. In the results it was found that those who were highly future oriented were less likely to be sexually experienced and had fewer sexual partners. Highly future oriented students were more likely to use alternate methods of reducing exposure to HIV. This study shows that future-oriented outlook enhances preventive behaviours. A positive association was found in high future-oriented thinking and participants' involvement in more preventive and safer health behaviour in diabetic patients (Dubey 2008) as well as better health and well-being among cancer, diabetic and myocardial infarction patients (Dubey 2003, 2012a, b). Intervention with cancer patients revealed that both optimistic look out and future-oriented thinking can be fostered (Dubey and Sharma 2006).

Another related concept thoroughly studied by the present researcher with as diverse groups as chronically ill patients, healthcare professionals, working women and people practicing yoga, is generalized control beliefs or perceived control (Dubey 2003, 2012a, b, 2013; Dubey and Shahi 2012). Perceived control means a person's self-assessment of control on various aspects of life as well as the ways and means to attain expected outcomes and to avoid unexpected ones. Steptoe et al. (1997) had explained the importance of perceived control and acknowledged that many of the health-related researches have especially focused on the control over aversive stimulation and on conditions in which the goal of control is the elimination of aversive events.

Control-related beliefs become crucial in the context of threatening traumatic events. Several investigations revealed that when individuals have prolonged traumatic health event and they come to believe that they have control over at least some aspects of that event, it leads to positive evaluation of quality of life and satisfaction with life. Perceived control predicted 10–31% variance in explaining quality of life in chronically ill patients and 68% variance in healthy individuals. Similarly, perceived control explained 26–42% variance in explaining satisfaction with life in chronically ill patients and 17–47% variance in healthy individuals (Dubey 2003). The studies with breast cancer patients (Taylor et al. 1984), men with AIDS (Reed et al. 1993) and heart disease patients (Taylor et al. 1991) revealed that the majority of patients felt that they had at least some or a high degree of control over their disease. These beliefs appear to be moderated by one's state of illness or prognosis. Thus, for example, asymptomatic breast cancer patients often assert that they have control over the disease itself and can prevent it from coming back (Taylor et al. 1984), whereas, men in the advanced stages of AIDS regard themselves as having a high degree of control over their day-to-day medical care and treatment, but only some degree of control over their overall course of illness. People high in feelings of perceived control are less likely to appraise events as threatening or negative. Patients who believe they can control illness are better off than those who do not see their illness as under their control (Dubey 2012a, b). They may believe that they can prevent the recurrence of disease through good health habits or by will power or by complying with the treatment regimen (Dubey 2013). Similar results have been obtained for patients suffering from rheumatoid arthritis (Affleck et al. 1987; Tennen et al. 1992) and post myocardial infarction patients (Helgeson 1992). When illness conditions are perceived as being modifiable and under one's personal control, the process of recovery from chronic disease is enhanced. Developing an internal locus of control would enhance the effectiveness of living with diabetes (Madhu et al. 1997; Sridhar and Madhu 2001). Dubey (2012a, b) examined the role of control beliefs, that is, the primary and perceived control in regularity and consistency in doing yogic practices with participants attending a yoga camp for a week. The control beliefs were assessed before starting the camp and after six months of the camp and found that only the participants high in control beliefs before the camp had continued with it on a regular basis. The regression analysis of the follow-up data (after six months) also confirmed that the contribution of perceived control and primary control towards health and well-being was 14 and 25 and 24 and 14%, respectively, considering participants who were regularly practicing yoga after attending the yoga camp. Awasthi and Mishra (2010) reported that women patients suffering with cancer with high social support have a stronger belief in 'self'-control than those with low social support, which suggests that social support can enhance their feeling of 'self-efficacy', which is a sign of positive psychological growth. There are some evidences which report that control beliefs can be modified in later stages of life too (Lachman 2006). Control beliefs play an important role in how people direct their own development during their life span.

Social-Cognitive Determinants of Health and Well-Being

People think about health, health-related problems and health practices very often. Sometimes if a person becomes ill, symptoms and bodily sensations are difficult to interpret. Then, beliefs and external information may be helpful in deciding whether a symptom is transitory or serious. So individual's ideas and beliefs about health and illness are important to describe health status. These cognitive determinants help us organize and make sense of incoming information from our bodies. Health beliefs and social learning theory are labelled as social cognitive theory which are applied in varying success in problems explaining, predicting and influencing health behaviour (Rosenstock et al. 1988).

The prevalence of beliefs and myths amongst cancer patients is a reflection of the level of knowledge in the community regarding cancer. Such beliefs influence the health-seeking behaviour of patients and may lead to delay in seeking medical care. Health behaviours and practices are influenced by individual's culturally determined systems of beliefs (Mishra and Awasthi 2004). The findings of Kishore et al. (2007) revealed that myths and misconceptions are widely prevalent among cancer patients in India. The perception regarding causation of cancer among cancer patients varied from curses, evil eye and spirits to past sins (Dubey 2003). Awasthi and Mishra (2008) reported that cancer patients held a stronger belief in supernatural causes as compared to those afflicted with diabetes. Sheikh and Furnham (2000) stated that culturally determined causal beliefs of mental distress contribute to attitudes towards seeking professional help for psychological problems for Asians. They reported that British Asians, Westerners and Pakistanis significantly differ in the causal attributions of mental distress. Although culture, as a variable, was not a significant predictor of a positive attitude to seeking professional help, causal beliefs of mental distress were significant predictors of attitudes to seeking help for the British Asian and the Pakistani groups. Beliefs were not significant predictors for attitudes to seeking help for the Western group (Sheikh and Furham 2000). However, the same is not true in Indian culture. Rural men and women of four major districts of eastern Utter Pradesh showed health beliefs both harmful as well as beneficial for them. For example, health and illness is God's will and the human being can't do anything; illness is the fruit of karma; women want to die before husband (as a *suhagin* or as a married woman); women's body is the home of diseases and illnesses; and they believed that disease can be treated by practising *Chua-chute* (untouchability), *nazar utarna* (ousting evil), *jadu-tona, jhar–phunk, jog–totka,* (black magic), *mannat mangna* (praying for a boon from God), along with going to doctors whether qualified or quacks (Dubey and Kumar 2012; Tripathi 2013).

As per the culture of the East, indigenous healing practices emphasize on supernatural causality including punishment from the spirit of God (Joshi 1988; Weiss et al. 1986), recovery from illness through sorcery, recuperation as God's will or the result of karma (Kohli and Dalal 1998; Dalal 2000). The rural women from low and medium socio-economic status of eastern Utter Pradesh believed that serious illnesses were results of supernatural causes i.e., wrath of any deity or witch or sorcerer who had been displeased. Hence, they worship, fast and go to traditional healers for '*nazar utarna*' or measures to avoid evil eyes (Dubey and Kumar 2012). The diabetic participants in a study in Kerala relied on biomedicine for treating diabetes, but frequently used Ayurvedic medicine and folk herbal remedies as supplements. They named 24 local plants and plant products that were employed to lower blood glucose levels. Knowledge of tried and tested local or regional remedies and their incorporation into individual and community healthcare practices are evidence of medical knowledge as cultural capital (Chacko 2003). A common sense understanding of the causes of illness is often a social construction derived from the cultural models of illness (Mishra 2008).

In our culture, decisions are taken by an individual but with the consent of the whole family (where the decisive role is played by eldest member of the family). This tendency goes further in community and at societal level. Therefore, it is suggestive that understanding and controlling of health behaviour and practices cannot be done without the cognizance of the role of family and community and the family is the best resource which made the sufferer perceive life's worth even facing life-threatening situations (Dubey and Agarwal 2008). In a study on rural women of eastern Uttar Pradesh, Dubey (2013) found that females had emphasized that generally for the family or health-related issues they are not being involved in decision making and sometimes if they are involved their arguments are not given due respect. Nevertheless, sometimes the males may consider issues raised by the elderly females of the family but this is mostly in case of reproductive health related matters not family resource-related issues. Many a times health-related decisions are influenced by the traditional norms, cultural beliefs and practices (Dubey and Kumar 2012; Dubey 2013). Studies on women showed that negative attitudes towards menopause were related to general symptom reporting and depression. Additionally, negative attitudes prior to menopause were related to subsequent symptom reporting during menopause (Avis and McKinlay 1991; Nosek et al.

2010). If a person has a positive attitude about any kind of illness he/she can actively cope with the illness (Dubey 2003). For example, people belonging to the type of families where exercise is practiced (Sallis et al. 1988) have positive attitude towards physical activity and perceive themselves as athletic or physically fit (Kendzierski 1990). Similarly, people who believe that people should take responsibility for their health are more likely to get involved in exercise programmes earlier than those who do not like exercising or believe in its benefits (Dishman 1982); exercise and fitness regimen if practiced during childhood leave lifetime implications (Blair et al. 1989). Tripathi (2013) found that attitude towards causal and control beliefs together explained 28% variance in satisfaction with life and 16% variance in quality of life on a sample of rural women.

Coping, Health and Well-Being

Coping is altering the thought and behaviour that people use to manage distress, in the context of a specific stressful encounter or situation (e.g. Moos 1974; Folkman and Lazarus 1980; Moos and Schaefer 1993). Coping generally refers to adaptive or constructive coping strategies to reduce stress. However, a few coping strategies can be considered maladaptive, as they intensify the stress. Maladaptive coping can thus be described, as non-coping. Moreover, the term coping commonly refers to reactive coping, i.e., the coping response follows the stressor.

Problem-solving coping entails efforts to do something constructive about stressful conditions that are harming, threatening or challenging for the individual. This coping strategy seems to transpire during childhood (Compass et al. 1991) and is of assistance across situations, like dealing with a chronic disease like cancer, diabetes or heart disease (Dubey 2003, 2012a, b; Dubey and Agarwal 2004, 2008; Dubey and Bajpai 2013) or workplace stress (Dubey and Shahi 2011) or family stress (Dubey and Shahi 2012). Application of active coping strategies by chronically ill patients leads them to actively follow a treatment regime and plan for a future course of action which bring relief and diminish uncertainty, which further encourage them to apply active coping strategies like planning, restraint coping, acceptance of the facts, etc. (Dubey 2003). Emotion-focused coping involves efforts to regulate emotions experienced because of stressful events. In other words, it involves releasing pent-up emotions, distracting oneself, managing hostile feelings, mediating or using systematic relaxation procedures. Emotion-focused coping is oriented towards managing the emotions that accompany the perception of stress. Emotion-focused coping skills develop in later childhood or early adolescents (Compass et al. 1991). Mishra and Dubey (2013) found that childless females opting for In Vitro-Fertilization (IVF) technique were applying emotion-focused coping strategies to overcome treatment-related stress as well as the social stigma of being childless. Actually, the nature of the event may be a factor to what coping strategies will be used (Vitaliono et al. 1990). When health problems are amenable to active efforts problem-focused coping is advantageous (Penley et al. 2002).

Health problems also lead people to seek social support (Vitaliono et al. 1990). In patients with chronic renal failure who are on dialysis the most commonly used coping strategies are emotion oriented, avoidance and isolated thoughts which correlate with stress levels (Kohli and Agrawal 2008). These findings suggest that a situation in which something constructive can be done will favour problem-focused coping, whereas those situations that simply must be accepted favour emotion-focused coping (Zakowski et al. 2001). Even managing the stressors of daily life can be benefited by emotional-approach coping which is especially beneficial for women (Stanton et al. 2000).

Coping strategy, named spirituality, and coping through religion is found helpful to women in two ways. By promoting internal resources (coping) women are able to come to terms with personal and social hardship, and obtain a feeling of well-being and calm. Studies with women both employees and homemakers, who are facing infertility problems or serious illness of a family member or dealing with day-to-day health problems, believe in spirituality and religion as beneficial coping means (Tripathi 2013; Dubey 2003, 2013; Dubey and Shahi 2012).

Dubey (2009) examined the psychosocial stress, negative mental state, life satisfaction, coping and health of employed and homemaker women and reported that in contrast to the general perception that employment leads to more psychosocial stress and poor well-being these findings showed that homemaker had more psychosocial stress on dimensions of economic constraints, marriage and health-related problems, adverse social and economic status as compared to their employed women counterparts. Homemakers reported more physical and other health-related symptoms, less satisfaction and more negative mental state as compared to employed women. The employed women were using significantly more active and humour-coping strategies as compared to homemakers. Dubey and Shahi (2012) explored the available social networks, identified the congruence/discrepancies in the social support desired and received while coping with stressors and health of the employed and the homemaker married women. The best social networks expressed by both groups of women were parents and friends followed by siblings and husband. The discrepancy in desired and received social support and employment status had significant effect in applying active coping strategies. The physical health was affected by the interaction of employment status and discrepancy in desired and received social support, whereas, for psychological health the effect of discrepancy in social support was observed.

Full Circles: Links in Psychological Resources, Coping, Health and Well-Being

Studies suggested links between health or illness beliefs and coping strategies. Internal causal health beliefs promote beliefs about one's ability to avoid future negative outcomes which is central in facilitating positive adjustment and well-being for women and chronically ill patients (Dubey 2003, 2012a, b). Internal causal health beliefs aid in coping by giving chronically ill patients meaningful explanation for their sufferings, helping them uphold a view of the world as a place where depressing events have identifiable causes. People who believe more in social, fatalistic and supernatural explanations for health and illness raises the level of personal energy to bear their own burden and cope effectively with chronic conditions (Furnham and Heaven 1999).

People with strong religious faith report greater life satisfaction, greater personal happiness and fewer negative consequences of traumatic life events. Religion promotes a sense of psychological well-being (Dubey 2003, 2012a, b; Tripathi 2013). However, it was found by Dubey and colleagues that sometimes a chronically ill patient feels that things are out of control and shows excessive dependence on prayer; in cases of such excessive dependence on prayer to make everything well make religion coping an adaptive or many a times a maladaptive coping strategy. Hence, those healthy people who have future-oriented outlook do not depend on God for removing all their difficulties and do not excessively pray to *Him* for this purpose (Dubey 2003, 2012a, b). Psychological resources like a sense of control, optimism and future oriented outlook along with a cohesive and healthy relationship in family and system maintenance in family was found to enhance the use of active coping strategies in chronically ill individuals (Dubey 2003, 2012a, b). Optimism significantly and negatively predicts two components of maladaptive coping strategies i.e., behavioural disengagement and venting of emotions for chronically ill patients (Dubey 2003). Effective coping strategies such as support from social networks and spirituality can reduce stress and promote physical and mental well-being, and improve health for women as well as for doctors (Dubey and Shahi 2011, 2012). Health has been identified as one of the most important factors related to life satisfaction (Dubey 2003) and use of active coping strategies were effective in promoting the level of satisfaction as a whole and also the present and future life satisfaction (Dubey and Agarwal 2007).

The health psychologists may help and give counseling to patients, doctors, students and women to develop resources that would help them to be optimistic, future oriented and positive even in adverse circumstances and guide them to use active coping strategies (Dubey and Sharma 2006; Dubey and Shahi 2012; Dubey and Bajpai 2013).

References

Affleck, G., Tennen, H., Pfeiffer, C., & Fifield, C. (1987). Appraisals of control and predictability in adapting to a chronic disease. *Journal of Personality and Social Psychology, 53,* 273–279.

Agarwal, A. (1993). Influence of prolonged deprivation, age and culture on the development of future orientation. *European Journal of Social Psychology, 14,* 451–453.

Agarwal, A., & Pandey, A. (1998). Coping with chronic disease: Role of psychosocial variables. *Psychological Studies, 43*(1&2), 58–64.

Agarwal, A., & Tiwari, S. (1988). Future orientation: A mediator in temporal coding. *International Journal of Psychology, 23,* 151–163.
Agarwal, A., & Tripathi, I. (2000). Chronic illness, symptoms and efficacy in children as related to some psychological characteristics of mothers. *Psychology and Developing Societies, 12*(1), 31–42.
Avis, N. E., & McKinlay, S. M. (1991). A longitudinal analysis of women's attitudes toward the menopause: Results from the Massachusetts Women's Health Study. *Maturitas, 13*(1), 65–79.
Awasthi, P., & Mishra, R. C. (2008). A comparative study of chronic illness beliefs of cancer and diabetic women. *Journal of Indian Health Psychology, 3*(1), 27–49.
Awasthi, P., & Mishra, R. C. (2010). Illness beliefs of women cancer patients and their relationships with social support. *Journal of the Indian Academy of Applied Psychology, 36*(2), 317–327.
Baker, D. W., Parker, R. M., Williams, M. V., & Clark, W. S. (1998). Health literacy and the risk of hospital admission. *Journal of General Internal Medicine, 13*(12), 791–798.
Blair, S. N., Clark, D. G., Cureton, K. J., & Powell, K. E. (1989). Exercise and fitness in childhood: Implications for a lifetime of health. *Perspectives in Exercise Science and Sports Medicine, 2,* 401–430.
Carver, C. S., Scheier, M. F., & Segerstrom, S. C. (2010). Optimism. *Clinical Psychology Review, 30*(7), 879–889.
Chacko, E. (2003). Culture and therapy: Complementary strategies for treatment of type 2 diabetes in an urban setting in Kerala, India. *Social Science & Medicine, 56*(5), 1087–1098.
Compass, B. E., Barnez, G. A., Malcarne, V., & Worshum, N. (1991). Perceived control and coping with stress: A development perspective. *Journal of Social Issues, 47,* 23–34.
Dalal, A. K. (2000). Living with a chronic disease: Healing and psychological adjustment in Indian Society. *Psychology Developing Societies, 12*(1), 67–81.
Diener, E. (1984). Subjective well-being. *Psychological Bulletin, 95,* 542–575.
Diener, E. (2000). Subjective well-being: The science of happiness, and a proposal for national index. *American Psychologist, 55,* 34–43.
Deiner, E., & Suh, E. M. (1997). Measuring quality of life: Economics, social and subjective indicators. *Social Indicators Research, 40,* 189–216.
Diener, E. S., Oishi, S., & Lucas, R. E. (2003). Personality, Culture, and subjective wellbeing: Emotional and cognitive evaluation of life. *Annual Review of Psychology, 54*, 403–25.
Dishman, R. K. (1982). Compliance/adherence in health-related exercise. *Health Psychology, 1,* 237–267.
Dubey, A. (2003). Role of some psychological variables in chronic illness. Unpublished doctoral dissertation. Department of Psychology, DDU Gorakhpur University, Gorakhpur.
Dubey, A. (2008). Future oriented thinking and wellbeing in diabetic patients. *Journal of Indian Psychology, 26*(1&2), 22–30.
Dubey, A. (2009). Does being employed have psychological consequences? *The Social Engineer, 12*(1&2), 41–50.
Dubey, A. (2012a). *Psychological perspectives on chronic illness*. New Delhi: Concept Publishing Company.
Dubey, A. (2012b). Perceived control as predictor of yogic practices and effects of yoga on health and wellbeing. *Journal of Psychology, 3*(2), 121–129.
Dubey, A. (2013). Psycho-social dynamics of health in women of rural Eastern Uttar Pradesh. Unpublished ICSSR funded project report. Department of Psychology, DDU Gorakhpur University, Gorakhpur.
Dubey, A., & Agarwal, A. (2004). Feeling well inspite of chronic illness. *Psychological Studies, 49,* 65–68.
Dubey, A., & Agarwal, A. (2007). Coping strategies and life satisfaction: Chronically ill patients' perspectives. *Journal of Indian Academy of Applied Psychology, 33*(2), 161–168.
Dubey, A., & Agarwal, A. (2008). Maintaining quality of life in adversity: A study on chronically ill patients. *Journal of Indian Health Psychology, 3*(1), 50–63.

Dubey, A., & Bajpai, L. (2013). Fostering emotional intelligence and coping with diabetes and evaluation of quality of life. *Indian Journal of Health and Well Being, 4*(5), 993–999.

Dubey, A., & Kumar, D. (2012). How health beliefs shape health practices, coping and well-being of women. In S. Ojha & S. Pandey (Eds.), *Positive psychology: Emerging issues* (Vol. 2, pp. 329–341). New Delhi: Shree Publisher and Distributors.

Dubey, A., & Shahi, D. (2012). Social networks, congruence in desired and received social support, coping and health of women. *Indian Journal of Health and Wellbeing*, *3*(2), 390–394.

Dubey, A., & Shahi, D. (2011). Psychological immunity and coping strategies: A study of medical professionals. *Indian Journal of Social Science Researches, 8*(1&2), 36–47.

Dubey, A., & Sharma, L. (2006). Cognitive behavioral intervention for cancer patients. *Psychological Studies, 51*(1 & 2), 212–216.

Dykema, J., Bergbower, K., & Peterson, C. (1995). Pessimistic explanatory style, stress, and illness. *Journal of Social and Clinical Psychology, 14,* 357–371.

Giltay, E. J., Kamphuis, M. H., Kalmijn, S., Zitman, F. G., & Kromhout, D. (2006). Dispositional optimism and the risk of cardiovascular death. The Zutphen elderly study. *Archives of Internal Medicine, 166*(4), 431–436.

Everson, S. A., Goldberg, D. E., Kaplan, G. A., Cohen, R. D., Pukkala, E., et al. (1996). Hopelessness and risk of mortality and incidence of myocardial infarction and cancer. *Psychosomatic Medicine, 58,* 113–121.

Folkman, S., & Lazarus, R. S. (1980). An analysis of coping in a middle, aged community sample. *Journal of Health and Social Behaviour, 21,* 219–239.

Furnham, A., & Heaven, P. (1999). *Personality and social behavior*. London: Arnold.

Grossmann, M. (2006). Education and nonmarket outcomes. In E. A. Hanushek & F. Welch (Eds.), *Handbook of the economics of education* (Vol. 1, pp. 578–633). Amsterdam: Elsevier BV.

Helgeson, V. S. (1992). Moderators of the relation between perceived control and adjustment to chronic illness. *Journal of Personality and Social Psychology, 63,* 656–666.

Hirsh, J. K. (2005). The role of positive psychology in the study and prevention of suicide. The President Column. Section on Clinical Emergencies and Crises, American Psychological Association.

India Literacy Project (ILP). (2000). (http://www.ilpc.org/) ILP, Washington DC, USA.

Joshi, P. C. (1988). Traditional medical system in the Central Himalayas. In: *The eastern anthropologists* (pp. 116–147). New York: Guilford Press.

Kendzierski, D. (1990). Exercise self schemata: Cognitive and behavioural correlates. *Health Psychology, 9,* 69–82.

Kishore, J., Ahmad, I., Kaur, R., & Mohanta, P. K. (2007). Beliefs and perceptions about cancers among patients attending radiotherapy OPD in Delhi, India. *Asian Pacific Journal of Cancer Prevention, 9,* 155–158.

Kohli, N., & Dalal, A. K. (1998). Psychological recovery of women with cervical cancer: The role of cultural beliefs. In: W. J. Lonner, D. L. Dinnel, D. K. Forgays, & S. Hayes (Eds.), Merging past, present, and future in cross-cultural psychology (pp. 348–364). Lisse, the Netherlands: Swets & Zeitlinger.

Kohli, S., & Agrawal, H. K. (2008). Psychological aspects of chronic renal failure. *Journal of Indian Health Psychology, 3*(1), 12–18.

Koivumaa-Honkanen, H., Honkanen, R., Viinamaki, H., Heikkila, K., Kaprio, J., & Koskenvuo, M. (2000). Self-reported life satisfaction and 20-year mortality in healthy Finnish adults. *American Journal of Epidemiology, 152,* 983–991.

Koivumaa-Honkanen, H., Honkanen, R., Viinamaki, H., Heikkila, K., Kaprio, J., & Koskenvuo, M. (2001). Life satisfaction and suicide: A 20-year follow-up study. *American Journal of Psychiatry, 158,* 433–439.

Kubzansky, L. D., Davidson, K. W., & Rozanski, A. (2005). The clinical impact of negative psychological states: Expanding the spectrum of risk for coronary artery disease. *Psychosomatic Medicine, 67*(Supplement 1), S10–S14.

Lachman, M. E. (2006). Perceived control over aging-related declines: Adaptive beliefs and behaviours. *Current Directions in Psychological Science, 15*(6), 282–286.

Lovallo, D., & Kahneman, D. (2003). Delusions of success: how optimism undermines executives' decisions. *Harvard Business Review*, 56–63.

Lynch, J. W., Kaplan, G. A., & Salonen, J. T. (1997). Why do poor people behave poorly? Variations in adult health behaviour and psychosocial characteristics, by stage of the socioeconomic life course. *Social Science and Medicine, 44,* 809–820.

Madhu, K., Veena, S., & Sridhar, G. R. (1997). Gender differences in quality of life among persons with diabetes mellitus in south India. *Diabetologia, 40*(Suppl 1), 2487–2632.

Mishra, M., & Agarwal, A. (2003). Coping and satisfaction with life in working women. In A. Agarwal & A. K. Saxena (Eds.), Psychological perspectives in environmental and developmental issues. New Delhi: Concept Publishing Company.

Mishra, K., & Dubey, A. (2013). Perceived psychosocial changes in life of women after marriage: A Narrative analysis. *International Journal of Social Science Tomorrow, 2*(9), 1–9.

Mishra, R. C. (2008). Health cognition and practices among the Kharwars of Naugarh region of Varanasi. In A. Shukla & R. C. Mishra (Eds.), *Culture cognition and behavior* (pp. 264–276). New Delhi: Concept Publishing Company.

Mishra, R. C., & Awasthi, P. (2004). Health psychology and community development. *Indian Journal of Community Psychology, 1,* 156–170.

Moos, R. H. (1974). Psychological techniques in assessment of adaptive behaviour. In G. V. Coelho, D. A. Hamberg, & J. E. Adams (Eds.), *Coping and adaptation* (pp. 334–99). New York: Basic Books.

Moos, R. H., & Schaefer, J. A. (1993). Coping resources and processes: Current concepts and measure. In L. Goldberger & S. Brezenitz (Eds.), *Handbook of stress: Theoretical and clinical aspects* (pp. 234–257). New York: Free Press.

Nes, L. S., & Segerstrom, S. C. (2006). Dispositional optimism and coping: A meta analytic review. *Personality and Social Psychology Review, 10*(3), 235–251.

Nosek, M., Kennedy, H.P., Beyene, Y., Taylor, D., lliss, C., & Lee, K. (2010). The effects of perceived stress and attitudes toward menopause and aging on symptoms of menopause. *Journal of Midwifery & Women's Health, 55*(4), 328–334.

Penley, J. A., Tamaka, J., & Weibe, J. S. (2002). The association of coping to physical and psychological health outcomes. A meta-analysis review. *Journal of Behavioural Medicine, 25,* 551–603.

Peterson, C., & Bossio, L. M. (2001). Optimism and physical well-being. In E. C. Chang, (Ed.), Optimism and pessimism: Implications for theory, research, and practice (pp. 127–145). Washington, DC: American Psychological Association.

Raina, B. L. (1990). *Health sciences in ancient India*. New Delhi: Common Wealth.

Rao, S. K. R. (1983). The conception of stress in Indian thought: The theoretical aspects of stress in Samkhya and Yoga Systems. *NIMHANS Journal, 2,* 115–121.

Reed, G. M., Taylor, S. E., & Kemeny, M. E. (1993). Perceived control and psychological adjustment in gay men with AIDS. *Journal of Applied Social Psychology, 23,* 791–824.

Rosenstock, I. M., Strecher, V. J., & Becker, M. H. (1988). Social learning theory and the health belief model. *Health Education Quarterly, 15*(2), 175–183.

Ross, C. E., & Wu, C. L. (1995). The links between education and health. *American Social Review, 60,* 719–745.

Rothspan, S., & Reed, S. J. (1996). Present versus future time perspective and HIV risk among heterosexual college students. *Health Psychology, 15*(2), 131–134.

Sallis, J. F., Patterson, T. L., Buono, M. J., Atkins, C. J., & Nader, P. R. (1988). Aggression of physical activity habits in Maxican-Americans and Anglo families. *Journal of Behavioural Medicine, 11,* 31–42.

Scheier, M. F., & Carver, C. S. (1987). Dispositional optimism and physical well being: The influence of generalized outcome expectancies on health. *Journal of Personality, 55,* 169–210.

Sharma, P. (1981). *Charak Samhita* (English Translation) Varanasi: Chaukhambha Sanskrit Series Office.

Sharma, S., & Misra, G. (2010). Health psychology: Progress and challenges. In: G. Misra (Ed.), *Psychology in India (Vol. 3)—Clinical and health psychology* (pp. 265–316). New Delhi: Pearson Education.

Sheikh, S., & Furham, A. (2000). A cross-cultural study of mental health beliefs and attitudes towards seeking professional help. *Social Psychiatry and Psychiatric Epidemiology, 35*(7), 326–334.

Sridhar, G. R., & Madhu, K. (2001). Stress in the cause and course of diabetes. *International Journal Diabetes in Developing Countries, 21,* 112–119.

Steptoe, A., Evans, O., & Fieldman, G. (1997). Perceived control over work: Psychophysiological response to self-paced and externally-paced tasks in an adult population sample. *International Journal of Psychophysiology, 25,* 211–220.

Sutton, S. (2004). Determinants of health-related behaviors: Theoretical and methodological issues. In S. Sutton, A. Baum, & M. Johnston (Eds.), *The Sage handbook of health psychology*. London: Sage.

Stanton, A. L., Kirk, S. B., Cameron, C. L., & Danoft-Burg, S. (2000). Coping through emotional approach: Scale construction and validation. *Journal of Personality and Social Psychology, 78,* 1150–1169.

Sumner, S. W. (1996). *Welfare, happiness, and ethics*. Oxford: Claredon Press.

Taylor, S. E., & Brown, J. D. (1988). Illusion and well being: A social psychological perspective on mental health. *Psychological Bulletin, 107*(2), 193–210.

Taylor, S. E., Helgeson, V. S., Reed, G. M., & Skokan, L. A. (1991). Self generated feelings of control and adjustment to physical illness. *Journal of Social Issues, 47,* 91–109.

Taylor, S. E., Lichtman, R. R., & Wood, J. V. (1984). Attributions, beliefs about control, and adjustment to breast cancer. *Journal of Personality and Social Psychology, 46,* 489–502.

Tennen, H., Affleck, G., Urrows, S., Higgins, P., & Mendola, R. (1992). Perceiving control, construing benefits and daily process in rheumatoid arthritis. *Canadian Journal of Behavioral Sciences, 24,* 186–203.

Tiwari, S., & Agarwal, A. (1989). Arousal of future orientation and attitude formation. *Indian Psychologists, 6*(1 & 2), 21–29.

Tripathi, K. M. (2013). Cognitive determinants of health and its relation to coping and well being of women. *Unpublished doctoral dissertation*. Department of Psychology, DDU Gorakhpur University, Gorakhpur, India.

Tripathi, K. M., & Dubey, A. (2013). Role of education in health and wellbeing of rural women. *Indian Journal of Social Science and organizational Behavior, 2*(1), 22–27.

Verma, S. K., & Verma, A. (1989). *Manual for PGI General Wellbeing Measure*. Lucknow: Ankur Psychology Agency.

Vitaliono, P. P., Maiuro, R. D., Russo, J., Katon, W. De, Wolfe, D., & Hall, G. (1990). Coping profiles associated with psychiatric, physical health, work and family problems. *Health Psychology, 9,* 348–376.

Weiss, M. G., Sharma, S. D., Gaur, R. K., Sharma, J. S., Desai, A., & Doongaji, D. R. (1986). Traditional concepts of mental disorder among Indian psychiatric patients: Preliminary report of work in progress. *Social Science and Medicine, 23*(4), 379–386.

Williams, M. V., Baker, D. W., Parker, R. M., & Nurss, J. R. (1998). Relationship of functional health literacy to patients' knowledge of their chronic disease: A study of patients with hypertension or diabetes. *Archives of Internal Medicine, 158,* 166–172.

World Health Organization. (1948). *Constitution of the World Health Organization*. Geneva, Switzerland: World Health organization Basic Documents.

Wills, T. A., Sandy, J. M., & Yaeger, A. M. (2001). Time perspective and early onset substance use: A model based on stress coping theory. *Psychology of Addictive Behavior, 15,* 118–125.

Zakowski, S. G., Hall, M. H., Klein, L. C., & Baum, A. (2001). Appraisal control, coping and stress in a community sample. A test of the goodness of fit hypothesis. *Analysis of Behavioural Medicine, 23,* 158–165.

Chapter 4
Psychology of Resilience

Amrita Deb

Psychology has traditionally focused more on the study of symptoms and disorders than on positive characteristics of individuals. The reason for this deficit-based approach may be traced to the aftermath of World War II (Seligman 2002) when the priority of psychologists was to 'repair damage' (Seligman and Csikszentmihalyi 2000) versus enhancing well-being. However, with Martin Seligman's presidential speech of the APA in 1998, where he drew attention to the fact that psychology is not just the study of pathology and damage, but also the study of strength and virtue, there began an effort to shift the attention from 'preoccupation only with repairing the worst things in life, to building positive qualities (Seligman and Csikszentmihalyi 2000, p. 5). This led to a series of studies on positive emotions, positive characteristics and positive institutions—all of which had not been priority areas in psychological research for a very long time. One of the areas that benefitted immensely from this movement is the area of psychological resilience.

Origin and Background of Resilience Research

The term 'resilience' is believed to have originated from the Latin word 'resilire' which means 'to recoil or leap back', and was typically used in the area of physical sciences and engineering to refer to the capacity to withstand strain without breaking or to recover to original form like a spring (Masten and Gewirtz 2006). Anthony (1974) presented the interesting analogy of three dolls made of glass, plastic and steel respectively to explain the concept. When struck by a hammer, the first doll shatters, the second is permanently damaged, and the third only emits a

A. Deb (✉)
Department of Liberal Arts, Indian Institute of Technology, Hyderabad, Telangana, India
e-mail: amrita@iith.ac.in

G. Misra (ed.), *Psychosocial Interventions for Health and Well-Being*,
https://doi.org/10.1007/978-81-322-3782-2_4

fine metallic sound, indicating its resilience to stress. While resilience was earlier described as 'bouncing back' from adversity (Luthar and Cicchetti 2000), the idea of 'bouncing forward' (Walsh 2002) came to be proposed later. Over the years, the construct has been operationalized in a variety of ways; however Fletcher and Sarkar (2013) observe that most definitions are based around the core concepts of adversity and positive adaptation. Simply defined, it is the phenomenon of displaying competence despite challenges. Recently, Bonanno et al. (2015) acknowledged that the term has taken on overlapping meanings and suggested that resilience studies must 'explicitly reference each of four constituent temporal elements: (a) baseline or preadversity functioning, (b) the actual aversive circumstances, (c) postadversity resilient outcomes, and (d) predictors of resilient outcomes" (p. 139).

Researchers have often referred to the concepts of risk, vulnerability and protective factors in order to provide a comprehensive understanding of resilience.

Risk and Protective Factors

Risk is defined as a psychosocial adversity that could maintain a problem condition and thus hinder functioning (Masten 1994). These may either work singly or in combination with other risk factors and may often pile up over time (Rutter 1987); this is referred to as cumulative risk. Adversities may occur in different forms such as illness, natural calamity or job stress and may cause different kinds of disturbances—short term, severe and chronic. Vulnerability to overwhelming obstacles is not unnatural, neither is it true that exposure to adversity would always and necessarily render us permanently damaged. Rather, these may make us stronger and better equipped to face further challenges ahead. However, not all individuals who are exposed to the same adversity exhibit similar levels of resilience. This difference is explained by how individuals use the protective factors available to them. The role of a protective factor is to buffer, interrupt or even prevent risk (Rutter 1987), thus playing a crucial part in the resiliency process. Like risk factors, they have a cumulative impact, that is, success in one area can serve as a springboard for success in other areas (Killian 2004). The critical feature of protective factors that is to be inferred is how it modifies one's response to a risk situation that in ordinary circumstances may lead to maladaptive outcome (Rutter 1987). Protective factors may range from internal buffers such as self-efficacy to external ones including strong relationships and community support.

Theoretical Models of Resilience

In their attempt to explain why some individuals are able to show competence despite adversities, researchers have proposed several theoretical models.

Antonovosky's (1979) Sense of Coherence Model and Kobasa's (1979) Hardiness Model may be one of the earliest attempts to explain positive adaptation. Grotberg's (1999) paradigm of resilience introduced the components of 'I have', 'I am', and 'I Can' to explain the mechanism of resilience in youth with depression while Kumpfer (1999) presented a person–environment transactional process that may lead to either resilient or maladaptive reintegration. Later, Richardson (2002) described a simple linear model that shows how individuals consciously or unconsciously go through the stages of biopsychospiritual homeostasis, disruption and integration that may result in either resilient reintegration, reintegration back to homeostasis, reintegration with loss, or dysfunctional reintegration. Interventions among adolescents were proposed through the youth resilience framework that highlights individual and sociocultural risk and protective factors (Ahern 2006; Rew and Horner 2003). Knight (2007) claims that the all-encompassing 3D-framework of resilience presenting the concept as a state, condition, and practice, can be applied in all contexts whereas van Breda's (2011) model that conceptualizes the workplace as a social system includes a range of environments such as schools, universities, hospitals, military, shops, welfare agencies, or factories and incorporates stressors, risk factors, protective factors and outcomes. All these models focus on complex transactional and developmental pathway systems (Kumpfer 1999) which are interrelated and interdependent (Killian 2004), thus influencing the interaction between the resilience factors and adversity. Researchers have often referred to these models in accordance with the contexts being assessed.

Conceptual and Methodological Constraints in Studying Resilience

Over the years, researchers have encountered several conceptual and methodological constraints in studying resilience. Even as they continued to systematically conduct empirical studies on resilience, researchers were simultaneously working on conceptualizing it in a better way. For instance, the terms 'invulnerable' and 'invincible' that were earlier used synonymously with resilience came to be rejected later as they refer to an absolute resistance to damage as if the individual was unscathed by the situation (Werner and Smith 1982). Furthermore, the initial conceptualization of resilience as a cluster of traits was later discarded in favour of the idea that this is a process that develops overtime by the interaction of the person with the environment (Masten 2001; Rutter 2012). While the concept continued to evolve over time, there were also attempts at providing distinctions between resilience and similar processes including adjustment, coping, competence and post-traumatic growth. Despite overlaps between many of these conceptualizations, it may be noted that researchers do agree on the assumption that resilience is understood to demonstrate positive outcome during adversity (Ungar 2008).

The assessment of the construct like its definition, has invited several controversies. One of the most discussed issues is regarding the criteria that may be used as a marker of resilience (Luthar and Cicchetti 2000; Masten 2001). Researchers recommend that the identification of resilience ought to involve judgements about the differences between the expected and observed outcomes (Masten 2001). These outcomes should preferably include both internal and external adaptation, as resilience relates to competent behaviour and not merely the absence of emotional distress. For instance, those who do not display obvious signs of mental suffering may be internalizing their symptoms thus showing apparent resilience (Luthar 2006). Internalized symptoms if left unattended can eventually derail apparently resilient trajectories (Luthar and Cicchetti 2000).

Furthermore, notions of overall resilience are considered to be of questionable utility, hence, Luthar (2006) recommends assessing it in terms of domain-specific competence such as academic, social or emotional. Researchers should also consider that certain factors can function as both risk and protective depending on the context (Rutter 1985) hence the assessment of resilience has to be derived from finding an interactive effect between them (M. Rutter, personal communication, April 19, 2007). Additionally, due to the varied manifestations of resilience in different scenarios, drawing overall conclusions becomes difficult. Rutter (2012) notes that the vast '...heterogeneity in people's responses to all manner of environmental adversities...' (p. 335) has proven to be a challenge for researchers. Hence, the criteria for positive adaptation must be set in accordance with the characteristics of the sample and adversity under scrutiny (Fletcher and Sarkar 2013).

Of the resilience tools that have been developed so far, the Connor–Davidson Resilience Scale, and Resilience Scale (Wagnild and Young 1993) are popular. Efforts are being made to study the psychometric properties of these instruments in different contexts; simultaneously, measures for specific populations such as gender minorities have been developed (Testa et al. 2015). Windle et al. (2011) methodological review in which 2979 studies were screened to select 19 resilience measures for a quality criteria appraisal, concluded that all 19 tools require further validation work. The authors suggest that all relevant validation statistics of tools be reported by future researchers. Also, resilience is a subjective concept and therefore, not simple to define; so researchers need to take into account individual perceptions (Masten 2001) while developing tools that can be used to assess resilience in different contexts.

Trajectory of Resilience Research

Resilience research is understood to have emerged in three waves: the first identifying individual resilience and factors, the second wave describing processes embedding resilience in developmental and ecological systems, the third aiming at highlighting interventions that foster resilience and finally, the fourth discovering resilience at cellular and neural levels (Masten 2007; O'Dougherty Wright et al. 2013). Initial resilience research including the Isle of Wight (Rutter 1987), Island of Kauai (Werner and Smith 1982) and Project Competence (Garmezy 1974) studies, had focused largely on children who despite growing up in adversity had showed good adjustment in later life. These landmark investigations laid the foundation for the future generation of resilience researchers who extended this work to include adults, families and communities, as well as different kinds of adversities. The construct is now applicable not only in case of severely critical situations such as natural calamity but also in case of everyday matters such as job stress and marital adjustment. Considering this, many resilience investigations have focused on stressors commonly encountered in transition from one life situation to another. Over time, investigators also began to show interest in the biological mechanisms involving resilience. The idea that exposure to adversities may either increase vulnerabilities through a sensitization effect or decrease vulnerabilities through a 'steeling effect' has been suggested (Rutter 2012, p. 337). Rutter cites immunization as an example where immunity is induced by administering a controlled dose of a modified version of the pathogen. The applicability of these results to psychosocial stressors and psychopathological outcomes in humans are being tested (Rutter 2012).

Recent Research on Resilience

A review of publications was conducted to specifically understand the current trend of research in the area. The search revealed that a large number of studies are being conducted on children, adolescents and women in the context of different adversities including multiple unfavourable childhood experiences among the war-affected youth (Panter-Brick et al. 2015) and body image issues in women (Snapp et al. 2012). Similarly, studies on specific samples such as older adults in same-sex relationships (Dziengel 2012) and Olympic champions (Fletcher and Sarkar 2012); certain adversities such as hurricane Sandy (Lowe et al. 2015), conflict-driven migration (Siriwardhana et al. 2014) and parental rejection and punishment behaviour (Petrowski et al. 2014) were recalled.

There is a remarkable trend that contemporary resilience researchers have been exploring novel areas by employing interesting approaches. For instance, Mazulyte et al. (2014) studied trauma experience, psychological resilience and dispositional optimism in three adult generations in Lithuania. Furthermore, Korstanje and Ivanov (2012) examined if tourism may be considered a resilient activity. Citing examples from museums, battlefields, masterpieces of art, cemeteries and other zones of disasters, the researchers explained how tourism works as a mechanism that society develops to intellectualize disasters. Researchers describe this as dark tourism, a process of psychological resilience that helps the community to understand the nature of disasters. Another interesting approach in this context was found in the work of Graham and Oswald (2010) who attempted to model psychological resilience in economics literature by discussing the implications of hedonic capital on resilience and hedonic adaptation. From the above discussion, it may be affirmed that resilience studies have now extended to a variety of samples and gained popularity across the globe; unlike even a decade earlier when most research publications were from America and focused on American samples, probably as it was the birthplace of positive psychology. In the present times, it is encouraging to find evidence of resilience research in Asian countries including Hong Kong, China, Japan, Afghanistan, Pakistan, Sri Lanka and India.

Resilience Research in India

Although resilience research is still in its initial stage, the phenomena of individuals showing remarkable recovery and sometimes high levels of functioning, despite been born into underprivileged backgrounds has been a recurrent theme of mythological tales, folklore, films, songs and literature in India. Prior to the positive psychology movement, studies that were conducted on the aftermath of adversity were largely based on the pathological framework. Later, most research was limited to resilience in the aftermath of natural calamities that struck India during that time such as tsunami and earthquake; while very few concentrated on resilience towards everyday stressors. Currently, there appears to be an urgent requirement for resilience scales for the Indian population. Barring a few measures such as Dash et al. (2006) and Annalakshmi and Abeer's (2011) Bharathiar University Resilience Scale, many tools used in Indian studies have been constructed as per non-Indian requirements.

In recent times, researchers in India have continued to focus strongly on the children and adolescent population reporting findings such as better mental health among resilient adolescents living in the international Jammu and Kashmir border (Sood et al. 2013), greater level of positive affect and life satisfaction among resilient students (Nath and Pradhan 2012; Singh and Yu 2010), and higher resiliency scores in participants subjected to intervention (Singh and Choubisa 2011). In a novel attempt, Kapur (2013) in the context of resilience among children, suggested the concept of Triguna with special focus on *satva* and declared it as '… the very essence of resilience…' (p. 263). The author affirms that *satva* is not only an inherited predisposition to resilience, but can also be developed by the individual. Kapur (2013) suggests that this concept along with Anna Freud's notion of developmental lines may be used in acquiring competencies that inspire effective functioning in times of adversity. Additionally, Indian researchers have also studied characteristics such as exhibition, impulsivity and understanding (Annalakshmi 2008), religious orientation (Annalakshmi and Abeer 2011; Bhushan 2010) and internal locus of control and positive self-concept (Herbert et al. 2013) along with resilience. Resilience has also been examined in the context of psychological symptoms. For example, Bhushan (2010) reported that religiosity appeared to enhance the effect of resilience in dealing with mental health issues among the Indian geriatric population. In studying adolescents, Deb and Arora (2011) found that academically resilient males reported better mental health than their less resilient counterparts; however, among females, no significant difference was reported in mental health of high and low resilience groups. Furthermore, Herbert et al's (2013) study on individuals with a parent diagnosed with schizophrenia found that coping mechanisms such as acceptance, religiosity and problem solving were used more by resilient adults as compared to less resilient participants. The most frequently reported protective factor in this study was a supportive relationship. Other studies focusing on relationships and resilience have been conducted, such as Harakraj's (2005) study on loss of a family member, and Ganth et al. (2013) investigation on infertility issues among couples. While the former study revealed open communication between family members, religion, support of relatives and friends, respect and trust between family members among the most frequently reported resiliency factors, the latter reported resilience and status of infertility as significant predictors of marital satisfaction. However, limited research was found in the area of organizational behaviour. Shahnawaz and Jafri's (2009) study revealed that public and private sector employees differed from each other in terms of all three dimensions of psychological capital, except resiliency. More recently, Arora and Rangnekar (2014) reported that career mentoring did not have any significant influence on career resilience despite psychosocial mentoring being a significant predictor of career resilience. This review depicts that resilience research is gradually expanding to different adversities as well as different samples in India. Kapur (2013) advocates that further exploration in integration and application of Indian and Western concepts in interpreting the complexity of resilience could help in understanding resilience holistically, both as theory and practice.

Application of Findings from Resilience Research

Despite the fact that resilience research has progressed considerably over the years, investigations aimed at discovering resilience factors have generally been more popular than intervention studies. Intervention studies have targeted young people (Annalakshmi and Abeer 2011; Grotberg 1999; Singh and Choubisa 2011), couples in troubled marriages (Ganth 2013) and sportspersons (Fletcher and Sarkar 2012) among others; however, certain populations and many specific adversities are yet to be focused upon.

Rees et al. (2015) observe that interventions often tend to adopt an over-inclusive approach, whereby several different strategies and techniques are included in the hope that something will be effective. The gap between intervention goals and empirical data supporting their efficacy may be attributed to differences in recipients' cultural values and dispositions in coping with stress, potential to increase stigma associated with mental health issues, and tendency to overestimate one's strengths or undermine the stressors perceived (Bonanno et al. 2011). Rees et al. (2015) suggest that the most powerful interventions will need to be drawn from theory and that the necessary groundwork needs to occur before meaningful interventions can be devised. Therefore, one must be careful in advocating a particular treatment unless its effectiveness has been independently evaluated (Werner 2005); for strategies that have proven successful in one context may not work in another. While most interventions involve training on awareness and practice of established positive psychology techniques, Masten (2001) recommends the use of risk-focused, asset-focused and process-focused strategies that may be customized as per the context.

Implications and Directions for Future Research

Although a wide array of literature is available on resilience studies, some areas demand more exploration. Researchers need to focus on specific adversities and samples, reassess measurement techniques and consider socio-cultural factors in interpretation of findings. In the context of samples under study, Bonanno et al. (2015) observe that 'the most complete body of evidence is available on individual psychological resilience in children and adults' and in 'contrast, the research on psychological resilience in families and communities is far more limited' (p. 139). Hence, it is recommended that efforts must be made to extend application widely across individual, family and community levels. At the individual level, researchers should consider not only specific adversities and resilience factors but also emerging trends including socio-cultural and technological phenomena which have influenced lifestyles as well personality characteristics. New age men, women and adolescents, for instance, may not react to adversities and display positive adaptation in the same manner that earlier generations did. At the family and community levels, there should be focus not only on traditional cultural elements but also on the unique characteristics of groups that are operative in specific adversities.

Considering samples of Indian investigations, it may be observed that resilience among children, adolescents and specific communities such as survivors of earthquake, floods and physical and mental illness have been explored to a reasonable extent. However, resilience among the geriatric population and at the workplace appears to have been largely overlooked by resilience researchers in India. Workplace resilience is a crucial area, not only because the employed people invest a considerable amount of time and energy at their workplace but also because global economic recession has a powerful effect on many companies and families (van Breda 2011). Rees et al. (2015) specifically point towards the absence of a model of individual workforce resilience that enables direct testing of the relationship between resilience and similar overlapping constructs such as self-efficacy. Possible correlates, antecedents and consequences of career resilience must be researched (Arora and Rangnekar 2014) as well.

With regard to adversities, it has been observed that while natural calamities such as war and everyday life situations such as academic challenges have received sufficient attention from resilience researchers, there is a range of everyday stressors such as failure in relationships and stress at work that need more exploration.

Similarly, further studies on resilience during illness and bereavement should be conducted. Participants in Mazulyte et al. (2014) reported that the most common traumatic event was the sudden, unexpected death of someone close. Hence, such life events which are deeply hurtful and unfortunately common should be considered priority areas for resilience research.

Resilience researchers have identified numerous distinct protective factors both internal and external over the years. However, it is also important to explore the interactive effect of these variables. Such outcome is depicted in Lowe et al. (2015) study on New York residents where both individual and community-level resources operated in tandem to shape resilience after hurricane Sandy. Similarly, many studies reveal sample characteristics that predict resilience; however, the underlying mechanisms are often left undetected. Sustained efforts are required in order to discover the process of interplay of personal and environmental resources during times of adversity among different populations.

Contradictory findings have been reported in the area of mental health of resilient individuals; and gender and resilience. Conner's (1992) definition of resilience as the capacity to absorb high levels of change while displaying minimal dysfunctional behaviour reflects that one does pay a price for showing resilience in certain areas of life. Those who display positive external adaptation may be internalizing their symptoms and thereby displaying what is referred to as apparent resilience or invulnerability (Luthar 1991). Thus, more detailed investigation is required in understanding how resilience in one area is carried on to other domains including mental health. Yet another area in which inconsistent findings have been reported is that of gender and resilience. While gender has been identified as a crucial aspect of resilience by highly regarded pioneers of resiliency research (Rutter 1987; Werner and Smith 1982), surprisingly, gender difference has rarely been the focus of resilience studies (Morales 2008). While it has been suggested that resilience may not be a function of gender after all and that males and females were equally likely to be resilient (Collishaw et al. 2007), it is also likely that gender differences in resilience change overtime (Sun and Stewart 2007). Petrowski et al. (2014) suggest that longitudinal data would be useful to draw conclusions on the gender-specific development of resilience.

With regard to assessment of resilience, a lot is yet to be accomplished. It has been observed that most studies have depended on self-reports of resilience. Efforts must be made to incorporate other tools of assessment including peer reports and biological measures; that can be used together to provide more conclusive evidence. Furthermore, since resilience is a dynamic phenomenon, longitudinal studies are required to track resilience outcomes overtime. Longitudinal data may be also useful in tracing the effect of interventions. Malhi (2012) observes that one of the major gaps in literature lies in assessment of resilient children. Since most methods currently being used have been modelled after adult stress inventories and completely disregard the child's perspective, Malhi insists that techniques that take into consideration the child's interpretations are required, as children possibly use different criteria than adults to define and assess risk. Furthermore, in understanding the subjective experience of resilience, it is important for future researches to focus more on examining cultural influences that impact individuals and societies. An example from Makkawi's (2012) qualitative exploratory study on 15 purposefully selected Palestinian female students may be cited in this regard where family support, female segregated schools, supportive female teachers, and resilient personal characteristics were cited as protective factors in relation to academic resilience. A few of these features would probably not function as protective factors if the study was to be replicated in a Westernized society. This emphasizes that cultural aspects play a vital role in the development of resilient traits. While larger samples in quantitative studies may lead us to more reliable results, unique features of the sample may be lost in this endeavour. Hence, qualitative methods may be required to understand the subtleties of the resilience process that are governed by unique socio-cultural contexts.

Researchers also recommend that resilience interventions be developed for different kinds of adversities and on different populations. For example, resilience interventions for certain occupational groups such as those working in palliative care settings where rates of compassion fatigue and burnout are high, (Rees et al. 2015) are vital concerns for resilience researchers. Additionally, researchers have expressed skepticism about the application of intervention techniques in resilience. While Greenberg (2006) points to the lack of integration of intervention strategies with findings in neuroscience, Jenson and Fraser (2011) point to the inconsistency of efforts to systematically apply the policies among vulnerable populations. This argument is supported by Hanewald (2011) who on the basis of a review of at-risk and resilient children reported a lack of evidence about the effectiveness of intervention programmes, despite the dedication of vast resources towards their implementation. Since, the definition of resilience varies according to the sample, setting, and variables under study (Ahern 2006) and the ways in which adversity is conceptualized at different stages of the lifespan and in relation to different groups of people is different (Daniel 2010), it is evident that without precise knowledge of these specifications, not only are interventions hampered but the understanding of the phenomena is also limited (Arrington and Wilson 2000). For example, Rajkumar et al. (2008) observed that survivors of the Tsunami valued their unique individual, social and spiritual coping strategies more than formal mental health services; hence they recommend that post-disaster interventions should be aimed more towards strengthening prevailing community coping strategies. In support, Ungar (2013) cites that in many cases, young people's resilience is the result of their quality engagement with adults more than a personal trait. The socio-ecological understanding of resilience avoids blaming young people who resort to maladaptive behaviour to survive and sets the onus on their families, schools and communities to make relationships with adults available that determines children's success. Rees et al. (2015) add that since resilience is a multidimensional construct, development of interventions aimed at enhancing individual resilience in the workplace would require more in-depth research information, for instance, on both stable traits such as neuroticism as well as more malleable intrapersonal factors including coping style. Additionally, future interventions could incorporate the principles of yoga, meditation, lifestyle changes that are expected to bring about changes in the self (Kapur 2013). O'Dougherty Wright et al. (2013) suggest that future research must aim to recognize conditions under which interventions may and may not work, identify the most cost-effective targets and timing for interventions, and explore natural reparative processes as well. Finally, in terms of the objectives of future studies, Shastri (2013) recommends that resilience research should not only detect 'at-risk' sample at a national, community or individual level; but should also identify the specific characteristics of these groups or individuals. This will be helpful in prevention of risk, intervention and policymaking.

In summary, it may be posited that further work must be continued with the aim of understanding how multiple levels of influence operate synergistically and how best biological, psychological, interpersonal, and cultural levels of analysis can be incorporated into our research and models for clinical intervention specifically among the most vulnerable children, youth and families in our communities (O'Dougherty Wright et al. 2013).

Diverse study designs and methodology restricts the cross-applicability of findings and makes definitive generalizations difficult ((Siriwardhana et al. 2014), therefore, resilience researchers from diverse backgrounds must join forces to maximize the utilization of findings obtained from different studies. Formation of resilience research organizations such as the recently established 'Resilio', will promote research and facilitate exchange of information, finally contributing towards building a resilient community. Additionally, speedy translation of findings from research into policy and practice is necessary.

Conclusion

Although the phenomena of resilience has been comprehended to a great extent, a lot still needs to be achieved in terms of application of this knowledge. Life is replete with instances of challenging situations that may not necessarily be physically life threatening or psychologically intimidating. Even routine events both positive and negative, such as being offered a new job, being reciprocated in love, or losing an emotionally valuable possession, could all be disruptive as they represent change. Although challenges do not always turn out to be catastrophic; accumulation of these relatively minor stressors might render the individual vulnerable towards other apparently trivial occurrences. Masten's (2001) reference to resilience as ordinary magic, stems from the observation that everyone has the capacity for it. It is thus, important for individuals to be aware of the protective systems in their lives by practicing resilient responses even in seemingly ordinary conditions. This will help to overcome unforeseen situations in life and to flourish under such challenges.

Acknowledgements I am thankful to Anindita Ghosh for her generous assistance.

References

Ahern, N. R. (2006). Adolescent resilience: An evolutionary concept analysis. *Journal of Pediatric Nursing, 21,* 175–185. https://doi.org/10.1016/j.pedn.2005.07.009.

Annalakshmi, N. (2008). The resilient individual: A personality analysis. *Journal of the Indian Academy of Applied Psychology, 34,* 110–118.

Annalakshmi, N., & Abeer, M. (2011). Islamic worldview, religious personality and resilience among Muslim adolescent students in India. *Europe's Journal of Psychology, 7*(4), 716–738.

Anthony, E. J. (1974). The syndrome of the psychologically invulnerable child. In E. J. Anthony & C. Koupernik (Eds.), *The child in his family: Children at psychiatric risk* (pp. 529–544). New York: Wiley.

Antonovosky, A. (1979). *Health, stress and coping.* California: Jossey-Bass Inc. Publishers.

Arora, R., & Rangnekar, S. (2014). Workplace mentoring and career resilience: An empirical test. *The Psychologist-Manager Journal, 17*(3), 205–220. https://doi.org/10.1037/mgr0000021.

Arrington, E. G., & Wilson, M. N. (2000). A re-examination of risk and resilience during adolescence: Incorporating culture and diversity. *Journal of Child and Family Studies, 9,* 221–230. https://doi.org/10.1023/A:1009423106045.

Bhushan, B. (2010). *Psychiatric profiling of the Indian geriatric population: Implication for possible interventions.* Paper presented at the Coping, Resilience and Hope Building, Asia Pacific Regional Conference, Brisbane 9–11 July 2010. Abstract retrieved from http://www.strengthsbasedpractice.com.au/coping_resilience_hope_building_conference_SPEAKERS_ABSTRACTS_1.htm.

Bonanno, G. A., Romero, S. A., & Klein, S. I. (2015). The temporal elements of psychological resilience: An integrative framework for the study of individuals, families, and communities. *Psychological Inquiry, 26*(2), 139–169. https://doi.org/10.1080/1047840X.2015.992677.

Bonanno, G. A., Westphal, M., & Mancini, A. D. (2011). Resilience to loss and potential trauma. *Annual Review of Clinical Psychology, 7,* 511–535. https://doi.org/10.1146/annurev-clinpsy-032210-104526.

Collishaw, S., Pickles, A., Messer, J., Rutter, M., Shearer, C., & Maughan, B. (2007). Resilience to adult psychopathology following childhood maltreatment: Evidence from a community sample. *Child Abuse and Neglect, 31,* 211–229. https://doi.org/10.1016/j.chiabu.2007.02.004.

Conner, D. R. (1992). *Managing at the speed of change: How resilient managers succeed and prosper where others fail.* New York: Villard Books.

Daniel, B. (2010). Concepts of adversity, risk, vulnerability and resilience: A discussion in the context of the child protection system. *Social Policy and Society, 9,* 231–241. https://doi.org/10.1017/S1474746409990364.

Dash, S., Dayal, A., & Lakshminarayana, R. N. (2006). Measuring resiliency in two states in India: The development of a valid and reliable instrument. In J. O. P. Diaz, R. S. Murthy, & R. Lakshminarayana (Eds.), *Advances in disaster mental health and psychological support* (pp. 147–152). New Delhi: Voluntary Health Association of India Press.

Deb, A., & Arora, M. (2011). Resilience and mental health: A study on adolescents in Varanasi. *Indian Journal of Health Psychology, 5*(2), 69–79.

Dziengel, L. (2012). Resilience, ambiguous loss, and older same-sex couples: The resilience constellation model. *Journal of Social Service Research, 38*(1), 74–88. https://doi.org/10.1080/01488376.2011.626354.

Fletcher, D., & Sarkar, M. (2012). A grounded theory of psychological resilience in Olympic champions. *Psychology of Sport and Exercise, 13,* 669–678. https://doi.org/10.1016/j.psychsport.2012.04.007.

Fletcher, D., & Sarkar, M. (2013). Psychological resilience: A review and critique of definitions, concepts, and theory. *European Psychologist, 18*(1), 12–23.

Ganth, D. B., Thiyagarajan, S., & Nigesh, (2013). Role of infertility, emotional intelligence and resilience on marital satisfaction among Indian couples. *International Journal of Applied Psychology, 3*(3), 31–37. https://doi.org/10.5923/j.ijap.20130303.01.

Garmezy, N. (1974). The study of competence in children at risk for severe psychopathology. In E. J. Anthony & C. Koupernick (Eds.), *The child in his family: Children at psychiatric risk* (pp. 77–97). New York: Wiley.

Graham, L., & Oswald, A. J. (2010). Hedonic capital, adaptation and resilience. *Journal of Economic Behavior & Organization, 76*(2), 372–384. https://doi.org/10.1016/j.jebo.2010.07.003.

Greenberg, M. (2006). Promoting resilience in children and youth: Preventive interventions and their interface with neuroscience. *Annals of the New York Academy of Sciences, 1094*(1), 139–150. https://doi.org/10.1196/annals.1376.013.

Grotberg, E. (1999). Countering depression with the five building blocks of resilience. *Reaching Today's Youth, 4*, 66–72. Retrieved June 21, 2013 from http://resilnet.uiuc.edu/library/grotb99.html.

Hanewald, R. (2011). Reviewing the literature on "at-risk" and resilient children and young people. *Australian Journal of Teacher Education, 36*(2), 16–29. https://doi.org/10.14221/ajte.2011v36n2.2.

Harakraj, N. (2005). *Resilience in Indian families in which a member has died.* (Unpublished masters dissertation). University of Zululand, South Africa.

Herbert, H. S., Manjula, M., & Philip, M. (2013). Resilience and factors contributing to resilience among the offsprings of parents with schizophrenia. *Psychological Studies, 58*(1), 80–88. https://doi.org/10.1007/s12646-012-0168-4.

Jenson, J. M., & Fraser, M. W. (2011). A risk and resilience framework for child, youth, and family policy. In J. M. Jenson & M. W. Fraser (Eds.), *Social policy for children and families: A risk and resilience perspective* (pp. 5–24). California: Sage Publications.

Kapur, M. (2013). Resilience and competence in childhood. In G. Misra (Ed.), *History of science, philosophy and culture in Indian civilization* (Vol. XIII, pp. 255–267). Part 3, Psychology and psychoanalysis New Delhi: Munshiram Manoharlal Publishers Private Ltd.

Killian, B. (2004). Risk and resilience. In R. Pharoah (Ed.), *A generation at risk? HIV/AIDS, vulnerable children and security in Southern Africa*. Institute for Security Studies: Pretoria.

Knight, C. (2007). A resilience framework: Perspectives for educators. *Health Education, 107*, 543–555.

Kobasa, S. C. (1979). Stressful life events, personality and health: An inquiry into hardiness. *Journal of Personality and Social Psychology, 37*, 1–11. https://doi.org/10.1037/0022-3514.37.1.1.

Korstanje, M. E., & Ivanov, S. (2012). Tourism as a form of new psychological resilience: The inception of dark tourism. *CULTUR - Revista de Cultura e Turismo, 6*(4), 56–71. https://doi.org/10.2139/ssrn.2168400.

Kumpfer, K. L. (1999). Factors and processes contributing to resilience: The resilience framework. In M. D. Glantz & J. L. Johnson (Eds.), *Resilience and development: Positive life adaptations* (pp. 179–224). New York: Kluwer Academic Publishers.

Lowe, S. R., Sampson, L., Gruebner, O., & Galea, S. (2015). Psychological resilience after hurricane Sandy: The influence of individual- and community-level factors on mental health after a large-scale natural disaster. *PLoS ONE, 10*(5), e0125761. https://doi.org/10.1371/journal.pone.0125761.

Luthar, S. S. (1991). Vulnerability and resilience: A study of highrisk adolescents. *Child Development, 62*(3), 600–616.

Luthar, S. S. (2006). Resilience in development: A synthesis of research across five decades. In D. Cicchetti & D. J. Cohen (Eds.), *Developmental Psychopathology: Risk, disorder, and adaptation* (pp. 740–795). New York: Wiley.

Luthar, S. S., & Cicchetti, D. (2000). The construct of resilience: Implications for intervention and social policy. *Development and Psychopathology, 12*, 857–885.

Mazulyte, E., Skeryte-Kazlauskiene, M., Eimontas, J., Gailiene, D., Grigutyte, N., & Kazlauskas, E. (2014). Trauma experience, psychological resilience and dispositional optimism: Three adult generations in Lithuania. *Psichologija, 49*, 20–33.

Makkawi, I. (2012). The psychology of resilience among Palestinian female students. *Global Journal of Community Psychology Practice, 3*(4). Retrieved May 20, 2013 from http://www.gjcpp.org/pdfs/2012-Lisboa-044-The%20Psychology%20of%20Resilience%20among%20Palestinian%20Female%20Students.pdf.

Malhi, S. (2012). Resilience in children: A review of literature. *The Undergraduate Journal of Psychology, 1*. Retrieved June 25, 2013 from http://www.inkblotjournal.com/wp-content/uploads/2012/05/24-28-Simritpal-Malhi-Resilience.pdf.

Masten, A. S. (1994). Resilience in individual development: Successful adaptation despite risk and adversity. In M. Wang & E. Gordon (Eds.), *Risk and resilience in inner city America: Challenges and prospects* (pp. 3–25). Hillsdale, New Jersey: Erlbaum.

Masten, A. S. (2001). Ordinary magic: Resilience processes in development. *American Psychologist, 56,* 227–238. https://doi.org/10.1037/0003-066X.56.3.227.

Masten, A. S. (2007). Resilience in developing systems: Progress and promise as the fourth wave rises. *Development and Psychopathology, 19,* 921–930. https://doi.org/10.1017/S0954579407000442.

Masten A. S., & Gewirtz, A. H. (2006). Resilience in development: The importance of early childhood. In R. E. Tremblay, R. G. Barr, & R. D. Peters (Eds.), *Encyclopedia on early childhood development* (pp. 1–6). Montreal, Quebec: Centre of Excellence for Early Childhood Development. Retrieved June 27, 2013 from http://www.child-encyclopedia.com/documents/Masten-GewirtzANGxp.pdf.

Morales, E. E. (2008). Academic resilience in retrospect: Following up a decade later. *Journal of Hispanic Higher Education, 7,* 228–248. https://doi.org/10.1177/1538192708317119.

Nath, P., & Pradhan, R. (2012). Influence of positive affect on physical health and psychological well-being: Examining the mediating role of psychological resilience. *Journal of Health Management, 14*(2), 161–174. https://doi.org/10.1177/097206341201400206.

O'Dougherty Wright, M. O., Masten, A. S., & Narayan, A. J. (2013). Resilience processes in development: Four waves of research on positive adaptation in the context of adversity. In S. Goldstein & R. B. Brooks (Eds.), *Handbook of resilience in children* (2nd ed., pp. 15–37). New York: Springer.

Panter-Brick, C., Grimon, M., Kalin, M., & Eggerman, M. (2015). Trauma memories, mental health, and resilience: A prospective study of Afghan youth. *Journal of Child Psychology and Psychiatry, 56*(7), 814–825. https://doi.org/10.1111/jcpp.12350.

Petrowski, K., Brähler, E., & Zenger, M. (2014). The relationship of parental rearing behavior and resilience as well as psychological symptoms in a representative sample. *Health and Quality of Life Outcomes, 12,* 95. https://doi.org/10.1186/1477-7525-12-95.

Rajkumar, A. P., Premkumar, T. S., & Tharyan, P. (2008). Coping with the Asian Tsunami: Perspectives from Tamil Nadu, India on the determinants of resilience in the face of adversity. *Social Science and Medicine, 67,* 844–853. https://doi.org/10.1016/j.socscimed.2008.05.014.

Rees, C. S., Breen, L. J., Cusack, L., & Hegney, D. (2015). Understanding individual resilience in the workplace: The international collaboration of workforce resilience model. *Frontiers in Psychology, 6*. Article 73. https://doi.org/10.3389/fpsyg.2015.00073.

Rew, L., & Horner, S. D. (2003). Youth resilience framework for reducing health-risk behaviors in adolescents. *Journal of Pediatric Nursing, 18,* 379–388. https://doi.org/10.1016/S0882-5963(03)00162-3.

Richardson, G. E. (2002). The metatheory of resilience and resiliency. *Journal of Clinical Psychology, 58,* 307–321. https://doi.org/10.1002/jclp.10020.

Rutter, M. (1985). Resilience in the face of adversity: Protective factors and resistance to psychiatric disorder. *British Journal of Psychiatry, 147,* 598–611. https://doi.org/10.1192/bjp.147.6.598.

Rutter, M. (1987). Psychological resilience and protective mechanisms. *American Journal of Orthopsychiatry, 57,* 316–331. https://doi.org/10.1111/j.1939-0025.1987.tb03541.x.

Rutter, M. (2012). Resilience as a dynamic concept. *Development and Psychopathology, 24,* 335–344. https://doi.org/10.1017/S0954579412000028.

Seligman, M. (2002). *Authentic happiness: Using the new positive psychology to realize your potential for lasting fulfilment*. New York: Free Press.
Seligman, M., & Csikszentmihalyi, M. (2000). Positive psychology: An introduction. *American Psychologist, 55,* 5–14. https://doi.org/10.1037/0003-066X.55.1.5.
Shahnawaz, M. G., & Jafri, M. H. (2009). Psychological capital as predictors of organizational commitment and organizational citizenship behaviour. *Journal of the Indian Academy of Applied Psychology, 35,* 78–84.
Shastri, P. C. (2013). Resilience: Building immunity in psychiatry. *Indian Journal of Psychiatry, 55*(3), 224–234. https://doi.org/10.4103/0019-5545.117134.
Singh, K., & Choubisa, R. (2011). Personality dimensions as predictors of happiness in Indian milieu: An empirical confirmation with different measurement approaches. *Indian Journal of Applied Psychology, 48,* 18–26.
Singh, K., & Yu, X. (2010). Psychometric evaluation of the Connor-Davidson Resilience Scale (CD-RISC) in a sample of Indian students. *Journal of Psychology, 1*(1), 23–30.
Siriwardhana, C., Sheik Ali, C., Roberts, B., & Stewart, R. (2014). A systematic review of resilience and mental health outcomes of conflict-driven adult forced migrants. *Conflict and Health, 8,* 13. https://doi.org/10.1186/1752-1505-8-13.
Snapp, S., Hensley-Choate, H., & Ryu, E. (2012). A body image resilience model for first-year college women. *Sex Roles, 67*(3–4), 211–221. https://doi.org/10.1007/s11199-012-0163-1.
Sood, S., Bakshi, A., & Devi, P. (2013). An assessment of perceived stress, resilience and mental health of adolescents living in border areas. *International Journal of Scientific and Research Publications, 3*(1), 176–179.
Sun, J., & Stewart, D. (2007). Age and gender effects on resilience in children and adolescents. *The International Journal of Mental Health Promotion, 9,* 16–25. https://doi.org/10.1080/14623730.2007.9721845.
Testa, R. J., Habarth, J., Peta, J., Balsam, K., & Bockting, W. (2015). Development of the gender minority stress and resilience measure. *Psychology of Sexual Orientation and Gender Diversity, 2*(1), 65–77. https://doi.org/10.1037/sgd0000081.
Ungar, M. (2008). Resilience across cultures. *British Journal of Social Work, 38,* 218–235. https://doi.org/10.1093/bjsw/bcl343.
Ungar, M. (2013). The impact of youth-adult relationships on resilience. *International Journal of Child, Youth and Family Studies, 3,* 328–336.
van Breda, A. D. (2011). Resilient workplaces: An initial conceptualization. *Families in Society, 92*(1), 33–40.
Wagnild, G. M., & Young, H. M. (1993). Development and psychometric evaluation of The Resilience Scale. *Journal of Nursing Measurement, 1,* 165–178.
Walsh, F. (2002). A family resilience framework: Innovative practice applications. *Family Relations, 51,* 130–137. https://doi.org/10.1111/j.1741-3729.2002.00130.x.
Werner, E. E. (2005). What can we learn about resilience from large scale longitudinal studies? In S. Goldstein & R. Brooks (Eds.), *Handbook of resilience in children* (pp. 91–106). New York: Kluwer Academic Publishers.
Werner, E. E., & Smith, R. S. (1982). *Vulnerable but invincible: A study of resilient children.* New York: McGraw-Hill.
Windle, G., Bennett, K. M., & Noyes, J. (2011). A methodological review of resilience measurement scales. *Health and Quality of Life Outcomes, 9*(8), 1–18. https://doi.org/10.1186/1477-7525-9-8.

Chapter 5
Understanding Resilience: Global Trends and Indian Research

Seema Mehrotra, Annalakshmi Narayanan and Ravikesh Tripathi

Rajan's name has come up today in the teachers' meeting as the most suitable candidate for best outgoing student award of the year. Not only has he done consistently well in academics, he has also demonstrated his initiatives in many activities. Only a handful of people, including rajan's class teacher who stood by him, know that he is the same rajan who was seen two years ago by his peers as an odd fellow, who did not speak the local language well, did not come as well dressed as other boys and was intermittently absent for long periods to help out his mother in earning the wages to look after the family and bear the expenses of his father's medical treatment. what may have been the internal factors and environmental forces that helped rajan rise against odds? is this a common story about the ordinary magic of resilience?

Introduction

In its most generic sense, resilience is a broad construct that refers to 'positive adaptation in any kind of dynamic system that comes under challenge or threat' (Masten and Obradovic 2006). The original usage of the term resilience as a construct first appeared in the field of material science and environmental studies, and was subsequently broadened to include human resilience. In the behavioural sciences literature, resilience was initially taken up for investigation in the context

S. Mehrotra (✉) · A. Narayanan
Department of Clinical Psychology, National Institute of Mental Health and Neurosciences, Bangalore, India
e-mail: drmehrotra_seema@yahoo.com

R. Tripathi
Institute of Behavioral Sciences, Gujarat Forensic Sciences University, Gandhinagar, Gujarat, India

G. Misra (ed.), *Psychosocial Interventions for Health and Well-Being*,
https://doi.org/10.1007/978-81-322-3782-2_5

of children's development (Garmezy 1974; Werner and Smith 1992; Rutter 1999) and then expanded to include the context of potentially traumatic events in adulthood as well as adverse experiences in general using a life span perspective. Rutter (2006) defined resilience as 'reduced vulnerability to environmental risk experiences, the overcoming of stress or adversity or a relatively good outcome despite risk experience'. The initial theorizing on resilience in psychology originated in the works of developmental psychologist and psychiatrists. Although resilience in response to adversity was often seen initially as an exceptional and rare phenomenon by researchers who tended to focus narrowly on risk factors; subsequent widening of attention tends to repeatedly indicate that resilience is not rare or uncommon. Masten (2001) spoke about the 'ordinary magic' to refer to the observations that many children survive very difficult home environments.

Beyond Risk and Protective Factors: Evolving Trends in Understanding Resilience in Children

It is now well understood that in the context of childhood, a focus on resilience requires attention on two essential factors, both of which need to be present, namely, exposure to risk or adversity and adaptive functioning. In risk assessment, the need to carefully examine the key feature of the risk, its severity, chronicity as well as the number of risk factors operating has been highlighted. Adaptive functioning has also been understood to be a multidimensional construct and is assessed in terms of competence in developmentally appropriate tasks, with the awareness that outcomes can fluctuate over time and across domains.

Zautra et al. (2010) argued that resilience needs to be examined in terms of recovering (bouncing back) from challenge as well as in terms of sustainability that refers to continuing forward with engagement in life tasks. They also highlighted how resilient resources should be examined separately from vulnerability or risk factors rather than treated as occupying the positive end on a single continuum of risk. It is worth mentioning protective factors here. Protective factors refer to processes that reduce the negative effects of adversity when risk factor is experienced (Rutter 1985). Similar to risk factors, these too operate at various levels such as individual, family and/or community levels and can change depending on the developmental phase as well as the nature of adversity. In contrast to protective factors, core resources (Masten et al. 2004) are conceptualized as resources that provide a foundation for resilience but are independent of risk experience.

Various basic models have been used to explain resilience in the context of risk. In the compensatory (main effects) model, the factors that neutralize exposure to risk are seen as having direct, independent and positive effects on outcomes irrespective of levels of risk. On the other hand, protective (moderating effects) models conceptualize factors or processes as having effects that depend on the level of risk, with a buffering effect being evident when the risk is high. The challenge model of resilience proposes that manageable degrees of adversity prepare an organism through development of an inoculation or steeling effects (similar to vaccination boosting one's immunity to a specific infection agent). Much more recently, there is increasing attention to models that involve gene-environment interactions and examine the moderating role of genes and personality on differential reactivity in the context of adversity. Thus, increasing attention is being paid to investigating the neurobiology of resilience (for example, genes as potential moderators of environmental risk and experiences as mitigators of genetic risk, role of early experiences in programming maladaptive stress systems and differential biological sensitivity to context).

According to Rutter (2007) the key element of the 'shift from risk/protective concepts to resilience is that the latter requires a move from variables to processes or mechanisms'. Masten and Wright (2010) highlighted that across models, resilience needs to be understood as a 'dynamic, interactional and inferential' concept in view of the fact that it refers to 'what happens during and following conditions that threaten the organism'. According to them, high functioning or adverse experiences by themselves cannot define resilience and studying resilience requires that the researchers 'define good adaptation and significant threat as well as any of the processes or resources' one hypothesizes to explain individual differences in outcomes.

A development in resilience research has been the recognition that 'positive adaptation despite adversity is never permanent; rather there is developmental progression, with new vulnerabilities and strengths emerging with changing life circumstances…' (Luthar 2006, p. 741) Resilience may be domain specific, especially in childhood and it is critical to consider context as well as the dynamic nature of risk and protective factors at different developmental stages.

Rutter (2013) enumerated several important features associated with resilience: (1) Resilience may arise from features that are not generally health promotive but are neutral or risky in absence of risk experience (e.g., adoption). (2) An important cognitive feature associated with resilience is the planning tendency and a sense of agency to deal with challenges which may be developed through experience of success in some domain or another. (3) Turning point effects can occur in adulthood resulting in discontinuity from the past and generation of new options for constructive changes. (4) Some risk factors can have steeling/strengthening effect if these occur in a manner and at a point when an individual can successfully cope with the same.

Examining Resilience in Adulthood

Conceptualization of resilience as a personality trait is a phenomenon which has often characterized resilience researchers focusing on adulthood period. Wagnild and Young (1993) defined resilience as a 'personality characteristic that moderates negative effects of stress and promotes adaptation…' Masten (1994) differentiated resilience (process-oriented) from resiliency (individual's internal traits). However, in recent times, several researchers have argued against the notion of resilience as a personality trait (resiliency). Taking a middle position, Luthar et al. (2000) argued that resilience attributes should be seen as shaped by life experiences rather than as predetermined. The researches that fail to focus on the subjective experiences and meanings of risk experiences and the active role of individuals as agents acting on the environmental influences have been criticized for providing an incomplete and impoverished picture about resilience processes (Gladstone et al. 2006). The need to view resilience as a process rather than a fixed attribute of a person, and treat it as an interactive concept that needs to be inferred rather than measured directly has been repeatedly emphasized by several researchers. (Garmezy et al. 1984; Rutter 1987). Current global trends indicate declining popularity of personality-based conceptualization of resilience.

Based on the nature of traumatic events that are typically encountered in adulthood; Bonanno (2004) defined resilience in adulthood as 'the ability of adults in otherwise normal circumstances who are exposed to an isolated and potentially highly disruptive event… to maintain relatively stable, healthy levels of psychological and physical functioning… as well as the capacity for generating experiences and positive emotions'. According to Bonanno et al. (2011), the heterogeneous responses to potentially traumatic events in adulthood can be described with the help of four prototypical trajectories—resilience, recovery, chronic distress and delayed distress. The resilience trajectory is characterized by transient symptoms, minimal impairment and relatively stable healthy functioning soon after traumatic event while recovery trajectory is differentiated from resilience and characterized by elevated symptoms and functional impairments following the event and a gradual return to normal functioning. The chronic distress trajectory, involves persistent elevated symptoms and functional impairment. Lastly, the delayed distress trajectory refers to elevated symptoms to begin with and gradual worsening over time. These researchers highlight that resilience is typically the modal outcome trajectory but with significant heterogeneities within the group of resilient individuals. It needs to be noted that persons identified as resilient using these criteria can experience mild to moderate transient stress reactions. A multitude of risk and protective factors may contribute to or subtract from the overall likelihood of a resilient outcome.

Resilience in Families and Communities

As a psychological construct, resilience has been examined more frequently in individuals and less frequently in larger social systems, such as families and communities. However, the studies on children growing in adverse circumstances have moved beyond deficit-based approach to examine risk and resilience in family as a functional unit using a systemic perspective rather than merely parental pathology or the child–parent dyad. The family resilience framework proposed by Walsh (1998, 2003) incorporates three domains of family functioning—family belief systems (making meaning of adversity, positive outlook and spirituality), organizational patterns (flexibility, connectedness, socioeconomic resources) and communication/problem solving approach (clarity, open emotional expression and collaborative problem solving). This attitude focuses on strengthening key processes and building resilience by affirming potentials. An additional category, namely, effective use of external support from social and community networks was added by Black and Lobo (2008) to describe family resilience. The concept of community resilience was elucidated by Norris et al. (2008) and defined as a process linking the network of adaptive capacities to adaptation after an adversity. They proposed that 'economic development', 'social capital', 'information and communication' and 'community competence' can be considered as the four primary adaptive capacities foster community resilience. Zautra et al. (2008) described the utility of a resilience perspective to develop a set of indicators of strong and healthy communities.

Emerging Trends in Resilience Research: Movement Towards Using a Social Ecological Perspective

Ungar (2011) highlighted how despite the shift in approach from traits of what were thought to be 'invulnerable children' to interactional processes in challenging environments; resilience researchers have often continued to limit their focus to a narrow set of traits and processes. A need for further shift in focus was argued for on the basis of accumulating evidence that 'resilience is less an individual trait and more a quality of a person's social and physical ecology'.

Resilience has been defined within the social ecological framework as referring to processes that are contextually and culturally specific functional adaptations to environmental challenges. In this framework, resilience is viewed as incorporating two processes—sequence of events whereby the individuals use internal and external developmental assets in the context of acute or chronic adversity to navigate new resources that can sustain well-being; capacity of the individual's social and physical ecology to provide the above-mentioned resources in culturally meaningful ways with the youth actively negotiating for whatever they might need to attain the functional standards of successful development as contextually defined. In other words, this view emphasizes that resilience is not just about an individual's behaviour but also an attribute of a person's environment and its capacity to respond to individual needs (Ungar 2008, 2011).

In an international mixed method study involving 11 countries and 14 sites, it was observed that resilient youth in adverse circumstances may adopt unique culturally specific pathways to resolve seven kinds of tensions that may be commonly experienced, namely, access to material resources, relationships, identity, cohesion, power and control, social justice, and cultural adherence (Ungar et al. 2007).

Ungar (2011) presented four basic principles in the social ecological framework of resilience in order to address the limitations that mark resilience research (1) *Decentrality:* This principle argues against a person-centered approach in which the responsibility for resilience outcome is placed on the victims of severely adverse environments. The key element of decentring is that the locus of change is seen to reside neither in the child nor in the environment but the processes through which the environments provide resources for the child growing up in adversity. In other words researchers need to recognize that in higher risk environments, resilience is influenced more by the availability and accessibility of culturally relevant social and physical resources than individual factors. (2) *Complexity:* Interactional patterns fluctuate as the person and the environment adapt continuously to one another and changes occur across contexts and time. This necessitates the development of contextually sensitive and temporally specific models of resilience. Complexity is beautifully illustrated by Ungar (2011) who asserted that 'many different starting points can lead to many different but equally desirable ends by many different processes relevant to different ecologies'. (3) *Atypicality*: More than examining predetermined outcomes in resilience, researchers need to attend to functionality of behaviours within a given context. This is because, in environments low in resources, atypical use of developmental resources may have adaptive significance. (4) *Cultural relativity*: This principle involves a sensitive understanding that standards of child development are variable across cultures and researchers need to take in account their cultural lens of observation.

Methodological Issues in Resilience Research

Resilience is a 'super ordinate' construct that is indirectly inferred from two component constructs subsumed under its definition: risk exposure and good adaptation (Kim-Cohen 2007, p. 272). Further, Rutter (2012) has pointed out that it is misleading to operationalize resilience in terms of generally superior functioning rather than as relatively better functioning compared with that manifested by those experiencing the same level of adversity. Assessment needs to entail functioning in developmentally appropriate multiple domains. It needs to be focused away from identifying presence of a psychiatric disorder as a manifestation of lack of resilience.

Windle et al. (2011) conducted a methodological systematic review of resilience measures using quality assessment criteria. Fifteen measures were identified and all except one were noted to be tapping availability of assets and resources that facilitate resilience and surmised that these are more useful for measuring the presence/absence of the resources leading to a resilient outcome rather than resilience per se, as an outcome. It was mentioned that only Brief Resilience Scale (Smith et al. 2008) focused on assessing resilience as an outcome (ability to bounce back). Only two of the measures were described as explicating item selection on a theoretical basis. The reviewers emphasized that in addition to individual resources, those at the level of family and community also need to be captured through assessment tools. Only five of the measures reviewed examined resilience across multiple levels. One of the measures was noted to have been extensively piloted in 11 countries. None of the measures defined minimal important change that becomes relevant in intervention programmes. The authors found lack of conceptually sound and psychometrically robust measure of resilience for children under 12 years of age to be glaring.

In addition to the questionnaire measures that form bulk of the resilience assessment tools, Ungar et al. (2007) have developed resilience interview guide which includes catalyst questions and probes. In addition, visual methods approaches have been developed by their Resilience Research Centre (Cameron et al. 2011). These visual methods have been developed/adapted for use across nations to obtain a culturally grounded and rich understanding of resilience processes. These involve videos of one day in the life of a thriving youth in challenging situations, a photo elicitation technique involving active engagement of the youth themselves and interviews providing scope for reflections. Using such methodologies, it was found that when youth in transition/adverse situations are provided culturally appropriate opportunities to assume responsibility for themselves and others and contribute in meaningful ways to their families and are acknowledged for the same, they are able to mitigate their risk and support their well-being through such experiences (Ungar et al. 2011). Such studies highlight the need for contextual sensitivity in resilience research, because in other contexts it is known that precocious (non-normative) contributions by youth may signify problems/dysfunction in the family.

Several criteria for methodological sound research studies on adult resilience following a potentially traumatic event were suggested by Bonanno (2012): (1) Temporal bounds of aversive events clearly operationalized, (2) Resilience operationalized as stable pattern of healthy functioning following the adverse event, (3) Resilience not equated with absence of pathology, (4) Use of measures at multiple points of time, (5) Initial measurement of outcome obtained close to the occurrence of adverse event.

Resilience Interventions

Resilience interventions in children can be in the form of universal programmes that aim at enhancing resilience capacity in all children; resilience promotion in vulnerable children or those experiencing chronic adversity; and programmes targeted at children exposed to one off traumatic event/disaster (Hunter 2012). Harvey (2007) highlighted school-wide methods for fostering resiliency in children. In the global international literature, resilience interventions in adulthood are seen with skepticism at least by some researchers (e.g. Bonanno et al. 2011). In general, interventions that aim to promote resilience on multiple levels and in multiple contexts have been shown to be more effective than those that target specific mechanisms of resilience or narrowly focus on risk reduction (Masten 2001). Rutter (2013) enumerated several prevention implications of resilience research. These include the following: (1) understanding the role of mental features such as planning, self-reflection and active personal agency (2) providing environments (universal experiences) that nurture the above-mentioned beneficial mental characteristics (3) being sensitive to inadvertent deskilling of participants by exercising non-optimal levels of control (4) using a life span approach while emphasizing early and middle childhood phase because this phase can partially shape subsequent experiences (5) developing ways of utilizing major turning point effects in adulthood.

Bonanno et al. (2011) raised concerns regarding several potential unwanted outcomes of universal resilience interventions such as misperception of risk and coping ability, increased sense of stigma, incompatibility with cultural values, mismatch between interventional goals and dispositional characteristics of the individuals or situational requirements, as well as almost exclusive focus on individuals to the neglect of their environments. On the whole, it appears that although several intervention programmes have been developed, these tend to focus on a broad range of protective factors that are assumed to facilitate resilience. Resilience intervention studies seem to have raised more questions than answers and several issues remain to be addressed in this nascent subfield. It appears that conceptual and methodological maturity in understanding and assessing resilience processes and outcomes across contexts and cultures is essential for developing and testing resilience-based interventions.

Waves of Resilience Research

Scholars tracing the evolution of research in human development have identified four waves of resilience research (Masten 2007; Masten and Wright 2010). The first wave of research revolved around describing and identifying resilience and contrasting those who did well under adverse circumstances from those who did poorly in terms of numerous variables. Moving beyond factors associated with resilience (the 'what' questions), the second wave of research focused on the processes/mechanisms underlying resilience (the 'how') questions. The third wave of research is said to be characterized by studies examining ways of resilience promotion through strengthening protective processes or factors. The hallmark of the fourth and the ongoing wave of research is its integrative focus with an attempt to integrate rapid advances in various fields such as genetics, neuro-behavioural development, etc. We also wish to add that the current trends are in addition characterized by rigorous efforts to examine resilience as an interactive concept and study resilient processes at multiple levels (biological, psychological, social). The research studies being carried out within the social ecological framework of resilience mentioned in the previous section exemplify the fourth wave research.

Studies on Resilience in India

People have always been intrigued by stories of the resilient who overcame adversity to succeed in life (Masten 2009). Individual characters in the Indian legends including Bhageeratha, Eklavya, Dhruva, Viswamitra, and Rama stand as ideal types of resilience and the resilient (Annalakshmi 2013). Indian psychologists have recognized Ramana Maharishi of Thiruvannamalai, India as the embodiment the extraordinary psychological resilience (Swaminathan and Rao 2010). However, examination of resilience as a scientific construct in the Indian psychological literature is a more recent phenomenon.

The Indian studies on resilience as a psychological construct are briefly reviewed in this section. These are discussed under the following subheads: assessment of resilience, risk and protective factors, personality and other correlates, resilience in special groups and intervention studies.

Assessment of Resilience

Attempts have been made to examine the applicability of one of the popular measures of resilience in Indian youth as well as to develop an indigenous measure of resilience.

The psychometric properties of the Connor–Davidson Resilience Scale (CD-RISC) have been explored in the Indian context on a sample of 256 students aged 16–29 years (Singh and Yu 2010). The Indian data failed to replicate the original five-factor solution reported for American samples. A four-factor structure emerged through exploratory factor analysis and these factors were named as hardiness, optimism, resourcefulness and purpose. The measure was noted to have adequate reliability and validity (concurrent and convergent) in the Indian sample. Resilience scores were positively correlated with life satisfaction, extroversion, openness, agreeableness, conscientiousness and positive affect. Researchers reiterated the observations noted in other studies that resilience items as on CD-RISC are likely to be differently understood by participants of Western and Eastern cultures.

Bharathiar University Resilience Scale was developed on a sample of 578 young adults (Annalakshmi 2009a). This 30-item scale measures seven domains of resilience including duration for getting back to normalcy, reaction to negative events, response to risk factors (specifically disadvantaged environment) in life, perception of effect of past negative events, defining problems, hope/confidence in coping with future and openness to experience and flexibility. The scale has been noted to have sound psychometric properties.

Risk and Protective Factors

Risk and protective factors of various kinds have been a subject of examination in several Indian studies. The risk and protective factors among the rural adolescent student population were examined in a large study (Annalakshmi 2010a). The sample for the study involved 1451 adolescent school students in rural schools in a district in South India. The study identified a number of risks for developmental adaptation. The risk, very widely prevalent in this sample, were belonging to a school in which majority of the students were from low-income families. The moderately prevalent risks included highly crowded classrooms, low socioeconomic background, poor student–teacher ratio, lack of clarity in rules and policies in school, insensitivity of the school to students' need and migration of schoolmates to other schools. Two percent of the sample was free from risks and 6.75% had only one risk factor whereas 5% of the sample had 11–19 risks. Multiple risks were common with more than three-fourth of the sample having two to 10 risks for their psychosocial development. Resilience was considered as achieving good outcomes despite high risk status. In this study, outcome was operationally defined as academic achievement in terms of marks earned and scores obtained on a measure of subjective well-being. Perceived family support for education, perceived significance of education and preference for a variety of vocations were found to be characteristic of resilient adolescents. Commitment to moderate *satvic* temperament, low aspirations for wealth, contribution to community, parental control with regard to recreation, parental monitoring of food habits, education and dressing and moderate degree of dominance over children served as protective factors.

Personality and Other Correlates of Resilience

A few studies on resilience have focused on personality correlates of resilience. A study of relationship between probabilistic orientation style of life and resilience on samples of postgraduate students and scientists revealed that probabilistic orientation and resilience were independent of one another among the groups studied (Annalakshmi 2007a). A study on a sample of postgraduate students aged 20–25 years showed that resilience was associated with low psychoticism, low neuroticism and high extraversion (Annalakshmi 2007b).

Resilience was associated with high need for affiliation, cognitive structure, dominance, endurance, exhibition, nurturance and understanding, and low need for impulsivity among young adult graduates (Annalakshmi 2008a). The relationship between risk taking, creativity and resilience was examined in a study using a sample of 181 young adults in the age group of 21–24 years (Annalakshmi 2008b). Creativity was found to be positively related to resilience while risk taking was negatively related to resilience. Creativity and risk taking had an interaction effect on resilience: The high creativity-low risk taking group had highest level of resilience and the high creativity–high risk taking group had the least level of resilience.

Garg and Rastogi (2009) examined the relationship between emotional intelligence and resilience in a sample of 140 postgraduate level and doctoral level students in a technology institute. Resilience was operationalized in terms of Stress Resiliency profile (Thomas and Tymon 2007). It was found that components of emotional intelligence jointly predicted 50% variance in deficiency focusing (habit of focusing on the negatives at the expense of the positives), 13% in necessitating (perceptions of task demands as inflexible) and 54% in low skills recognition (tendency to underestimate one's competence). These three criterion variables form the subscales on stress resiliency profile and are conceptualized as interpretative habits that influence stress.

The psychological correlates of resilience among the engineering college students belonging to scheduled castes and scheduled tribes were explored by Annalakshmi (2010b). The survey involved a stratified sample of 1008 students drawn from four districts in Tamil Nadu. Student alienation and learned helplessness were negatively correlated with academic resilience. Past academic achievement, positive attitude towards education, powerful other dimensions of the locus of control, academic self-concept and study habits positively predicted academic resilience.

A few investigations have focused on cognitive correlates of resilience. Resilience was found to be related to causal attributions in a study on 11th graders (Annalakshmi 2010c). Resilient adolescents perceived cause of events to be originating from within them and perceived higher degree of volitional influence that can be exerted over a cause. Resilience was unrelated to stability and external control dimensions of causal attributions.

Relationship between resilience and cognitive styles in terms of field dependence and field independence (FD-FID) was examined in a study using a sample of 112 high school students in the age group 15–16 years (Annalakshmi 2009b). Resilience as a whole was unrelated to FD-FID cognitive style. Field independence was found to be positively related to personal competence. Another study on 114 high school students aged 15–16 years revealed that resilience is associated with a preference for complex rather than simple explanations for human behavior and higher usage of metacognitions concerning explanations (Annalakshmi 2009c). The relationship between resilience and approach–avoidance motivation was investigated on a sample of 200 graduate students (Annalakshmi 2011a). The resilient were not only less inhibited but also were less responsive to rewards.

Tankha and Gill (2007) examined resilience as a trait along with other related variables in a study utilizing 120 first-year college students. They noted that females had higher scores than males on resilience. The study, in addition, highlighted the importance of family environment in understanding academic achievement in this group. Family type was examined as correlate of resilience in another Indian study (Gupta and Singh 2011).

A few studies have examined the relationship of resilience with religiosity or spirituality. The relationship between resilience and spiritual intelligence was explored in a study of 200 Christian adolescents (Annalakshmi and Tony 2011). Resilience was positively related to consciousness, graceful living, in alignment with the sacred sense of meaning in life and transcendence and truthful living. That was reflected in open acceptance, forgiveness, curiosity and love for all creation. In another investigation, Islamic rituals (religious practice and ritual behaviour indicative of the manifestation of one's religious worldview) and *Mu'amalat* (religiously guided behaviours towards one's family, fellow human beings and the rest of creation including animals and the natural environment) were associated with resilience in a sample of 204 Muslim adolescents (Narayanan and Mohammed 2011). Interestingly, resilience was not associated with Islamic worldview indicating that mere knowledge of the Islamic worldviews did not help resilience.

The role of resilience as a mediator of positive outcomes has also been the subject of inquiry. Nath and Pradhan (2012) examined the relationship of resilience with positive affect, physical health and psychological well-being in a sample of 146 engineering, research and management students. Resilience as assessed by 'Ego Resiliency Scale' (Block and Kremen 1996) was found to mediate the association between positive affect and physical health and psychological well-being.

Resilience in Special Groups

A few Indian studies have examined resilience as a construct in the context of significant adversity such as disability or illness or specific groups in the community.

Assessments and observations in Andaman and Nicobar islands, in an early phase post Tusnami disaster in 2005 indicated that 5–8% of the population was suffering from significant mental health problems. This study noted high resilience in joint family systems of the tribal Nicobarese during this phase (Math et al. 2006). Rajkumar et al. (2008) conducted focus group discussions nine months after the tsunami with two groups of fishermen, two groups of housewives, a group of village leaders and a group of young men in four villages of Nagapattinam, Tamil Nadu that were affected by Tsunami. The study revolved around understanding determinants of resilience in the face of disaster. Despite a lack of complete reconstruction of their lives, participants were engaged in reconstructing the meaning for the causes and the aftermath of the disaster using their cultural idiom. Survivors were noted to value their unique individual, social and spiritual coping strategies more than formal mental health services. According to researchers, the narratives demonstrated that collective response to massive trauma need not necessarily result in social collapse but may also facilitate positive effects. They recommend that interventions after disaster should be grounded in ethno-cultural beliefs and practices and should be aimed at strengthening community coping strategies being in use.

Forty undergraduate college students from India and Japan who were experiencing bereavement related to death of a close person though campus suicides were recruited for a study on resilience following a traumatic event. The role of cognitive emotional processes in coping was explored in the above-mentioned context. Resilience was assessed through Wagnild and Young's (1993) resilience measure. Positive reappraisal was noted to mediate the relationship between resilience and proactive coping. On the other hand, negative thoughts about the self, mediated the association between resilience and proactive and reflective coping. Indians scored significantly higher than Japanese young adults on resilience (Bhushan et al. 2011).

Lisha (2012) conducted a study that utilized an interpretative phenomenological analysis (IPA) for exploring resilience in persons with locomotor handicap. Six individuals between 30 and 40 years of age who were identified (through snowball sampling) to be doing well despite the handicap were interviewed and the transcripts were subjected to interpretive phenomenological analysis. It was found that the pattern of social interaction, assertiveness, family support, individual relationship, and optimism served as inner protectors of resilience among these individuals. The phenomenological nature of psychological resilience was observed to be not confined to individual traits, as it included social connectedness with fellow human beings and presence of support.

Annalakshmi and Ragitha (2012) using a purposive sample of 80 hearing impaired and 89 non-impaired adolescents found that those high on resilience in this sample differed in their emotional processing styles compared to those low on resilience. The sample was drawn from two government schools situated in Thrissur, Kerala. Highly resilient adolescents used impoverished emotional experience to a significantly lesser extent than the low resilience group in their processing of emotion.

The pattern of family factors that facilitate an effective and sustainable positive adaptation in the presence of chronic disease such as Turners Syndrome were explored in a study by Jha et al. (2012). The level of cognitive and emotional functioning of the child as well as family functioning in terms of stress and coping pattern were assessed in relation to chronic illness. This assessment was followed by a psychological intervention along with the pharmacological management and occupational therapy. Promoting the strengths of the child while he/she was undergoing the negative experience and at the same time encouraging the adaptability and coping strategies of the family members, and also providing opportunities to seek help were relevant to the well-being of children with such a medical condition. The findings suggest that caring relationships, positive expectations and opportunity for meaningful relationships provided by the family, school and community can reinforce the child's ability to handle adversities.

Parenting a child with intellectual disability could be associated with both positive and negative experiences. Recently, resilience of parents and its relationship with the impact of child's disability was examined by Rajan and John (2016). The study participants included 121 parents living with a child diagnosed with intellectual disability for a minimum of 2 years. Parental perceptions regarding the child's disability could influence their resilience. Positive parental perceptions of the disability were found to be associated with the experience of greater resilience.

The impact of role model on resilience was explored by Kurien (2012) using a sample of 502 adolescent students belonging to low socioeconomic status. The highly resilient adolescents were high on academic achievement, even when educational risk and intelligence were controlled. Role models also had an impact on academic resilience.

A cross-sectional study compared students belonging to different communities, namely, Scheduled Tribes, Scheduled Caste, Most Backward Class, Backward Class, and Other Class with regard to resilience in addition to a host of other factors (Annalakshmi 2012). The sample included 333 adolescent students, boys and girls, studying in a government college in Tamil Nadu. Students from different communities did not differ from one another on resilience or perceived discrimination, caste identity, probabilistic orientation, and social desirability. However, it is interesting to note that resilience explained varying proportion of variance in active coping in different community groups.

Deb and Arora (2012) attempted to examine resilience in adolescence preparing for highly competitive engineering/Medical entrance examinations in various coaching centers in Varanasi. Two hundred adolescents experiencing high academic adversity were chosen from a larger group of 566 adolescents. A median split procedure based on scores on a resilience measure was used to form high and low resilience subgroups. Higher resilience subgroup showed better academic performance than their counterparts. Males also scored higher than females on resilience in this study. The researchers reported that the chances of high resilience subgroup adolescents being successful in competitive examinations (selection to one's target institute) were 120% greater than that of low resilience subgroup participants.

Herbert et al. (2013) examined resilience and its correlates in offsprings of parents with schizophrenia. The sample comprised 45 adults who had one parent diagnosed with schizophrenia. Presence of good support system, use of problem-focused coping and positive self-concept were found to be the key factors associated with resilience. The authors using the Connor Davidson Resilience Scale for this study reported that 60 and 24% of their sample exhibited medium and high levels of resilience respectively.

Saraf et al. (2013) utilized narrative analysis with interview data from cervical cancer survivors. They observed that meaning making was strongly mediated by faith in God and increased religiosity which in turn facilitated hope and resilience in the context of adaptation to a life-threatening illness.

Sood et al. (2013) examined stress, resilience and mental health of adolescents living at international border areas of Jammu and Kashmir. The study involved a random sample of adolescents from villages falling within a radius of 5 km from the border. Individuals low on resilience as assessed on the Wagnild and Young Resilience scale were significantly different from the high resilient counterparts on two of the five subscales of the measure used for mental health assessment; with the former being higher on loss of emotional control and lower on positive affect than the latter.

Somasundaram and Devamani (2016) examined the relationship between resilience, social support and hopelessness among cancer patients (n = 60). It was found that resilience was significantly associated with lower levels of hopelessness and higher levels of perceived social support.

Factors associated with resilience in spouses of men with alcohol dependence were examined in a sample of 80 patients and their spouses attending outpatient psychiatric services (Sreeja Sreekumar and Varghese 2016). Higher resilience was associated with a shorter duration and lower severity of dependence, absence of domestic violence and involvement in external support groups. The study highlights the role of contextual factors in resilience.

Intervention for Promoting Resilience

Several Indian studies have focused on developing intervention programmes to improve resilience among different sections of the population.

A major research project examined the plausibility of fostering academic resilience among students belonging to a lower socioeconomic section of the population studying in a college in rural regions through psychological intervention adopting a two-group experimental design (Annalakshmi 2011b). Three hundred students, including both males and females, participated in this study. The intervention programme, evolved to enhance resilience among rural college students, included inputs to maximize cognitive social learning. It provided scaffolding for development of the participants by providing an environment that supports development of resilience. The intervention included introducing to the participants certain psychological concepts relevant to resilience-potential and discussing the possibilities of applying them for furthering individual resources to do better despite adversities. The concepts included in this study were conscientiousness, self-concept, creativity, locus of control, level of aspiration, study skills and academic attitudes. The intervention designed to foster resilience, including academic resilience was delivered to the participants in seven sessions spread over a span of 3.5 months. Conscientiousness and openness of the participants increased after the intervention programme. The participants also showed higher internal locus of control in dealing with their academic venture, better study skills, and a more positive attitude towards education, an enhanced level of creativity.

A psychological intervention for enhancing the 'resilient-self' among students with hearing impairment was designed and evaluated using an experimental paradigm (Ragitha 2012). The intervention provided exercises for improving their physical, social, academic, and transpersonal self-concepts. The strategies adopted included conceptual teaching, storytelling and self-reflection. The sample included 109 adolescent students. The experimental group was administered the intervention for 15 weeks (one session per week). The intervention was delivered by the investigator who was qualified and well versed in sign language. Comparisons of the groups revealed that the intervention has been efficacious in improving the resilient-self of the participants as well as improving academic achievement among the participants.

An investigation exclusively focused on promoting academic resilience among Muslim adolescent students who were facing risks for achievement in the context of marginalization and poverty. The academic achievement was operationally defined in this investigation as the mean of the marks earned by the participants in two consecutive examinations conducted by the school in all the subjects relative to the risks faced by him/her for education reckoned by the Educational Risk Survey (Abeer 2013). The intervention designed for enhancing individuals' academic resilience included exercises to promote various competencies relevant to academics including goal-setting skills, study skills, emotional competence, interpersonal competence, academic help-seeking and moral competence. The intervention was delivered in eight sessions spread over a period of eight weeks. The competence-focused intervention helped to facilitate goal-setting skills, study skills, increased cognitive reappraisal and decreased expressive suppression strategies, increased interpersonal competence, self-disclosure, conflict resolution, assertive influence, help seeking, approach orientation as well as resilience.

Karthik and Mythili (2012) attempted to use an intervention to promote resilience among girls studying in a government higher secondary school in Chennai that serve the poorest of the poor in the city. The Wagnild and Young (1993) Resilience Scale was administered to 106 students studying in 8th and 9th standards. Thirty girls each (showing low level of resilience) were identified using a cutoff score of 130 on the scale and assigned to the experimental group and control group, respectively. The intervention programme designed to promote resilience was administered on twice a week basis for five weeks. It included yogic relaxation, SWOT analysis and training on perseverance, positive attitude, time management and goal-setting exercises. The components were planned so as to develop the core characteristics of resilience equanimity, perseverance, meaning, self-reliance and existential aloneness as indicated by the author of the resilience measure. The experimental group showed significant improvement on resilience scores as compared to the control group, at the end of the intervention period.

An intervention integrating Probabilistic Orientation, Gratitude Exercise, and Loving-Kindness Meditation was conceived to promote resilience, academic achievement and well-being among institutionalized adolescents and was tested for its efficacy using a two-group experimental design (Lijo 2012). The module of the intervention was evidence-based. The evidences supporting the inputs were primarily drawn from the findings of positive development programs for youth (Catalano et al. 2004). This intervention programme of eight weeks' duration resulted in improvement on the probabilistic orientation, forgiveness, gratitude, as well as resilience in these adolescents. The positive impact of the intervention persisted a follow-up assessment carried out three months after the conclusion of the intervention.

The Penn Resiliency Program (PRP) aims at reducing risk factors for depression and improving resiliency in early adolescence. Its utility in an Indian study was examined by Sankaranarayanan and Cycil (2014). Utilizing a sample of 58 fifth-grade children in an urban Indian setting, they found that the intervention group manifested a significant reduction in pessimistic attributional style and an increase in optimistic orientation as compared to the control group, while controlling for baseline scores.

Critique

The high universal appeal of the concept of resilience has come with its price in terms of the multiplicity of meanings associated with the term. In fact, this observation led Rutter (1999) to use the phrase the 'millennium Rorschach' in a lighter vein, to describe the state of affairs in which individuals project their own idiosyncratic meanings to the concept of resilience, with several of these meanings bearing little resemblance to each other. Kumpfer (1999) observed that there are numerous challenges to be overcome in the research on resilience. Some of these include lack of consensus on definitions of resilience and absence of unbiased definitions of successful outcomes, locating appropriate measures, and understanding transactional, bi directional, non-linear data. Resilience research has included virtually all possible intra-personal and external variables, transactional and mediating or moderating factors that may affect life adaptation (Kumpfer 1999). There has also been confusion between mechanisms underlying resilience and resilience as an outcome. In fact, Gordon and Song (1994) voiced that resilience may not be a single construct but a 'complex of related processes that deserve to be identified and studied as discrete constructs'.

Each of the above issues of concerns seems to be applicable when Indian research on resilience is reviewed. There is lack of clarity on what exactly is being assessed from one study to another owing to insufficient efforts to explicate the way resilience is being defined in a given study. This can at times create significant challenges in interpretation of findings and drawing of conclusions. There is an urgent need for researchers to clearly explain their operationalization of resilience in individual studies.

Kumpfer (1999) described five major types of resilience research. These included retrospective, single sample/cross-sectional studies, retrospective, cross-sectional multivariate studies, short-term transactional and longitudinal studies, long-term prospective developmental studies without control group and prospective multisample studies. Majority of the Indian studies are cross-sectional in nature and though these have attempted to examine multiple variables, conceptual overlaps or redundancies are at times difficult to rule out and the rationale for choice of variables often needs a stronger articulation.

Based on the nature of studies reviewed, it appears that resilience has been more often conceptualized and examined as an individual-level trait factor and sometimes as an outcome but research-on-process issues is conspicuous by its rarity in the Indian context. The dominant trend seems more characteristic of the first wave of resilience research described in the global literature. Personality factors may be important in resilient outcomes but these should ideally be assessed prior to the occurrence of potentially traumatic events. Self-report measures of resilient traits are unlikely to capture the whole picture of resilience and, moreover, these should not be treated as a proxy for resilient outcomes. When resilience related personality traits are assessed in the absence of adversity/trauma, it becomes difficult to understand resilient processes or outcomes as these may emerge in the context of coping with adversity. Repeated assessments of functioning are required to discern the trajectory of responses to potentially traumatic events (Bonanno (2012). There is a clear dominance of self-report measures and single-point assessments in the Indian literature and an exploration of alternative methods is sorely needed. Resilience measures should not automatically be assumed to be valid proxy measures of resilient outcomes (Bonanno et al. 2011). Bonanno (2012) in an elegant commentary on uses and abuses of the resilience construct pointed out several problems in this field of research. He highlighted how the developmental literature has focused mostly on chronic adversities to the neglect of acute potentially traumatic events while the case is reversed with the adult literature on resilience. Moreover, he brought to attention the pitfalls of studying resilience in the absence of actual significant stressor/adversity. In the Indian literature that was reviewed, several studies have examined resilience as a construct without any well-defined adverse-context. This can be considered an issue of concern as it poses challenges in drawing inferences. In few of the Indian studies that have used samples of participants in a context characterized by adversity; the nature of adversities examined have mostly been chronic ones. Resilience in the context of potentially traumatic events has been a rather neglected topic.

An important point of concern in resilience research is the manner in which good outcomes are defined and operationalized. According to the developmental perspective, good outcomes mean much more than absence of problems. Positive adaptation need to include internal functioning (e.g., psychological well-being) and external functioning (e.g., doing well at work). Competence that broadly refers to effective functioning in terms of age-appropriate tasks is by nature multidimensional and the levels of competence often vary across domains. At times children may manifest resilience in behavioural terms but could be experiencing internal distress (Luthar 2006). Similarly, they may show differential functioning in different domains (e.g., scholastic tasks versus emotional functioning). Awareness of this issue plays an important role in how outcomes may be conceptualized, measured and focused upon individual studies and needs can be taken in consideration in a much more consistent and rigorous fashion in future studies by Indian researchers. Moreover, there is a need for studies that examines resilience at multiple levels of analysis. In the international literature too, the need to understand resilience as a heterogeneous, multilevel process involving individual, family and community-level risk as well as protective factors has been stressed upon (Hunter 2012).

There have been a few Indian studies that have used the broad construct of resilience in the context of interventions. Here again, there is a need to clearly delineate processes that are targeted and outcomes that are being examined. The use of a socioecological framework and a focus beyond individuals to transactional processes within one's sociocultural environment can not only deepen the understanding of resilience as an emergent phenomenon in our cultural context but also inform approaches to interventions for strengthening resilience-facilitating properties of the environments.

Conclusion

The field of resilience research across the globe has witnessed significant milestones from a focus on risk factors to protective factors, from attention to understanding the constituent factors to unraveling processes and mechanisms, and from restricting the field of inquiry to individuals to capturing the dynamic environment of individuals. Indian researchers interested in the field of resilience need to strive hard towards enhancing conceptual clarity and methodological rigour in order to make further strides in the field.

References

Abeer, M. K. C. (2013). *An intervention for promoting academic resilience among young adult students belonging to a minority community* (Doctoral Dissertation, Bharathiar University, Coimbatore).

Annalakshmi, N. (2007a). Probabilistic orientation and resilience. *Journal of the Indian Academy of Applied Psychology, 33*(2), 267–272.

Annalakshmi, N. (2007b). Resilience in relation to extraversion-introversion, psychoticism, and neuroticism. *Indian Journal of Psychometry and Education, 38*(1), 51–55.

Annalakshmi, N. (2008a). The resilient individual a personality analysis. *Journal of Indian Academy of Applied Psychology, 34,* 110–118.

Annalakshmi, N. (2008b). Effect of creativity and risk taking on resilience. *Behavioural Scientist, 9*(1), 15–22.

Annalakshmi, N. (2009a). Bharathiar university resilience scale. In H. Purohit & A. Wagh (Eds.), *Research methodology—Tools and techniques* (pp. 105–121). New Delhi: Sri Publishers.

Annalakshmi, N. (2009b). Resilience among high and low field-independents. *Indian Journal of Clinical Psychology, 36*(2), 39–45.

Annalakshmi, N. (2009c). Resilience, metacognition and complexity. *Journal of Indian Academy of Applied Psychology, 35,* 112–118.

Annalakshmi, N. (2010a). *Enhancing resilience of rural adolescent students under risk.* Report of the Major Research Project submitted to the Indian Council for Social Science Research (ICSSR), New Delhi.

Annalakshmi, N. (2010b). *Psychological dynamics of academic resilience among SC/ST students in higher education in Tamil Nadu.* Report of the Major Research Project submitted to the Centre for Educational Research, Madurai Kamaraj University (CER-MKU), Tamil Nadu.

Annalakshmi, N. (2010c). Causal attributions of the high and low resilient adolescents. *Indian Journal of Positive Psychology, 1*(1–2), 21–23.

Annalakshmi, N. (2011a). Resilience, behavior approach and inhibition among adolescents. *Journal of Indian Academy of Applied Psychology, 37,* 119–127.

Annalakshmi, N. (2011b). *Fostering academic resilience among rural low socioeconomic college students.* Report of the Major Research Project submitted to the University Grants Commission (UGC), New Delhi.

Annalakshmi, N. (2012). Perceived discrimination and active coping among socially marginalized and non-marginalized college students in India. In A. Sobrun-Maharaj, F. Rossen, S. Parackal, S. Nayar, E. Ho, D. Newcombe, Y. Ratnasabapathy, J. Hand, & S. Ameratunga (Eds.), *Social Environment, Migration, and Health: Proceedings of the Fifth International Asian and Ethnic Minority Health and Wellbeing Conference* (pp. 73–84). Auckland, New Zealand: University of Auckland.

Annalakshmi, N. (2013). Constructs of resilience in the Indian context. In S. Saini & N. Goyal (Eds.), *Positive psychology in the light of Indian traditions*. New Delhi: Arihant Publications.

Annalakshmi, N., & Ragitha, R. (2012). Hearing impairment, resilience and emotional processing styles. *Indian Journal of Clinical Psychology, 39*(1), 54–60.

Annalakshmi, N., & Tony, P. J. (2011). Spiritual intelligence and resilience among Christian Youth in Kerala. *Journal of the Indian Academy of Applied Psychology, 37*(2), 263–268.

Bhushan, B., Kumar, S., & Harizuka, S. (2011). Bereavement, cognitive-emotional processing, and coping with the loss: A study of Indian and Japanese students. *Journal of Social Work in End-of-Life & Palliative Care, 7,* 263–280.

Black, K., & Lobo, M. (2008). A conceptual review of family resilience factors. *Journal of Family Nursing, 14,* 33–55.

Block, J., & Kremen, A. M. (1996). IQ and ego-resiliency: Conceptual and empirical connections and separateness. *Journal of Personality and Social Psychology, 70,* 349–361.

Bonanno, G. A. (2004). Loss, trauma, and human resilience: Have we under-estimated the human capacity to thrive after extremely aversive events? *American Psychologist, 59,* 20–28.

Bonanno, G. A. (2012). Uses and abuses of the resilience construct: Loss, trauma, and health-related adversities. *Social Science and Medicine, 74,* 753–756.

Bonanno, G. A., Westphal, M., & Mancini, A. D. (2011). Resilience to loss and potential trauma. *Annual Review of Clinical Psychology, 7,* 11–125.

Cameron, C. A., Theron, L., Ungar, M., & Liebenberg, L. (2011). Adapting visual methodologies to identify youth protective processes in negotiating resilience across cultures and contexts. *Australian Community Psychologist, 23*(2), 68–84.

Catalano, R. F., Berglund, M. L., Ryan, J. A. M., Lonczak, H. S., & Hawkins, J. D. (2004). Positive youth development in the united states: Research findings on evaluations of positive youth development programs. *The Annals of the American Academy of Political and Social Science, 591*(1), 98–124.

Deb, A., & Arora, M. (2012). Resilience and academic achievement among adolescents. *Journal of the Indian Academy of Applied Psychology, 38,* 93–101.

Garg, P., & Rastogi, R. (2009). Emotional intelligence and stress resiliency: A relationship study. *International Journal of Educational Administration, 1,* 1–16.

Garmezy, N. (1974). The study of competence in children at risk for severe psychopathology. In E. J. Anthony & C. Koupernik (Eds.), *The child in his family: Children at psychiatric risk* (3rd ed., Vol. III, pp. 77–97). New York: Wiley.

Garmezy, N., Masten, A. S., & Tellegen, A. (1984). The study of stress and competence in children: A building block for developmental psychology. *Child Development, 55*(97), 111.

Gladstone, B. M., Boydell, K. M., & McKeever, P. (2006). Recasting research into children's experiences of parental mental illness: Beyond risk and resilience. *Social Science and Medicine, 62,* 2540–2550.

Gordon, E. W., & Song, L. D. (1994). Variations in the experience of resilience. In M. C. Wang & E. W. Gordon (Eds.), *Educational resilience in inner-city America: Challenges and prospects* (pp. 27–43). Hillsdale, NJ: Erlbaum.

Gupta, L., & Singh, R. (2011). Impact of family type on resilience. *Indian Journal of Positive Psychology, 2*(1), 17–20.

Harvey, V. S. (2007). Schoolwide methods for fostering resiliency. *Principal Leadership (High School Ed.), 7*(5), 10–14.

Herbert, H., Manjula, M., & Philip, M. (2013). Resilience and factors contributing to resilience among the offsprings of parents with schizophrenia. *Psychological Studies, 58,* 80–88.

Hunter, C. (2012). *Is resilience still a useful concept when working with children and young people?* (CFCA Paper No. 2). Australian Institute of Family Studies, Melbourne.

Jha, M., Sharma, V., & Singh, T. B. (2012). Factors influencing resilience in a child suffering with Turners syndrome: Psychological perspective. *Indian Journal of Positive Psychology, 3*(2), 124–127.

Karthik, L. R. M., & Mythili, T. (2012). Psychological intervention with early adolescent girls. *Journal of School Social Work, 9*(6), 21–25.

Kim-Cohen, J. (2007). Resilience and developmental psychopathology. *Child and Adolescent Psychiatric Clinics of North America, 16,* 271–283.

Kumpfer, K. L. (1999). Factors and processes contributing to resilience: The resilience framework. In M. D. Glantz & J. L. Johnson (Eds.), *Resilience and development: Positive life adaptions* (pp. 179–224). New York: Kluwer Academic/Plenum Publishers.

Kurien, N. (2012). Impact of resilience and role model influence on academic achievement of low socio-economic status adolescent students. *Indian Journal of Positive Psychology, 3*(3), 250–254.

Lijo, K. J. (2012). *Promoting resilience through fostering probabilistic orientation, forgiveness and gratitude in institutionalized adolescents: An experimental study* (Doctoral Dissertation, Bharathiar University, Coimbatore).

Lisha, S. (2012). *Factors of resilience among physically disabled-an interpretative phenomenological analysis* (M.Phil. Dissertation, Bharathiar University, Coimbatore).

Luthar, S. S. (2006). Resilience in development: A synthesis of research across five decades. In D. Cicchetti & D. J. Cohen (Eds.), *Developmental psychopathology: Risk, disorder and adaptation* (2nd ed., Vol. 3, pp. 739–795). Hoboken, NJ: Wiley.

Luthar, S. S., Cicchetti, D., & Becker, B. (2000). The construct of resilience: A critical evaluation and guidelines for future work. *Child Development, 71,* 543–562.

Masten, A. S. (1994). Resilience in individual development: Successful adaptation despite risk and adversity. In M. C. Wang & E. Gordon (Eds.), *Educational resilience in inner-city America: Challenges and prospects* (pp. 3–25). Hillsdale, New Jersey: Lawrence Erilbaum Associates Inc.

Masten, A. S. (2001). Ordinary magic: Resilience processes in development. *American Psychologist, 56,* 227–238.

Masten, A. S. (2007). Resilience in developing systems: Progress and promise as the fourth wave rises. *Development and Psychopathology, 19,* 921–930.

Masten, A. S. (2009). Ordinary magic: Lessons from research on resilience in human development. *Education Canada, 49*(3), 28–32.

Masten, A. S., Burt, K. B., Roisman, G. I., Obradovic, J., Long, J. D., & Tellegen, A. (2004). Resources and resilience in the transition to adulthood: Continuity and change. *Development and Psychopathology, 16,* 1071–1094.

Masten, A. S., & Obradovic, J. (2006). Competence and resilience in development. *Analysis of the New York Academy of Sciences, 1094,* 13–27.

Masten, A. S., & Wright, O. M. (2010). Resilience over the life span: Developmental perspectives on resistance, recovery, and transformation. In J. W. Reich, A. J. Zautra, & J. S. Hall (Eds.), *Handbook of adult resilience* (pp. 213–237). New York: Guilford Publications Inc.

Math, S. B., Girimaji, S. C., Benegal, V., Uday Kumar, G. S., Hamza, A., & Nagaraja, D. (2006). Tsunami: psychosocial aspects of Andaman and Nicobar islands. Assessments and intervention in the early phase. *International Review of Psychiatry, 18*(3), 233–239.

Narayanan, A., & Mohammed, A. (2011). Islamic worldview, religious personality and resilience among Muslim adolescent students in India. *Europe's Journal of Psychology, 7*(4), 716–738.

Nath, P., & Pradhan, R. K. (2012). Influence of positive affect on physical health and psychological well-being: Examining the mediating role of psychological resilience. *Journal of Health Management, 14,* 161–174.

Norris, F. H., Stevens, S. P., Pfefferbaum, B., Wyche, K. F., & Pfefferbaum, R. L. (2008). Community resilience as a metaphor, theory, set of capacities, and strategy for disaster readiness. *American Journal of Community Psychology, 41,* 127–150.

Ragitha, R. (2012). *Psychological intervention for enhancing resilient—Self among students with hearing impairment* (Doctoral dissertation, Bharathiar University, Coimbatore).
Rajan, A. M., & John, R. (2016). Resilience and impact of children's intellectual disability on Indian parents. *Journal of Intellectual Disabilities,* 1744629516654588.
Rajkumar, A. P., Premkumar, T. S., & Tharyan, P. (2008). Coping with the Asian tsunami: Perspectives from Tamil Nadu, India on the determinants of resilience in the face of adversity. *Social Science and Medicine, 67,* 844–853.
Rutter, M. (1985). Resilience in the face of adversity, protective factors and resistance to psychiatric disorder. *British Journal of Psychiatry, 147,* 598–611.
Rutter, M. (1987). Psychosocial resilience and protective mechanisms. *American Journal of Orthopsychiatry, 57,* 316–331.
Rutter, M. (1999). Resilience as the millennium Rorschach: Response to Smith and GorrellBarnes. *Journal of Family Therapy, 21,* 159–160.
Rutter, M. (2006). Implications of resilience concepts for scientific understanding. *Annals of the New York Academy of Sciences, 1094,* 1–12.
Rutter, M. (2007). Resilience, competence, and coping. *Child Abuse and Neglect, 31,* 205–209.
Rutter, M. (2012). Resilience as a dynamic concept. *Development and Psychopathology, 24,* 335–344.
Rutter, M. (2013). Annual research Review: Resilience: Clinical implications. *Journal of Child Psychology and Psychiatry, 54*(4), 474–487.
Sankaranarayanan, A., & Cycil, C. (2014). Resiliency training in Indian children: a pilot investigation of the Penn Resiliency Program. *International Journal of Environmental Research and Public Health, 11*(4), 4125–4139.
Saraf, S., Singh, T. B., & Khurana, S. (2013). Cervical cancer survivors: Meaning in life. *Psychological Studies, 58,* 144–152.
Singh, K., & Yu, X. (2010). Psychometric evaluation of the Connor-Davidson Resilience Scale (CD-RISC) in a Sample of Indian Students. *Journal of Psychology, 1*(1), 23–30.
Smith, B. W., Dalen, J., Wiggins, K., Tooley, E., Christopher, P., & Bernard, J. (2008). The brief resilience scale: Assessing the ability to bounce back. *International Journal of Behavioural Medicine, 15,* 194–200.
Somasundaram, R. O., & Devamani, K. A. (2016). A comparative study on resilience, perceived social support and hopelessness among cancer patients treated with curative and palliative care. *Indian Journal of Palliative Care, 22*(2), 135–140.
Sood, S., Bakshi, A., & Devi, P. (2013). An assessment of perceived stress, resilience, and mental health of adolescents living in border areas. *International Journal of Scientific and Research Publications, 3,* 1–4.
Sreeja Sreekumar, T. P., & Varghese, P. J. (2016). Factors associated with resilience in wives of individuals with alcohol dependence syndrome. *Indian Journal of Psychiatry, 58*(3), 307.
Swaminathan, G., & Rao, R. S. B. R. (2010). Going beyond psychopathology—Positive emotions and psychological resilience. *Indian Journal of Psychiatry, 52,* 6–8.
Tankha, G., & Gill, P. (2007). A comparative study of gender and academic achievement on resilience and its linked measures. *Indian Journal of Clinical Psychology, 34,* 55–61.
Thomas, K. W., & Tymon, W. G., Jr. (2007). Stress resiliency profile: A measure of interpretive styles that contribute to stress. In C. P. Zalaquett & R. J. Wood (Eds.), *Evaluating stress: A book of resources.* Lanham, MD: Scarecrow Press.
Ungar, M. (2008). Resilience across cultures. *British Journal of Social Work, 38*(2), 218–235.
Ungar, M. (2011). The social ecology of resilience: Addressing contextual and cultural ambiguity of a nascent construct. *American Journal of Orthopsychiatry, 81,* 1–17.
Ungar, M., Brown, M., Liebenberg, L., Othman, R., Kwong, W. M., Armstrong, M., et al. (2007). Unique pathways to resilience across cultures. *Adolescence, 42,* 287–310.
Ungar, M., Theron, L. C., & Didkowsky, N. (2011). Adolescents' precocious and developmentally appropriate contributions to their families' wellbeing and resilience in five countries. *Family Relations, 60*(2), 231–246.

Wagnild, G. M., & Young, H. M. (1993). Development and psychometric evaluation of the resilience scale. *Journal of Nursing Measurement, 1,* 165–178.

Walsh, F. (1998). *Strengthening family resilience*. New York: Guilford Press.

Walsh, F. (2003). Family resilience: A framework for clinical practice. *Family Process, 42,* 1–18.

Werner, E. E., & Smith, R. S. (1992). *Overcoming the odds: High–risk children from birth to adulthood*. New York: Cornell University Press.

Windle, G., Bennett, K. M., & Noyes, J. (2011). A methodological review of resilience measurement scales. *Health and Quality of Life Outcomes, 9,* 8–18.

Zautra, A. J., Hall, J. S., & Murray, K. (2008). Community development and community resilience: An integrative approach. *Community Development, 39,* 1–18.

Zautra, A. J., Hall, J. S., & Murray, K. E. (2010). Resilience: A new definition of health for people and communities. In J. W. Reich, A. J. Zautra, & J. S. Hall (Eds.), *Handbook of adult resilience* (pp. 3–34). New York: Guilford.

Chapter 6
Perspectives on Posttraumatic Growth

Braj Bhushan

History is full of stories of people witnessing positive changes after suffering and trauma. Published literature in psychology and allied disciplines have consistently reported evidence for 'constructive confrontation' (Schaefer and Moos 1992), 'positive changes in outlook' (Joseph et al. 1993), 'benefit finding' (Affleck and Tennen 1996; Davis et al. 1998; Taylor 1983), 'stress related growth' (Park et al. 1996), 'posttraumatic growth (PTG)' (Tedeschi and Calhoun 1996), 'perceived benefit' (McMillen and Fisher 1998), 'thriving' (Abraido-Lanza et al. 1998), 'positive by-products' (McMillen et al. 2001), and positive adaptation (Linley 2003) and 'growth through adversity' (Joseph and Linley 2005) in the aftermath of a traumatic life event. Of them 'posttraumatic growth' is the commonly used terminology by most researchers. Tedeschi et al. (1998) have conceptualized posttraumatic growth as 'a significant beneficial change in cognitive and emotional life that may have behavioral implications as well" (p. 3). Further, it involves 'such fundamental changes or insights about living that it does not appear to be merely another coping mechanism' (p. 3).

Understanding Posttraumatic Growth

It is true that a large number of people remain unaffected by traumatic events (Bonanno 2004, 2005). However, here the focus is on those who report one or the other type of change after experiencing some type of trauma in their life. As known to everyone, the initial focus was on the identification of symptoms of posttraumatic stress disorder (PTSD), but since last two decades or so the positive outcome of trauma (posttraumatic growth or PTG) has also attracted attention of researchers. In this context two

B. Bhushan (✉)
Department of Humanities & Social Sciences, Indian Institute of Technology, Kanpur, India
e-mail: brajb@iitk.ac.in

G. Misra (ed.), *Psychosocial Interventions for Health and Well-Being*,
https://doi.org/10.1007/978-81-322-3782-2_6

developments are worth mentioning. First, a group of researchers felt the need to redefine posttraumatic stress arguing that posttraumatic reactions are 'normal reactions experienced by people in response to stressful and traumatic situations, indicative of need for cognitive-emotional processing, rather than an abnormal state of mind' (Joseph and Williams 2005, p. 426). Second, 30–90% of the people experiencing traumatic life events were found to report PTG (Tedeschi et al. 1998).

Empirical research gives three different perspectives on trauma and PTG. Studies have reported negative (Evers et al. 2001), positive (Lev-Wiesel and Amir 2003) and no correlation (Powell et al. 2003; Solomon et al. 1999; Ursano et al. 1986) between the symptoms of distress and growth. As evident here, the first perspective suggests negative correlation between distress and growth. The other perspective suggests a two-dimensional response to traumatic stressors where growth and distress coexist. It has been advocated that distress and growth coexist and PTG emerges as a byproduct of posttraumatic struggle and not the trauma itself (Tedeschi and Calhoun 1995, 2004). However, high score on one does not necessitate low score on the other. Hence, these two outcomes remain unrelated though they exist in the same individual at the same time. Morris et al. (2005) also found coexistence of trauma and growth. Further, perceived severity of trauma was found to be associated with higher growth. The third perspective lends support to positive correlation between distress and PTG. This view argues benefit finding and growth as a function of traumatic life experiences. Empirical support for this viewpoint has been extended by many researchers (Hussain and Bhushan 2011a; Pargament et al. 1998; Park et al. 1996; Snape 1997).

Mostly, researchers have either examined PTSD or PTG in their studies barring few who have simultaneously examined both (Linley et al. 2008; Salsman et al. 2009). The relationship between the two posttraumatic outcomes—posttraumatic stress and posttraumatic growth have also been examined. Based on their study of survivors of fires, earthquakes and floods, Saccinto et al. (2013) have reported positive relationship between avoidance and intrusion-hyperarousal symptoms and PTG. Examining the different roles of peri and post trauma experiences, they found that peritraumatic panic predicted both, posttraumatic intrusion-hyperarousal symptoms as well as PTG. On the other hand, posttraumatic intrusion-hyperarousal symptoms mediated the relationship between peritraumatic panic symptoms and posttraumatic growth. Measuring direct as well as indirect exposure to ongoing terrorism, Palmer et al. (2012) have reported positive relationship of exposure of family members to terror to PTS and PTG, both. They further found that PTS mediated the indirect relationship between subjective exposure and PTG. This endorses the importance of emotional suffering in PTG.

It is well understood that PTG is moving beyond the pre-trauma state rather than returning to the baseline. Few variables such as gender, perceived stress and trauma severity have been reported to predict positive (PTG) and negative (PTSD) outcomes in the same direction. On the other hand, few variables such as personality, mood, social support and coping behaviour have been reported to show mixed or opposite directionality. Hence, understanding the trajectory of posttraumatic growth seems to be important. This chapter is a small attempt to do so.

Survivors of a catastrophic event largely report positive change in their self-perception. They also report such changes in their relationships with others. Above all, they report change in their life philosophy as well. In terms of self-perception, one feels stronger despite vulnerability following the trauma. Openness, increased compassion and greater valuing of loved ones are the changes visible in the interpersonal relationship. Change in life philosophy gets reflected in increase in religiosity/spirituality, change in life priorities and appreciation of each and every day of one's life. Few studies have tried to relate PTG and severity of trauma. This is typically referred to as dose-response. Researchers have contested that trauma severity and PTG has an inverted U-shaped relationship with moderate trauma leading to high level of PTG than low or high level of trauma. This has been found in veterans of the Vietnam War (Fontana and Rosenheck 1998) and survivors of 11 September 2001 terrorist attacks in New York (Butler et al. 2005).

However, one also has to factor in other findings and viewpoints. It has been argued that human response to extreme stress has a mixture of resilience and vulnerability. Some researchers did not find relationship among PTG, well-being, flourishing and distress (Chan and Rhodes 2013). Another viewpoint contests that growth is possible only when individuals are deeply involved in translating growth cognitions to growth actions. Hobfoll et al. (2007) have talked about action-focused growth saying that 'positive benefit in posttraumatic growth' was found 'only when individuals were deeply involved in translating growth cognitions to growth actions' (p. 345).

Comparable Constructs

Literature in psychology is full of theories that explain human adaptive capability. The dispositional optimism by Carver and Scheier (1999), internal locus of control by Rotter (1966), self-efficacy by Bandura (1982), hardiness by Kobasa (1979) and Antonovsky's sense of coherence (1987), all of them have relevance to posttraumatic outcomes. Let us succinctly look at the constructs that are close to PTG. The 'wholist framework' of Valent (1999) explains trauma and its outcome in terms of process, parameters and depth where process describes nature of the trauma, parameters elucidates its context and depth explicates its effect. Tennen and Affleck (1998) has explained the role of optimism in posttraumatic growth. Dispositional optimism has been found to positively correlate with enhanced coping and adjustment (Carver 1998). Locus of control (Rotter 1966) describes contingency between behaviour and outcome inasmuch as internal locus of control contingency envisage problem-focused coping, thus facilitating positive adaptation in a traumatic situation. Maercker and Herrle (2003) studied the survivors of the February 1945 Dresden bombing and found that those experiencing PTG were the ones who had high internal locus of control. Self-efficacy is defined as the 'belief in one's capability to organize and execute the course of action required to manage prospective situations' (Bandura 1997, p. 2). The self-efficacy theory (Bandura 1982) talks about one's belief in own capabilities. This belief encourages coping behaviour. Kobasa's theory of hardiness (Kobasa 1979) and Antonovsky's (1987) sense of coherence have also been found to foster better adaptation to traumatic life experiences.

Westphal and Bonanno (2007) have pointed out that the researchers 'implicitly or explicitly equate PTG with resilience or even consider PTG superior to resilient outcomes' (p. 420). Rutter (1985) opined that 'the promotion of resilience does not lie in an avoidance of stress, but rather in encountering stress at a time and in a way that allows self confidence and social competence to increase through mastery and appropriate responsibility' (p. 608).

Medical sociologist Aaron Antonovsky (1923–1994) developed the construct 'sense of coherence'. Based on his work on Holocaust survivors he propounded the theory of salutogenesis (Antonovsky 1987) which talks about association between stress, health and coping. According to him sense of coherence is 'a global orientation that expresses the extent to which one has a pervasive, enduring though dynamic feeling of confidence that (1) the stimuli deriving from one's internal and external environments in the course of living are structured and predictable, and explicable; (2) the resources are available to one to meet the demands posed by these stimuli; and (3) these demands are challenges, worthy of investment and engagement' (Antonovsky 1987, p. 19). In terms of assessment, sense of coherence scale has three subscales—comprehensibility, manageability and meaningfulness. Comprehensibility measures the extent to which one can derive sense from the adversity whereas manageability is the degree of perception of the available resources and its worth in meeting the challenges. Finally, meaningfulness reflects the feeling of worthiness in the engagement with the posed challenges. It is important to note that two of the constructs, hardiness and self-efficacy, do find place in sense of coherence.

According to Waysman et al. (2001) 'those who view themselves as in charge of their fate (control), who are committed to meaningful goals and activities (commitment), and who view their stress as a surmountable challenge are more likely in the long run to integrate the trauma into their lives and to enjoy a satisfactory level of adjustment' (p. 545).

Distinct Nature of PTG Studies

PTG studies are unique in certain ways. If you look at the nature of sample chosen for studying PTG, you would find almost all types of distressing experiences covered by them. For instance, life-threatening ailments such as cancer and HIV/AIDS have been very well studied with all inherent variations. Researchers have studied PTG in a wide range of cancer patients such as prostate cancer (Kinsinger et al. 2006), testicular cancer (Rieker et al. 1989), melanoma (Dirksen 1995) and bone marrow transplant (Tallman et al. 2007; Widows et al. 2005). Stanton et al. (2006) reviewed studies on PTG in cancer patients published between 1960 and 2004. They found prevalence of PTG varying between 53 (Taylor et al. 1984) and 83% (Sears et al. 2003) in breast cancer patients and 95% of adult survivors of childhood cancer (Wasserman et al. 1987). Similarly, Tallman et al. (2007) found that the constituents of growth (perceived benefit finding) by prostate cancer survivors were life perspective, relationships, self-perception, health, new directions and religious/spiritual changes.

Besides ailments, many other unique human experiences have also been carried out by researchers. Study of military combat, prisoner of wars (POWs), political imprisonments, refugee displacement and other types of rare life experiences have also been researched by psychologists. Table 6.1 broadly summarizes the traumatic life events studied by PTG researchers.

There are many studies reporting posttraumatic stress in soldiers citing multiple stressors and their effect. Researchers have reported PTG in the soldiers who served during World War II, Korean War, Gulf War I, Vietnam War and Israeli operations, just to mention a few. The deployment experiences of soldiers have been found to correlate with PTG. Johnson et al. (2007) studied deployment conditions (pre-deployment, deployment and post-deployment) and their effect on posttraumatic growth in a sample of Gulf War I veterans. They found that post-deployment conditions predicted certain aspects of PTG. Perceived threat appeared as the strongest predictor of appreciation of life. Another post-deployment variable, social support, predicted relating to others and personal strength dimensions of growth. Studies investigating combat exposure and PTG have reported mixed findings. The findings are bidirectional in a sense that some researchers argue that higher combat exposure leading to growth while some argue the opposite. Combat exposure also

Table 6.1 Summary of empirical research on posttraumatic growth

Traumatic life event	Researchers
Bereavement	Davis et al. (1998)
Bone marrow transplantation	Fromm et al. (1996)
Breast cancer	Cordova et al. (2001), Taylor (1983), Weiss (2002)
Childhood sexual abuse	McMillen et al. (1995)
Refugees and immigrants	Weiss and Berger (2006), Powell et al. (2003)
Gulf War I Veterans	Johnson et al. (2007)
Prisoners of war	Solomon and Dekel (2007)
Relief workers	Bhushan and Kumar (2012)
Chronic illness	Abraido-Lanza et al. (1998)
Disaster	McMillen et al. (1997)
HIV infection	Updegraff et al. (2002)
Military combat	Fontana and Rosenheck (1998)
Myocardial infarction	Affleck et al. (1987)
Parenting child with leukaemia	Best et al. (2001)
Refugees	Hussain and Bhushan (2011a, b, 2013), Powell et al. (2003)
Sexual assault	Frazier et al. (2001)
Shipwreck	Joseph et al. (1993)

has inbuilt perceived threat associated with it and some researchers contest that this is also associated with PTG (Fontana and Rosenheck 1998). Cordova et al. (2001) have reported association between growth and higher degree of life threat. It has been advocated that when one faces mortality, he/she re-evaluates and redefines life goals and priorities. This, in turn, result into PTG (Tedeschi and Calhoun 1995).

Interestingly, there are studies reporting growth and accepting war exposure as an important developmental milestone (Dohrenwend et al. 2004; Elder et al. 1991; Gade 1991). Studying World War II and Korean War veterans, Aldwin et al. (1994) observed linear relationship between combat and positive outcomes such as coping and perspective on life.

Psychologists have also studied ex-prisoners of war (POWs) and the effect of such experiences. Studies have mostly focused on PTSD (Sutker and Allain 1996; Tennant et al. 1997), anxiety and depression (Engdahl et al. 1991), hypochondria (Klonoff et al. 1976), alcoholism (Beebe 1975) and other negative outcomes. But this is only one half of the story. Solomon and Dekel (2007) examined the Israeli ex-POWs for both, PTSD and PTG and found evidence for PTG on all five dimensions of PTGI. Studies have reported positive changes in ex-POWs. 90% of the American air-force officers held as POWs in Vietnam reported positive changes as a result of captivity (Sledge et al. 1980). These changes included greater understanding of self and others and change in priorities in life. Similar positive experiences have been reported by Israeli ex-POWs and war veterans (Solomon et al. 1999).

The sufferings associated with participation in political movements have not been very well studied in psychology. Researchers have argued that traumatic stress during political activities is likely to increase 'psychological preparedness' for trauma (Basoglu et al. 1997; Ehlers et al. 2000). Maercker and Zöllner (2004) studied East German former political prisoners and found that 72% of them reported examples of PTG following their imprisonment.

Besides combat, the other rare human experience studied by PTG researchers is of the Holocaust survivors. In a unique study Lev-Wiesel a and Amir (2003) examined 97 Holocaust child survivors born after 1930 in Israel to understand the relationship between posttraumatic symptoms, perceived social and personal resources, and posttraumatic growth. The findings indicated inverse relationship between PTSD symptoms and personal resources. The dimensions of PTG were also positively correlated with arousal. The researchers concluded that those exhibiting arousal of PTSD symptoms might experience better growth. Further, social support also affected the level of new possibilities of PTG.

The other unique group studied by researchers is the refugees. Refugees are defined as people who 'owing to a well-founded fear of being persecuted for reasons of race, religion, nationality, membership of a particular social group or political opinion, is outside the country of his nationality, and is unable to, or owing to such fear, is unwilling to avail himself of the protection of that country' (The 1951 Refugee Convention). These special groups of human beings have also attracted the attention of psychologists working on PTG. Powell et al. (2003) studied PTG in the refugees settled in Sarajevo, Bosnia and Herzegovina. The recent studies have reported PTG in people experiencing refugee-related torture and trauma prior to migrating to Australia (Barrington and Shakespeare-Finch 2013a), Tibetan refugees staying in Dharamshala (Hussain and Bhushan 2011b, 2013) and refugee citizens of Cote d'Ivoire living in asylum in Liberia (Gregory and Prana 2013).

One can see the wide range of rare human experiences covered under the ambit of PTG research.

Indian Studies on PTG

Although the nuances of PTG can very well be seen in the Indian religious traditions, culture and literature, survey of the scientific literature in psychology reveal that not many researchers have shown interest in studying PTG in India. Search through EBSCO in October 2013 shows only five publications pertaining to PTG from India (Bhushan and Kumar 2012; Hussain and Bhushan 2011a, b, 2013; Thombre et al. 2010). Bhushan and Kumar (2012) had examined PTG in Tsunami relief volunteers. Thombre et al. (2010) examined PTG in 61 cancer patients from the city of Pune. Hussain and Bhushan (2011a, b, 2013) examined PTG in the Tibetan refugees staying in Dharamshala.

During our study of the Tibetan refugees (Hussain and Bhushan 2011a), we realized that the traumatic experiences of this population had very distinctive features. Besides survival, trauma and deprivation/uncertainty, ethnic concern such as ethnic discrimination and destruction of the place of worship were also major source of trauma for them (Hussain and Bhushan 2009). The uniqueness of this group has also been reported by other researchers (Terheggen et al. 2001). Our qualitative investigation of Tibetan refugees using semi-structured interviews (Hussain and Bhushan 2013) showed that irrespective of uninterrupted encounter with trauma, people report positive experiences learnt from adverse life experiences. We found three major themes related to PTG—change in outlook, personal strength, and meaningful relationships. Changes in outlook comprised themes such as acceptance, responsibility, compassion, and optimism. Increased intimacy and meaningfulness in relationship were other reported changes. Personal strength included themes such as self-reliance, self as survivor, and experience of success and achievement. Their narratives clearly reflected the deep impression of the law of karma on their thought and behaviour.

PTG as a Cognitive Output

It has been argued that PTG is an outcome of cognitive and emotional struggle. It has also been argued that the variation in cognitive or affective processing after a traumatic event predispose the survivors to PTSD (Tolin and Foa 2006). The type of coping strategy adopted after stressful life experiences is also supposed to be mediated by cognitive emotional processing strategy (Hussain and Bhushan 2011b) which offer the coping function (Garnefski et al. 2001, 2002). The Janus-face model of PTG talks about two coexisting components—a self-transcending constructive component and a self-deceptive illusory component. As elucidated by Zöllner and Maercker (2006a), with the passage of time the constructive component grow while the illusory component diminishes. This allows successful coping to happen.

As mentioned above, Hobfoll et al. (2007) have emphasized on the relationship between action and PTG by endorsing action as the key to PTG. According to them 'PTG may serve the role of a cognitive coping strategy following extreme stress, but not translate to actual change in positive posttraumatic functioning' (Hobfoll et al. 2007, p. 361). Some researchers consider PTG as a cognitive process not necessarily leading to action. However, the possibility of action is not overruled in the cognitive framework (Maercker and Zöllner 2004; Zöllner and Maercker 2006b).

Ruminative thoughts and their impact on behaviour has also been examined. According to Martin and Tesser (1996) rumination is 'a class of conscious thoughts that revolve around a common instrumental theme and that recur in the absence of immediate environmental demands requiring the thought' (p. 7). Rumination has been conceptualized as chronic past oriented self-focus that is mostly associated with neurotic personality. Elaborating individual differences in attention to the negative and positive aspects of events, Noguchi et al. (2006) have suggested that self-reported attention to negative information is positively associated to negative affectivity, neuroticism and behavioural inhibition system and inversely related to optimism. On the other hand, self-reported attention to positive information correlates to positive effect, extraversion, behavioural approach system and optimism. Attention bias, whether positive or negative, is an indicator of our cognitive processing style. It shows our tendency to selectively attend either negative or positive aspects of any life event.

It can be assumed that negative attention bias may adversely affect trauma-related rumination, thus predicting PTSD symptoms whereas positive attention bias is likely to exert positive influence on rumination resulting in PTG. This makes it evident that the valence of attention bias and hence the cognitive processing style might help plot the trajectory of the negative (PTSD) and positive (PTG) outcomes of a traumatic event. Chan et al. (2011) found positive correlation between cancer related positive rumination and PTG. Lepore (2001) have reported that the cognitive processing of cancer mediated adjustment of the individuals to the disease. Calhoun et al. (2000), Calhoun and Tedeschi (2006) have advocated co-occurrence of intrusive and deliberate rumination inasmuch as in the first case one recollects the negative experiences of the traumatic event but in the second case one deliberately ruminates and derives sense out of the traumatic event. According to Mansell (2000), acquisition of new information or voluntary appraisal modifies lower order attention bias, thus influencing changes in higher order schema.

Cognitive theories (Segerstrom et al. 2003; Watkins 2008) suggest that the valence of thought is crucial for determining the effect of rumination. The cognitive processes underlying posttraumatic outcomes signify that ruminative thoughts determine the negative as well as the positive effect. Repetitive recollection of stressor and negative appraisal of it is proven to be one of the sources of PTSD (Ehlers and Clark 2000). On the other hand, rumination is needed to rebuild the schemas that get shattered by the traumatic experience (Tedeschi and Calhoun 2004). Calhoun et al. (2000) and Calhoun and Tedeschi (1998) advocate that rumination is essential to actively think and derive meaning out of what had happened and this is important for PTG. Several researchers have endorsed that premeditated event-related rumination with focus on the positive aspects foster PTG (Bower et al. 1998; Calhoun et al. 2000; Taku et al. 2008; Watkins 2008).

However, besides cognitive component PTG needs to be understood and examined with respect to emotional, social and behavioural components.

Correlates of PTG

Researchers have examined many variables for their possible association with PTSD as well as PTG. Studies show that PTSD symptoms are correlated to negative self-cognitions (Bryant and Guthrie 2007), negative global beliefs (Dunmore et al. 1999), pessimistic attributional style (McCormick et al. 1989), neuroticism and introversion (Lauterbach and Vrana 2001) whereas PTG is correlated to optimism, hope and extraversion (Zoellner and Maercker 2006). In an interesting research, Bayer-Topilsky et al. (2013) found positive religious coping and living status without a partner as predictors of PTG, optimism expectations, social support and other religious factors did not relate to PTG. Meta-analytic studies have identified optimism, social support, religiosity/spirituality, coping styles, especially acceptance coping, reappraisal coping, religious coping and seeking support coping, as strong correlates of PTG. Among them, optimism and social support have moderate effect whereas coping styles such as positive reappraisal and religious coping have high association with PTG. Looking at the relationship of PTG and these factors and their predictive power in terms of the effect size, acceptance coping has small, social support has medium, optimism and spirituality has moderate, and religious coping and positive reappraisal coping have a strong predictive power. Of these factors, here the focus would be only on religious orientation, social support and gender. The selection of these correlates is guided by the importance of these factors in the Indian setting.

Religious Orientation

In our day-to-day interaction, religiosity and spirituality are interchangeably used. However, psychologists establish distinction between them. Where belief on any kind of worship is considered as an indicator of religiosity, spirituality refers to a broad array of personal experiences that does not require obligations, commitments and practices that are typically coupled with religiosity. Religion has been defined as a 'system of beliefs, practices, customs and ceremonies rooted in a culture; a view of the individual's relationship to the universe; a moral and ethical code; and a community of adherents providing social relationships' (Sacks 1985, p. 27) whereas spirituality engages one in 'transcendental values, meaning, experience, and development; for knowledge of an ultimate reality; for a belongingness and relatedness with the moral universe and community; and for union with immanent, supernatural powers that guide people and the universe for good or evil' (Siporin 1985, p. 199). As defined by Wink and Dillon (2002) 'spirituality connotes the self existential search for ultimate meaning through an individualized understanding of the sacred' (p. 79). Researchers have made further distinction between practice-oriented and seeking-oriented spirituality (Wuthnow 1998). Similarly, religiosity has also been classified as intrinsic and extrinsic religious orientation. The former is self-transcendental whereas the later is self-oriented in nature (Allport and Ross 1967). Besides these two dimensions, quest religion has also been talked about. Quest religion refers to 'the degree to which a person's religion involves an open ended, responsive dialogue with existential questions raised by the contradictions and tragedies of life' (Batson and Ventis 1982).

Empirical research on PTG has largely not shown interest in looking at spirituality and religiosity separately. Studies confirm that religious and spiritual beliefs can grow following trauma and are helpful in overcoming the traumatic experience (Khouzam 2000; Park et al. 1996; Rudnick 1997). The qualitative as well as quantitative data indicate religious belief as a catalyst of the process of PTG (Emmons et al. 1998; Fallot 1997). Based on the meta-analysis of 103 studies, Prati and Pietrantoni (2009) have endorsed the relationship between spirituality and religious coping and PTG.

While measuring religious involvement in the context of PTG, different dimensions of religiosity has been assessed by different researchers. Most of the researchers have used intrinsic and extrinsic religiosity as variables in their study (Hall et al. 1994). Park et al. (1996) have reported strong association between intrinsic religiosity and PTG. Some researchers have defined intrinsic religiosity as an end in itself (Maltby and Lewis 1996). Calhoun et al. (2000) found that two aspects of quest religion—readiness to face existential questions and openness to religious change—were associated with PTG. Considering the fact that intrinsic, extrinsic and quest religion are all global indicators of religion, it remained a challenge to measure religiosity and trace the pathway to PTG.

Schuster et al. (2001) surveyed American people after 11 September 2001 terrorist attacks. They found that 90% of their sample showed increased inclination towards their religious faith. In an interesting study, Ullman (1982) compared converts and religiously affiliated non-converts and found that converts recollected more childhood trauma describing their childhood and adolescence less happy. As anticipated, human beings do elicit diverse behaviour. In the aftermath of traumatic experience, some people show loss of religious commitment with increased cynicism (Schwartzberg and Janoff-Bulman 1991) while some do not show any change (Overcash et al. 1996). Siegel and Schrimshaw (2000) assessed stress-related growth in women who were either HIV positive or were living with AIDS. These women reported spirituality as a means of finding meaning in life, initially by holding God responsible for not safeguarding them and then by deepening their faith which gave a sense of peace.

Let us examine the issue of assessment of religiosity/spirituality that has been used in PTG studies. Studies attempting quantitative assessment of PTG have mostly used The Posttraumatic Growth Inventory (PTGI) (Tedeschi and Calhoun 1995, 1996). This is a 21-item measure with five subscales—appreciation of life, relating to others, new possibilities, personal strength and spiritual change. In fact, the 'spiritual change' subscale of the PTGI consists of two items. The first one states that 'I have a stronger religious faith' and the second one states 'A better understanding of spiritual matters'. Many researchers consider this as an abrupt combination that needs to be resolved (cf. Hill and Pargament 2003). Development of RCOPE (Pargament et al. 2000) was important in this aspect as it measured both the positive and negative aspects of religious coping. This tool considers working collaboratively with God and considering death as a passage to heaven as positive religious coping, whereas questioning religious beliefs and feeling punished by God as negative religious coping. Pargament et al. (1998) found association between PTG and religious coping, both positive as well as negative. However, this study did not detail as to which positive and negative subscales were correlated with PTG. The correspondence between PTG and religious coping (the subscales of RCOPE) has been given by Koenig et al. (1998). They found correlation between all the 12 aspects of positive and six of the nine aspects of negative religious coping with PTG. However, the correlation coefficients of negative religious coping were weaker, less consistent and sometimes negative. Pargament et al. (2000) findings also corroborated these findings.

It has been accepted that 'religion or spirituality can provide a unifying philosophy of life and serve as an integrating and stabilizing force that provides a framework for interpreting life's challenges and provides a resolution to such concerns as suffering, death, tragedy and injustice' (Emmons et al. 1998, p. 175). It seems that in the process of deriving meaning in life one also develops greater existential awareness (Yalom and Lieberman 1991), thus becoming more religious/spiritual. Traumatic events are also instrumental in developing one's faith.

Social Support

Social support is another variable of importance for two reasons, one it is supposed to influence coping in the aftermath of a crisis and two, it is something that can be built or strengthened in the system to maximize benefit to the victims and survivors. It is also important as it defines the inherent nature of collectivist cultures. Social support has been identified as a significant environmental resource that positively affects outcomes after a life crisis (Schaefer and Moos 1998; Tedeschi and Calhoun 2004). As stated by Tedeschi and Calhoun (2004), 'supportive others can aid in posttraumatic growth by providing a way to craft narratives about the changes that have occurred, and by offering perspectives that can be integrated into schema change' (p. 8). Almedom (2005) has categorically stated that the type, time and level of social support available to the survivors might determine outcomes of a traumatic event.

Social support influences coping behaviour finally leading to personal growth. Acceptance and reappraisal coping are likely to be affected by the available support. On one hand acceptance help adapt to situations that cannot be changed whereas on the other hand positive reappraisal of the event is the beginning of PTG (Schaefer and Moos 1998; Zöllner and Maercker 2006a, b).

Gender

Many studies have reported gender difference in PTG with women reporting higher levels of growth compared to men (Park et al. 1996; Tedeschi and Calhoun 1996). These findings have largely remained consistent irrespective of the nature of trauma and tool used to measure it. For instance, gender difference have been reported for cancer, HIV/AIDS, terrorism, and natural disasters (Bellizzi 2004; Jang 2006; Milam 2004; Milam et al. 2005). In terms of usage of tool, Park et al. (1996) used the Stress-Related Growth Scale (SRGS) whereas Tedeschi and Calhoun (1996) had administered the Posttraumatic Growth Inventory (PTGI). However, the findings of all these studies endorsed difference between males and females.

Studies attempting meta-analysis to examine this gender difference have also confirmed it. For instance, the meta-analysis by Helgeson et al. (2006) found the level of posttraumatic growth in women slightly higher than the men with a small effect size ($r = 0.08, p < 0.001$). Vishnevsky et al. (2010) also performed a meta-analysis with 16,076 participants drawn from 70 studies. They also found moderate gender difference ($g = 0.27$, 95% CI = 0.21 − 0.32) with women reporting more PTG compared to men. It may be interesting to note that these studies largely included trauma such as cancer, bereavement, terrorism, natural disaster and mixed nature of trauma and were conducted on samples drawn from the United States of America, United Kingdom, Australia and Turkey. What was also interesting was the fact that the reported level of PTG increased with a rise in the mean age of the women sample.

One of the reasons cited in studies is that women engage more in ruminative thoughts. The other explanation is that they perceive the severity of traumatic events more and this could lead to more self-reported growth (Tedeschi and Calhoun 1996).

Many researchers have examined the occurrence of PTG in women-specific experiences. Studying PTG in 60 women who were around 33 years of age and had experienced intimate partner violence, Cobb et al. (2006) found that despite negative psychological outcomes they reported PTG. Their mean PTG score on PTGI was higher than the reported mean scores by survivors of breast cancer (Weiss 2002) or victims of violent crime (Peltzer 2000). Other studies pertaining to intimate partner violence have also reported similar findings (Draucker 2001; McCann and Pearlman 1990). Another study examining changes in 22 women who had terminated their relationship due to abusive violence also found increased interpersonal relationship, self-awareness and religiosity besides few other changes (Senter and Caldwell 2002). Such studies have also reported relationship between severity of abuse and appreciation of life dimension of PTG. Konrad (2006) found that mothers of children who acquired disabilities reconstructed meaning of care giving and compassion in the aftermath of this experience, thus reporting PTG. It is important to note that in this study none of the mothers reported PTSD. Konrad (2006) has nicely summarized it stating that 'PTG does not diminish or contradict the burden and suffering experienced by caregivers, nor is it meant to silence the very real and difficult emotions brought about by bearing witness to a child's struggles and distress. Rather, it is meant to add to the complexity, richness, and fuller appreciation of our understanding of the caregiver experience' (p. 109). Amongst breast cancer survivors PTG have also been studied by researchers. On one hand (Naidich and Motta 2000) PTSD was reported in 20% women with breast cancer whereas PTG was in the range of 53% (Taylor et al. 1984) to 84% (Collins et al. 1990). The reported growth is mostly in terms of appreciation of life, change in priorities, improvement in relationship, and positive changes in religious beliefs.

It is important to note that there are few studies reporting no gender difference or opposite relationship (Hooper 2003; Polatinsky and Esprey 2000). Some researchers have observed that women also perceive threat and loss of control more than men including intense fear, intrusion, avoidance, panic and anxiety (Olff et al. 2007). This predisposes them to a higher prevalence rate of PTSD.

We have already talked about PTG with reference to rumination. Some studies have shown that women engage more in premeditated and threatening rumination (Treynor et al. 2003). As premeditated rumination is more productive in nature than threatening rumination, they experience more posttraumatic stress as well as report more PTG (Janoff-Bulman 2006; Tedeschi and Calhoun 2004). Another important factor could be the predominant coping style. Women show increased likelihood of using emotion-focused coping (de Ridder 2000). This could, in turn, be instrumental in facilitating PTG. The association between PTG and emotion-focused coping strategies, including positive reappraisal, acceptance, and denial has been reported (Helgeson et al. 2006) by researchers. Problem and emotion-focused coping has also been found to correlate with PTG (Prati and Pietrantoni 2009).

Assessment of PTG

The current trend of assessment examines a construct using statistical methods and in few cases it is also supplemented by neuropsychological evidences. Let us examine PTG in the light of these two methods.

Psychometric Viewpoint

Development of an appropriate measure is always a difficult task, especially when it is supposed to be administered across cultures. This is true for the assessment of PTG as well. Several psychometric tools have been developed to measure 'growth'. This includes Benefit Finding Scale (Mohr et al. 1991; Tomich and Helgeson 2004), Perceived Benefit Scale (McMillen and Fisher 1998), Posttraumatic Growth Inventory (PTGI) (Tedeschi and Calhoun 1996), Stress Related Growth Scale (SRGC) (Park et al. 1996), Thriving Scale (Abraido-Lanza et al. 1998) and Changes in Outlook Questionnaire (Joseph et al. 2005). Few researchers have used open-ended measures (Bower et al. 1998). For some reasons most of the studies on PTG have either used the PTGI or SRGC. Between them also, PTGI has been mostly used by researchers. Both, Benefit Finding Scale and Perceived Benefit Scale assess a range of 'benefits' but not all of them are associated with post-traumatic growth. Changes in Outlook Questionnaire is the most recent measure compared to the rest. It measures positive as well as negative changes. The open-ended measures have not been extensively validated. It is equally important to know the nature of sample on which these PTG measures were administered to develop the tool. PTGI was built with undergraduate students (Tedeschi and Calhoun 1996), Perceived Benefit Scale with adults involved in church activities (McMillen and Fisher 1998) and Thriving Scale with Latinas suffering from chronic illness (Abraido-Lanza et al. 1998). The very difference in the nature of the sample could have affected the structural conceptualization of the construct.

The PTGI (Tedeschi and Calhoun 1996) is the most widely used tool to assess PTG. This 21-item measure has five subscales—appreciation of life, relating to others, new possibilities, personal strength and spiritual change. With respect to the factor structure of the measures of PTG, Joseph et al. (2004) have argued that these measures have used eigen values-greater-than-one criterion for determining the number of components. As large number of variables lead to larger eigen value (Zwick and Velicer 1986), scree test seem a more reliable indicator (Cattell 1966). The five-factor model of PTGI was an outcome of principal components analysis used while developing it and many researchers have accepted this without redoing the factor analysis (e.g., Peltzer 2000; Polatinsky and Esprey 2000). Powell et al. (2003) analysed the factor structure and found that PTGI items loaded on three factors—changes in self/positive life attitude, philosophy of life and relating to others. Morris et al. (2005) conducted a study on 219 Australian participants and used exploratory factor analyses with principal components analysis (with varimax rotation) to find out the factor structure of PTGI. The findings were similar to the original scale with the items mostly falling into the same five dimensions. Morris et al. (2005) have argued that replication of factor structure irrespective of rotation method and additional items (the researchers had added three items pertaining to spiritual change) conforms the robustness of PTGI as a psychological tool. Barrington and Shakespeare-Finch (2013b) performed confirmatory factor analysis and found adequate five-factor fit.

However, there are exceptions. Polatinsky and Esprey's (2000) study did not support the five factors structure of PTGI. They also did not find sex difference in PTG. Studies examining construct validity of PTGI have reported conflicting results (Weinrib et al. 2006; Frazier and Kaler 2006; Smith and Cook 2004). Further, the factor structure of PTGI need not be the same in different cultures (Ho et al. 2004; Taku et al. 2007; Weiss and Berger 2006).

The other concern related to PTGI is the wording of the instructions. The instructions given to participants ask them to recall a specific crisis and then respond whether changes on any of the items in the five areas was caused by that event or not. Some researchers contest that linking PTGI items to a specific crisis causes positive bias in the respondents whereby they overestimate their growth. Taylor (1983) described this process as self-enhancing thinking. The alternative to this could be responding to items by revisiting recent changes in one's life rather than anchoring it to a specific event. Smith and Cook (2004) adopted two methods to measure PTG using PTGI. In the first case, participants were asked to identify a specific stressful event and respond to the items of PTGI whereas in the second case participants were asked to rate the positive changes experienced over the last four years. This study yielded satisfactory reliability and construct validity. The findings also indicated that PTG reports were higher when the responses were not linked to a specific event. One of the noteworthy observation of this study was that when items of PTGI are responded with respect to a specific event the degree of growth is underestimated 'to a small but significant degree' (Smith and Cook 2004, p. 356), especially on two dimensions—'personal strength' and 'relating to others'.

It is evident that researchers have assessed PTG using retrospective self-reports in their studies adopting cross-sectional designs. Cohen et al. (1998) have suggested that the self-reported level of PTG should be analysed with some amount of skepticism. Bonnano (2005) has pointed out that self-reports might reflect real changes or it could be a reattribution while looking backward during the process of recovery. Hence, PTG might echo self-protective and self-enhancing processes (McFarland and Alvaro 2000; Wilson and Ross 2001). Joseph (2011) has argued that 'distinction needs to be made between experiences that survivors themselves perceive to be growthful and changes that are growthful in a way consistent with theory and empirical evidence on what constitutes positive functioning' (p. 844).

An inherent problem with the self-report measures is a possible disparity between questionnaire and the real outcomes. Although there are arguments that actual as well as perceived change after the trauma contribute to reported PTG (Ransom et al. 2008), few researchers endorse the need for additional validation

(Tomich and Helgeson 2004). It has been argued that the scores on the questionnaires might not correspond to actual growth (Frazier and Kaler 2006; Ransom et al. 2008) and the growth scores of self-reported questionnaires might reflect 'illusory perceptions of temporal change' (McFarland and Alvaro 2000, p. 340) to some extent. However, this inherent limitation of self-report measures does not completely defy the existence of PTG. In order to validate the concept of growth, Park et al. (2006) and Weiss (2002) compared the obtained scores on self-reported measures of PTG with the reports from significant others and found moderate correlation between self-reports and informant reports.

The other concern related to PTGI is the inclusion of religiosity. In fact, the 'spiritual change' subscale of the PTGI consists of two items—'A better understanding of spiritual matters' and 'I have stronger religious faith'. This implies that when total score is used for statistical analyses it implies higher religious coping by default. Hence, PTGI total score confound with the measures of religious coping. Considering religiosity and spirituality within the ambit of PTG has another problem, the direction of change. It has been observed that in the aftermath of tragedy and suffering some people reconcile their religious beliefs thus deepening their faith whereas some challenge it. In their study of PTG amongst the survivors of September 11 attack in New York, Poulin et al. (2009) found that of the 1382 participants 9.3% reported increase in religious benefits. Although the reported benefit is perceived as growth, it does not necessarily mean deepening of the faith. Challenging one's own religious belief and thus lessening of faith is also growth (Shaw et al. 2005). An atheist might consider such perceived growth as illusion. According to Joseph (2011), 'it cannot be universally agreed whether increased religiosity and spirituality, is a positive or a negative outcome' (p. 845). Psychometrically speaking, assessment of religious and spiritual change needs to be measured without assuming linear relationship between its increase and positive functioning.

However, religiosity has been found to foster PTG. The other measure used to assess religiosity/spirituality in PTG studies is RCOPE (mentioned above). Moussa and Bates (2011) have reported that various subscales of the RCOPE (Pargament et al. 2000) correlate with PTG.

Neuropsychological Viewpoint

Studies exploring the neuropsychological correlates of PTG are sparse. Studying PTG in survivors of severe traffic accidents, Rabe et al. (2006) found correlation between EEG alpha power asymmetry of the left frontal brain and the PTGI score. Further, anterior asymmetry was associated with different dimensions of PTGI. Four dimensions of PTGI, namely, new possibilities, changed relationships, appreciation of life and personal strength were associated with relative activities of the left fronto-central areas of the brain. Relative left frontal activity is considered an indication of goal-directed approach tendencies (Davidson 1995).

Hence, it can be construed that there are neuropsychological evidence in favour of PTG as a cognitive-motivational process that reflects in the form of new perspectives. It is also important to note that the spiritual change dimension did not show significant correlation.

Looking Forward

Having discussed these issues, findings and concern, it is equally important to examine the new areas of exploration in the field of PTG. An unanswered question related to PTG is the issue of temporality. Although a wide range of trauma-inducing situations have been studied for their negative and positive effects, there is still no consensus on the time needed after the event to experience such positive changes. Polatinsky and Esprey (2000) have reported positive correlation between time since trauma and PTG. In their study of bereaved parents they found that two factors of PTGI, namely New Possibilities and Appreciation of Life, was highly correlated with the time passed since the trauma. It has also been argued that for certain events growth might take relatively less time to get reflected whereas in certain other events (such as child abuse) growth requires substantial time to be evident (McMillen et al. 1995). In terms of temporality, Helgeson et al. (2006) found that the strength of PTG and positive outcomes was high after a passage of at least two years since the traumatic event. The days to come are likely to answer this and many other issues.

References

Abraido-Lanza, A. F., Guier, C., & Colon, R. M. (1998). Psychological thriving among Latinas with chronic illness. *Journal of Social Issues, 54,* 405–424.

Affleck, G., & Tennen, H. (1996). Construing benefits from adversity: Adaptational significance and dispositional underpinnings. *Journal of Personality, 64,* 899–922.

Affleck, G., Tennen, H., Croog, S., & Levine, S. (1987). Causal attribution, perceived benefits, and morbidity after a heart attack: An 8-year study. *Journal of Consulting and Clinical Psychology, 55,* 29–35.

Aldwin, C. M., Levenson, M. R., & Spiro, A. (1994). Vulnerability and resilience to combat exposure: Can stress have lifelong effects? *Psychology and Aging, 9,* 34–44.

Allport, G. W., & Ross, J. M. (1967). Personal religious orientation and prejudice. *Journal of Personality and Social Psychology, 5,* 432–443.

Almedom, A. M. (2005). Resilience, hardiness, sense of coherence, and posttraumatic growth: All paths leading to "light at the end of the tunnel"? *Journal of Loss and Trauma, 10,* 253–265.

Antonovsky, A. (1987). *Unraveling the mystery of health: How people manage stress and stay well.* San Francisco, CA: Jossey-Bass.

Bandura, A. (1982). Self-efficacy mechanism in human agency. *American Psychologist, 37,* 122–147.

Bandura, A. (1997). *Self-efficacy: The exercise of control.* New York: Freeman.

Barrington, A., & Shakespeare-Finch, J. (2013a). Posttraumaticgrowth and posttraumatic depreciation as predictors of psychological adjustment. *Journal of Loss & Trauma, 18,* 429–443.

Barrington, A. J., & Shakespeare-Finch, J. (2013b). Working with refugee survivors of torture and trauma: An opportunity for vicarious post-traumatic growth. *Counselling Psychology Quarterly, 26,* 89–105.

Basoglu, M., Mineka, S., Paker, M., Aker, T., Livanou, M., & Gök, S. (1997). Psychological preparedness for trauma as a protective factor in survivors of torture. *Psychological Medicine, 27,* 1421–1433.

Batson, C. D., & Ventis, W. L. (1982). *The religious experience: A social psychological perspective*. New York: Oxford University Press.

Bayer-Topilsky, T., Itzhaky, H., Dekel, R., & Marmor, Y. N. (2013). Mental health and posttraumatic growth in civilians exposed to ongoing terror. *Journal of Loss & Trauma, 18,* 227–247.

Beebe, G. W. (1975). Follow up studies of World War II and Korean War prisoners: Morbidity, disability, and maladjustment. *American Journal of Epidemiology, 10,* 400–422.

Bellizzi, K. M. (2004). Expressions of generativity and posttraumatic growth in adult cancer survivors. *International Journal of Aging and Human Development, 58,* 267–287.

Best, M., Streisand, R., Catania, L., & Kazak, A. E. (2001). Parental distress during pediatric leukemia and Posttraumatic Stress Symptoms (PTSS) after treatment ends. *Journal of Pediatric Psychology, 26,* 299–307.

Bhushan, B., & Kumar, J. S. (2012). A study of posttraumatic stress and growth in the tsunami relief volunteers. *Journal of Loss & Trauma, 17,* 113–124.

Bonnano, G. (2004). Loss, trauma, and human resilience: Have we underestimated the human capacity to thrive after extremely aversive events? *American Psychologist, 59,* 20–28.

Bonnano, G. (2005). Resilience in the face of potential trauma. *Current Directions in Psychological Science, 14,* 135–138.

Bower, J. E., Kemeny, M. E., Taylor, S. E., & Fahey, J. L. (1998). Cognitive processing, discovery of meaning, CD4 decline, and AIDS-related mortality among bereaved HIV-seropositive men. *Journal of Consulting and Clinical Psychology, 66,* 979–986.

Bryant, R. A., & Guthrie, R. M. (2007). Maladaptive self-appraisals before trauma exposure predict posttraumatic stress disorder. *Journal of Consulting and Clinical Psychology, 75,* 812–815.

Butler, L. D., Blasey, C. M., Azarow, J., McCaslin, S. E., Garlan, R. W., Chen, X.-H., et al. (2005). Posttraumatic growth following the terrorist attacks of September 11, 2001: Cognitive, coping, and trauma symptom predictors in an internet convenience sample. *Traumatology, 11,* 247–267.

Calhoun, L. G., Cann, A., Tedeschi, R. G., & McMillan, J. (2000). A correlational test of the relationship between posttraumatic growth, religion, and cognitive processing. *Journal of Traumatic Stress, 13,* 521–527.

Calhoun, L. G., & Tedeschi, R. G. (1998). Posttraumatic growth: Future directions. In R. G. Tedeshci, C. L. Park, & L. G. Calhoun (Eds.), *Posttraumatic growth: Positive changes in the aftermath of crisis* (pp. 215–238). Mahwah, NJ: Lawrence Erlbaum Associates, Publishers.

Calhoun, L. G., & Tedeschi, R. G. (2006). The foundations of posttraumatic growth: an expanded framework. In L. G. Calhoun & R. G. Tedeschi (Eds.), *Handbook of posttraumatic growth* (pp. 3–23). New Jersey: Lawrence Erlbaum Associates Inc.

Carver, C. S. (1998). Resilience and thriving: Issues, models, and linkages. *Journal of Social Issues, 54,* 245–266.

Carver C. S., & Scheier, M. F. (1999). Optimism. In C. R. Snyder (Ed.), *Coping: The psychology of what works* (pp. 182–204). New York: Oxford University Press.

Cattell, R. B. (1966). The scree test for the number of factors. *Multivariate Behavioural Research, 1,* 140–161.

Chan, M. W. C., Ho, S. M. Y., Tedeschi, R. G., & Leung, C. W. L. (2011). The valence of attentional bias and cancer-related rumination in posttraumatic stress and posttraumatic growth among women with breast cancer. *Psycho-Oncology, 20,* 544–552.

Chan, C. S., & Rhodes, J. E. (2013). Religious coping, posttraumatic stress, psychological distress, and posttraumatic growth among female survivors four years after hurricane Katrina. *Journal of Traumatic Stress, 26,* 257–265.

Cobb, A. R., Tedeschi, R. G., Calhoun, L. G., & Cann, A. (2006). Correlates of posttraumatic growth in survivors of intimate partner violence. *Journal of Traumatic Stress, 19,* 895–903.

Cohen, L. H., Hettler, T. R., & Pane, N. (1998). Assessment of posttraumatic growth. In R. G. Tedeschi, C. L. Park, & L. G. Calhoun (Eds.), *Posttraumatic growth: Positive changes in the aftermath of crisis* (pp. 23–42). Mahwah, NJ: Erlbaum.

Collins, R., Taylor, S., & Skohan, L. (1990). A better world or a shattered vision? Changes in perspectives following victimization. *Social Cognition, 8,* 263–285.

Cordova, M. J., Cunningham, L. L. C., Carlson, C. R., & Andrykowski, M. (2001). Posttraumatic growth following breast cancer: A controlled comparison study. *Health Psychology, 20,* 176–185.

Davidson, R. J. (1995). Cerebral asymmetry, emotion, and affective style. In R. J. Davidson & K. Hugdahl (Eds.), *Brain asymmetry* (pp. 361–387). Cambridge, MA: MIT Press.

Davis, C. G., Nolen-Hoeksema, S., & Larson, J. (1998). Making sense of loss and benefiting from the experience: Two construals of meaning. *Journal of Personality and Social Psychology, 75,* 561–574.

de Ridder, D. (2000). Gender, stress and coping: Do women handle stressful situations differently from men? In L. Sherr & J. St. Lawrence (Eds.), *Women, health and the mind* (pp. 115–135). Chichester, UK: Wiley.

Dirksen, S. R. (1995). Search for meaning in long-term cancer survivors. *Journal of Advanced Nursing, 21,* 628–633.

Dohrenwend, B., Neria, Y., Marshall, R., Lewis-Fernandez, R., Turner, J., Turse, N., et al. (2004). Positive tertiary appraisals and posttraumatic stress disorder in U.S. male veterans of the war in Vietnam: The roles of positive affirmation, positive reformulation, and defensive denial. *Journal of Consulting and Clinical Psychology, 72,* 417–433.

Draucker, C. B. (2001). Learning the harsh realities of life: Sexual violence, disillusionment, and meaning. *Health Care for Women International, 22,* 67–84.

Dunmore, E., Clark, D. M., & Ehlers, A. (1999). Cognitive factors involved in the onset and maintenance of posttraumatic stress disorder (PTSD) after physical or sexual assault. *Behaviour Research and Therapy, 37,* 809–829.

Ehlers, A., Boos, A., & Maercker, A. (2000). Predictors of chronic PTSD following political imprisonment: The role of mental defeat, alienation, and perceived permanent change. *Journal of Abnormal Psychology, 109,* 45–55.

Ehlers, A., & Clark, D. M. (2000). A cognitive model of posttraumatic stress disorder. *Behaviour Research and Therapy, 38,* 319–345.

Elder, G., Gimbel, C., & Ivie, R. (1991). Turning points in life: The case of military service and war. *Military Psychology, 3,* 215–231.

Emmons, R. A., Colby, P. M., & Kaiser, H. A. (1998). When losses lead to gains: Personal goals and the recovery of meaning. In P. T. P. Wong & P. S. Fry (Eds.), *The human quest for meaning: A handbook of psychological research and clinical applications* (pp. 163–178). Mahwah, NJ: Lawrence Erlbaum.

Engdahl, B. E., Page, W. F., & Miller, T. W. (1991). Age, education, maltreatment, and social support as predicators of chronic depression in former prisoners of war. *Social Psychiatry and Psychiatric Epidemiology, 26,* 63–67.

Evers, A. W. M., Kraaimaat, F. W., Van Lankveld, W., Jongen, P. J. H., Jacobs, J. W. G., & Bijlsma, J. W. J. (2001). Beyond unfavorable thinking: The illness cognition questionnaire for chronic diseases. *Journal of Consulting and Clinical Psychology, 69,* 1026–1036.

Fallot, R. D. (1997). Spirituality in trauma recovery. In M. Harris & C. Landis (Eds.), *Sexual abuse in the lives of women diagnosed with serious mental illness* (pp. 337–355). Amsterdam, Netherlands: Harwood Academic Publishers.

Fontana, A., & Rosenheck, R. (1998). Psychological benefits and liabilities of traumatic exposure in the war zone. *Journal of Traumatic Stress, 11,* 485–505.

Frazier, P., Conlon, A., & Glaser, T. (2001). Positive and negative life changes following sexual assault. *Journal of Consulting and Clinical Psychology, 69,* 1048–1055.

Frazier, P. A., & Kaler, M. E. (2006). Assessing the validity of self reported stress-related growth. *Journal of Consulting and Clinical Psychology, 74,* 859–869.

Fromm, K., Andrykowski, M. A., & Hunt, J. (1996). Positive and negative psychosocial sequelae of bone marrow transplantation: Implications for Quality of Life assessment. *Journal of Behavioral Medicine, 19,* 221–240.

Gade, P. (1991). Military service and the life-course perspective: A turning point for military personnel research. *Military Psychology, 3,* 187–199.

Garnefski, N., Kraaij, V., & Spinhoven, Ph. (2001). Negative life events, cognitive emotion regulation and depression. *Personality and Individual Differences, 30,* 1311–1327.

Garnefski, N., Kraaij, V., & Spinhoven, Ph. (2002). *Manual for the use of the cognitive emotion regulation questionnaire*. Leiderdorp, The Netherlands: DATEC.

Gregory, J. L., & Prana, H. (2013). Posttraumatic growth in Côte d'Ivoire refugees using the companion recovery model. *Traumatology, 19,* 223–232.

Hall, T. W., Tisdale, T. C., & Brokaw, B. F. (1994). Assessment of religious dimensions in Christian clients: A review of selected instruments for research and clinical use. *Journal of Psychology and Theology, 22,* 395–421.

Helgeson, V. S., Reynolds, K. A., & Tomich, P. L. (2006). A meta-analytic review of benefit finding and growth. *Journal of Consulting and Clinical Psychology, 74,* 797–815.

Hill, P. C., & Pargament, K. I. (2003). Advances in the conceptualization and measurement of spirituality and religion: Implications for physical and mental health research. *American Psychologist, 58,* 64–74.

Ho, S. M. Y., Chan, C. L. W., & Ho, R. T. H. (2004). Posttraumatic growth in Chinese cancer survivors. *Psycho-Oncology, 13,* 377–389.

Hobfoll, S. E., Hall, B. J., Canetti-Nisim, D., Galea, S., Johnson, R. J., & Palmieri, P. A. (2007). Refining our understanding of traumatic growth in the face of terrorism: Moving from meaning cognitions to doing what is meaningful. *Applied Psychology, 56,* 345–366.

Hooper, L. M. (2003). Parentification, resiliency, secure adult attachment style, and differentiation of self as predictors of growth among college students. *Dissertation Abstracts International: Section B: The Sciences and Engineering, 64,* 1493.

Hussain, D., & Bhushan, B. (2009). The development and validation of Refugee Trauma Experience Inventory. *Psychological Trauma: Theory, Research, Practice, and Policy, 1,* 107–117.

Hussain, D., & Bhushan, B. (2011a). Cultural factors promoting coping among Tibetan refugees: a qualitative investigation. *Mental Health, Religion & Culture, 14,* 575–587.

Hussain, D., & Bhushan, B. (2011b). Posttraumatic stress and growth among Tibetan refugees: The mediating role of cognitive-emotional regulation strategies. *Journal of Clinical Psychology, 67,* 720–735.

Hussain, D., & Bhushan, B. (2013). Posttraumatic growth experiences among Tibetan refugees: A qualitative investigation. *Qualitative Research in Psychology, 10,* 204–216.

Jang, L. (2006). The 9–21 earthquake: A study of the effects of Taiwanese cultural factors on resilience. *Dissertation Abstracts International: Section A: Humanities and Social Sciences, 66,* 2723.

Janoff-Bulman, R. (2006). Schema-change perspectives on posttraumatic growth. In L. G. Calhoun & R. G. Tedeschi (Eds.), *Handbook of posttraumatic growth: Research and practice* (pp. 81–99). Mahwah, NJ: Erlbaum.

Johnson, R. J., Hobfoll, S. E., Hall, B. J., Canetti-Nisim, D., Galea, S., & Palmieri, P. A. (2007). Posttraumatic growth: Action and reaction. *Applied Psychology: An International Review, 56,* 428–436.

Joseph, S. (2011). Religiosity and posttraumatic growth: A note concerning the problems of confounding in their measurement and the inclusion of religiosity within the definition of posttraumatic growth. *Mental Health, Religion & Culture, 14,* 843–845.

Joseph, S., & Linley, P. A. (2005). Positive adjustment to threatening events: An organismic valuing theory of growth through adversity. *Review of General Psychology, 9,* 262–280.

Joseph, S., Linley, P. A., Andrews, L., Harris, G., Howle, B., Woodward, C., et al. (2005). Assessing positive and negative changes in the aftermath of adversity: Psychometric evaluation of the Changes in Outlook Questionnaire. *Psychological Assessment, 17,* 70–80.

Joseph, S., Linley, P. A., & Harris, G. J. (2004). Understanding positive change following trauma and adversity: Structural clarification. *Journal of Loss and Trauma, 10,* 83–96.

Joseph, S., & Williams, R. (2005). Understanding posttraumatic stress: Theory, reflections, context and future. *Behavioural and Cognitive Psychotherapy, 33,* 423–441.

Joseph, S., Williams, R., & Yule, W. (1993). Changes in outlook following disaster: The preliminary development of a measure to assess positive and negative responses. *Journal of Traumatic Stress, 6,* 271–279.

Khouzam, H. R. (2000). Religious mediation and it's effect on posttraumatic stress disorder in a Korean War veteran. *Clinical Gerontologist, 22,* 125–131.

Kinsinger, D. P., Penedo, F. J., Antoni, M. H., Dahn, J. R., Lechner, S., & Schneiderman, N. (2006). Psychosocial and sociodemographic correlates of benefit-finding in men treated for localized prostate cancer. *Psycho-Oncology, 15,* 954–961.

Klonoff, H., Clark, C., Horgan, J., Kramer, P., & McDougall, G. (1976). The MMPI profile of prisoners of war. *Journal of Clinical Psychology, 32,* 623–627.

Kobasa, S. C. (1979). Stressful life events, personality and health: An inquiry into hardiness. *Journal of Personality and Social Psychology, 37,* 1–11.

Koenig, H. G., Pargament, K. I., & Nielsen, J. (1998). Religious coping and health status in medically ill hospitalised older adults. *Journal of Nervous and Mental Disease, 186,* 513–521.

Konrad, S. C. (2006). Posttraumatic growth in mothers of children with acquired disabilities. *Journal of Loss and Trauma, 11,* 101–113.

Lauterbach, D., & Vrana, S. (2001). The relationship among personality variables, exposure to traumatic events, and severity of posttraumatic stress symptoms. *Journal of Traumatic Stress, 14,* 29–45.

Lepore, S. J. (2001). A social-cognitive processing model of emotional adjustment to cancer. In A. Baum & B. Andersen (Eds.), *Psychosocial interventions for cancer* (pp. 99–118). Washington, DC: American Psychological Association.

Lev-Wiesel, R., & Amir, M. (2003). Posttraumatic growth among holocaust child survivors. *Journal of Loss & Trauma, 8,* 229–237.

Linley, P. A. (2003). Positive adaptation to trauma: Wisdom as both process and outcome. *Journal of Traumatic Stress, 16,* 601–610.

Linley, P., Joseph, S., & Goodfellow, B. (2008). Positive changes in outlook following trauma and their relationship to subsequent posttraumatic stress, depression, and anxiety. *Journal of Social and Clinical Psychology, 27,* 877–891.

Maercker, A., & Herrle, J. (2003). Long-term effects of the Dresden bombing: Relationships to control beliefs, religious coping, and personal growth. *Journal of Traumatic Stress, 16,* 579–587.

Maercker, A., & Zöllner, T. (2004). The Janus face of posttraumatic growth: Towards a two component model of posttraumatic growth. *Psychological Inquiry, 15,* 41–48.

Maltby, J., & Lewis, C. A. (1996). Measuring intrinsic and extrinsic orientation toward religion: Amendments for its use among religious and non-religious samples. *Personality and Individual Differences, 21,* 937–946.

Mansell, W. (2000). Conscious appraisal and the modification of automatic processes in anxiety. *Behavioural and Cognitive Psychotherapy, 28,* 99–120.

Martin, L. L., & Tesser, A. (1996). Clarifying our thoughts. In R. S. Wyer (Ed.), *Ruminative thought: Vol. 9. Advances in social cognition* (pp. 189–209). Mahwah, NJ: Erlbaum.

McCann, I. L., & Pearlman, L. A. (1990). *Psychological trauma and the adult survivor: Theory, therapy and transformation.* New York: Brunner/Mazel.

McCormick, R. A., Taber, J. I., & Kruedelbach, N. (1989). The relationship between attributional style and posttraumatic stress disorder in addicted patients. *Journal of Traumatic Stress, 2,* 477–487.

McFarland, C., & Alvaro, C. (2000). The impact of motivation on temporal comparisons: Coping with traumatic events by perceiving personal growth. *Journal of Personality and Social Psychology, 79,* 327–343.

McMillen, J. C., & Fisher, R. H. (1998). The perceived benefits scales: Measuring perceived positive life changes after negative events. *Social Work Research, 22,* 173–187.
McMillen, C., Howard, M. O., Nower, L., & Chung, S. (2001). Positive by-products of the struggle with chemical dependency. *Journal of Substance Abuse Treatment, 20,* 69–79.
McMillen, J. C., Smith, E. M., & Fisher, R. H. (1997). Perceived benefit and mental health after three types of disaster. *Journal of Consulting and Clinical Psychology, 65,* 733–739.
McMillen, C., Zuravin, S., & Rideout, G. (1995). Perceived benefits from child sexual abuse. *Journal of Consulting and Clinical Psychology, 63,* 1037–1043.
Milam, J. E. (2004). Posttraumatic growth among HIV/AIDS patients. *Journal of Applied Social Psychology, 34,* 2353–2376.
Milam, J. E., Ritt-Olson, A., Tan, S., Unger, J., & Nezam, E. (2005). The September 11th 2001 attacks and reports of posttraumatic growth among a multiethnic sample of adolescents. *Traumatology, 11,* 233–246.
Mohr, D. C., Dick, L. P., Russo, D., Pinn, J., Boudewyn, A. C., Likosky, W., et al. (1991). The psychosocial impact of multiple sclerosis: Exploring the patient's perspective. *Health Psychology, 18,* 376–382.
Morris, B. A., Shakespeare-Finch, J., Rieck, M., & Newbery, J. (2005). Multidimensional nature of posttraumatic growth in an Australian population. *Journal of Traumatic Stress, 18,* 575–585.
Moussa, M. M., & Bates, G. W. (2011). A preliminary investigation of Lebanese students' strategies for coping with stressful events. *Mental Health, Religion, & Culture, 14,* 489–510.
Naidich, J. B., & Motta, R. W. (2000). PTSD-related symptoms in women with breast cancer. *Journal of Psychotherapy in Independent Practice, 1,* 35–54.
Noguchi, K., Gohm, C. L., & Dalsky, D. J. (2006). Cognitive tendencies of focusing on positive and negative information. *Journal of Research in Personality, 40,* 891–910.
Olff, M., Langeland, W., Draijer, N., & Gersons, B. P. R. (2007). Gender differences in posttraumatic stress disorder. *Psychological Bulletin, 133,* 183–204.
Overcash, W., Calhoun, L. G., Cann, A., & Tedeschi, R. G. (1996). Coping with crises: An examination of the impact of traumatic events on religious beliefs. *Journal of Genetic Psychology, 157,* 455–464.
Palmer, G. A., Graca, J. J., & Occhietti, K. E. (2012). Confirmatory factor analysis of the posttraumatic growth inventory in a veteran sample with posttraumatic stress disorder. *Journal of Loss & Trauma, 17,* 545–556.
Pargament, K. I., Koenig, H. G., & Perez, L. M. (2000). The many methods of religious coping: Development and initial validation of the RCOPE. *Journal of Clinical Psychology, 56,* 519–543.
Pargament, K. I., Smith, B. W., Koenig, H. G., & Perez, L. M. (1998). Patterns of positive and negative religious coping with major life stressors. *Journal for the Scientific Study of Religion, 37,* 710–724.
Park, C. L., Cohen, L. H., & Murch, R. L. (1996). Assessment and prediction of stress-related growth. *Journal of Personality, 64,* 71–105.
Park, C. L., Mills-Baxter, M. A., & Fenster, J. R. (2006). Posttraumatic growth from life's most traumatic event: Influences of elder's current coping and adjustment. *Traumatology, 11,* 297–306.
Peltzer, K. (2000). Trauma symptom correlates of criminal victimization in an urban community sample. *Journal of Psychology in Africa, 10,* 49–62.
Polatinsky, S., & Esprey, Y. (2000). An assessment of gender differences in the perception of benefit resulting from the loss of a child. *Journal of Traumatic Stress, 13,* 709–718.
Poulin, M. J., Silver, R. C., Gil-Rivas, V., Holman, E. A., & McIntosh, D. N. (2009). Finding social benefits after a collective trauma: Perceiving societal changes and well-being following 9/11. *Journal of Traumatic Stress, 22,* 81–90.
Powell, S., Rosner, R., Butollo, W., Tedeschi, R. G., & Calhoun, L. G. (2003). Posttraumatic growth after war: A study with former refugees and displaced people in Sarajevo. *Journal of Clinical Psychology, 59,* 71–83.
Prati, G., & Pietrantoni, L. (2009). Optimism, social support, and coping strategies as factors contributing to posttraumatic growth: A meta-analysis. *Journal of Loss & Trauma, 14,* 364–388.

Rabe, S., Zöllner, T., Maercker, A., & Karl, A. (2006). Neural correlates of posttraumatic growth after severe motor vehicle accidents. *Journal of Consulting and Clinical Psychology, 74,* 880–886.

Ransom, S., Sheldon, K. M., & Jacobsen, P. B. (2008). Actual change and inaccurate recall contribute to posttraumatic growth following radiotherapy. *Journal of Consulting and Clinical Psychology, 76,* 811–819.

Rieker, P. P., Fitzgerald, E. M., Kalish, L. A., et al. (1989). Psychosocial factors, curative therapies, and behavioral outcomes. A comparison of testis cancer survivors and a control group of healthy men. *Cancer, 64,* 2399–2407.

Rotter, J. B. (1966). Generalized expectancies for internal versus external control of reinforcement. *Psychological Monographs, 80,* 1–28.

Rudnick, A. (1997). Psychotherapeutic effects of religion. *Psychosomatics, 38,* 576–578.

Rutter, M. (1985). Resilience in the face of adversity: Protective factors and resistance to psychiatric disorder. *British Journal of Psychiatry, 147,* 598–611.

Saccinto, E., Prati, G., Pietrantoni, L., & Pérez-Testor, C. (2013). Posttraumaticstress symptoms and posttraumatic growth among Italian survivors of emergency situations. *Journal of Loss & Trauma, 18,* 210–226.

Sacks, J. M. (1985). Religious issues in psychotherapy. *Journal of Religion and Health, 24,* 26–30.

Salsman, J., Segerstrom, S., Brechting, E., Carlson, C., & Andrykowski, M. (2009). Posttraumatic growth and PTSD symptomatology among colorectal cancer survivors: A 3-month longitudinal examination of cognitive processing. *Psycho-Oncology, 18,* 30–41.

Schaefer, J. A., & Moos, R. H. (1992). Life crisis and personal growth. In B. N. Carpenter (Ed.), *Personal coping: Theory, research and application* (pp. 149–170). Westport, CT: Praeger.

Schaefer, J., & Moos, R. (1998). The context for posttraumatic growth: Life crises, individual and social resources, and coping. In R. Tedeschi, C. Park, & L. Calhoun (Eds.), *Posttraumatic growth: Positive changes in the aftermath of crisis* (pp. 99–126). Mahwah, NJ: Erlbaum.

Schuster, M. A., Stein, B. D., Jaycox, L. H., Collins, R. L., Marshall, G. N., Elliot, M. N., et al. (2001). A national survey of stress reactions after the September 11th, 2001 terrorist attacks. *New England Journal of Medicine, 345,* 1507–1512.

Schwartzberg, S. S., & Janoff-Bulman, R. (1991). Grief and the search for meaning: Exploring the assumptive worlds of bereaved college students. *Journal of Social and Clinical Psychology, 10,* 270–288.

Sears, S. R., Stanton, A. L., & Danoff-Burg, S. (2003). The yellow brick road and the emerald city: Benefit finding, positive reappraisal coping, and posttraumatic growth in women with early-stage breast cancer. *Health Psychology, 22,* 487–497.

Segerstrom, S. C., Stanton, A. L., Alden, L. E., & Shortridge, B. E. (2003). A multidimensional structure for repetitive thought: what's on your mind, and how, and how much? *Journal of Personality and Social Psychology, 85,* 909–921.

Senter, K. E., & Caldwell, K. (2002). Spirituality and the maintenance of change: A phenomenological study of women who leave abusive relationships. *Contemporary Family Therapy, 24,* 543–564.

Shaw, A., Joseph, S., & Linley, P. A. (2005). Religion, spirituality, and posttraumatic growth: A systematic review. *Mental Health, Religion, & Culture, 8,* 1–11.

Siegel, K., & Schrimshaw, E. W. (2000). Perceiving benefits in adversity: Stress-related growth in women living with HIV/AIDS. *Social Science and Medicine, 51,* 1543–1554.

Siporin, M. (1985). Current social work perspectives on clinical practice. *Clinical Social Work Journal, 13,* 198–217.

Sledge, W. H., Boydstun, J. A., & Rabe, A. J. (1980). Self-concept changes related to war captivity. *Archives of General Psychiatry, 37,* 430–443.

Smith, S. G., & Cook, S. L. (2004). Are reports of posttraumatic growth positively biased? *Journal of Traumatic Stress, 17,* 353–358.

Snape, M. C. (1997). Reactions to a traumatic event: The good, the bad, and the ugly? *Psychology, Health and Medicine, 2,* 237–242.

Solomon, Z., & Dekel, R. (2007). Posttraumatic stress disorder and posttraumatic growth among Israeli ex-POWs. *Journal of Traumatic Stress, 20,* 303–312.

Solomon, Z., Waysman, M., & Neria, Y. (1999). Positive and negative changes in the lives of Israeli former prisoners of war. *Journal of Social and Clinical Psychology, 18,* 419–435.

Stanton, A. L., Bower, J. E., Low C. A. (2006). Posttraumatic growth after cancer. In: L. G. Calhoun, R. G. Tedeschi (Eds.), Handbook of posttraumatic growth: Research and practice. Mahwah, NJ: Erlbaum.

Sutker, P. B., & Allain, A. N. (1996). Assessment of PTSD and other mental disorders in World War II and Korean Conflict POW survivors and combat veterans. *Psychological Assessment, 8,* 18–25.

Taku, K., Calhoun, L. G., Cann, A., & Tedeschi, R. G. (2008). The role of rumination in the coexistence of distress and posttraumatic growth among bereaved Japanese university student. *Death Studies, 32,* 428–444.

Taku, K., Calhoun, L. G., Tedeschi, R. G., Gil-Rivas, V., Kilmer, R. P., & Cann, A. (2007). Examining posttraumatic growth among Japanese university students. *Anxiety Stress and Coping, 20,* 353–367.

Tallman, B. A., Altmaier, E., & Garcia, C. (2007). Finding benefit from cancer. *Journal of Counselling Psychology, 54,* 481–487.

Taylor, S. E. (1983). Adjustment to threatening events: A theory of cognitive adaptation. *American Psychologist, 38,* 1161–1173.

Taylor, S. E., Lichtman, R., & Wood, J. (1984). Attributions, beliefs about control, and adjustment to breast cancer. *Journal of Personality and Social Psychology, 46,* 489–502.

Tedeschi, R. G., & Calhoun, L. G. (1995). *Trauma and transformation: Growing in the aftermath of suffering*. Thousand Oaks, CA: Sage.

Tedeschi, R. G., & Calhoun, L. G. (1996). The posttraumatic growth inventory: Measuring the positive legacy of trauma. *Journal of Traumatic Stress, 9,* 455–471.

Tedeschi, R. G., & Calhoun, L. G. (2004). Posttraumatic growth: Conceptual foundations and empirical evidence. *Psychological Inquiry, 15,* 1–18.

Tedeschi, R. G., Park, C. L., & Calhoun, L. G. (1998). Posttraumatic growth: Conceptual issues. In R. G. Tedeschi, C. L. Park, & L. G. Calhoun (Eds.), *Posttraumatic growth: Positive changes in the aftermath of crisis* (pp. 1–17). Mahwah, NJ: Erlbaum.

Tennant, C. C., Fairley, M., Dent, O. F., Sulway, M. R., & Broe, G. A. (1997). Declining prevalence of psychiatric disorder in older former prisoners of war. *Journal of Nervous and Mental Disease, 185,* 686–689.

Tennen, H., & Affleck, G. (1998). Personality and transformation in the face of adversity. In R. G. Tedeschi, C. L. Park, & L. G. Calhoun (Eds.), *Posttraumatic growth: Positive changes in the aftermath of crisis* (pp. 65–98). Mahwah, NJ: Erlbaum.

Terheggen, M. A., Stroebe, M. S., & Kleber, R. J. (2001). Western conceptualizations and eastern experience: A cross-cultural study of traumatic stress reactions among Tibetan refugees in India. *Journal of Traumatic Stress, 14,* 391–403.

Thombre, A., Sherman, A. C., & Simonton, S. (2010). Posttraumatic growth among cancer patients in India. *Journal of Behavioral Medicine, 33,* 15–23.

Tolin, D. F., & Foa, E. B. (2006). Sex differences in trauma and posttraumatic stress disorder: A quantitative review of 25 years of research. *Psychological Bulletin, 132,* 959–992.

Tomich, P. L., & Helgeson, V. S. (2004). Is finding something good in the bad always good? Benefit finding among women with breast cancer. *Health Psychology, 23,* 16–23.

Treynor, W., Gonzalez, R., & Nolen-Hoeksema, S. (2003). Rumination reconsidered: A psychometric analysis. *Cognitive Therapy and Research, 27,* 247–259.

Ullman, C. (1982). Cognitive and emotional antecedents of religious conversion. *Journal of Personality and Social Psychology, 43,* 183–192.

Updegraff, J. A., Taylor, S. E., Kemeny, M. E., & Wyatt, G. E. (2002). Positive and negative effects of HIV infection in women with low socioeconomic resources. *Personality and Social Psychology Bulletin, 28,* 382–394.

Ursano, R. J., Wheatley, R. D., Sledge, W., Rabe, A., & Carlson, E. (1986). Coping and recovery styles in the Vietnam era prisoner of war. *Journal of Nervous and Mental Disease, 174,* 707–714.

Valent, P. (1999). *Trauma and fulfillment therapy: A wholist framework.* Philadelphia, PA: Brunner/Mazel.

Vishnevsky, T., Cann, A., Calhoun, L. G., Tedeschi, R. G., & Demakis, G. J. (2010). Gender differences in self-reported posttraumatic growth: A meta-analysis. *Psychology of Women Quarterly, 34,* 110–120.

Wasserman, A. L., Thompson, E. I., Wilimas, J. A., & Fairclough, D. L. (1987). The psychological status of survivors of childhood/adolescent Hodgkin's disease. *American Journal of Diseases of Children, 141,* 626–631.

Watkins, E. R. (2008). Constructive and unconstructive repetitive thought. *Psychological Bulletin, 134,* 163–206.

Waysman, M., Schwarzwald, J., & Solomon, Z. (2001). Hardiness: An examination of its relationship with positive and negative long term changes following trauma. *Journal of Traumatic Stress, 14,* 531–548.

Weinrib, A. Z., Rothrock, N. E., Johnsen, E. L., & Lutgendorf, S. K. (2006). The assessment and validity of stress-related growth in a community-based sample. *Journal of Consulting and Clinical Psychology, 74,* 851–858.

Weiss, T. (2002). Posttraumatic growth in women with breast cancer and their husbands: An intersubjective validation study. *Journal of Psychosocial Oncology, 20,* 65–80.

Weiss, T., & Berger, R. (2006). Reliability and validity of a Spanish version of the posttraumatic growth inventory. *Research on Social Work Practice, 16,* 191–199.

Westphal, M., & Bonanno, G. A. (2007). Posttraumatic growth and resilience to trauma: Different sides of the same coin or different coins? *Applied Psychology: An International Review, 56,* 417–427.

Widows, M. R., Jacobsen, P. B., Booth-Jones, M., & Fields, K. K. (2005). Predictors of posttraumatic growth following bone marrow transplantation for cancer. *Health Psychology, 24,* 266–273.

Wilson, A. E., & Ross, M. (2001). The frequency of temporal-self and social comparisons in people's personal appraisals. *Journal of Personality and Social Psychology, 78,* 928–942.

Wink, P., & Dillon, M. (2002). Spiritual development across the adult life course: Findings from a longitudinal study. *Journal of Adult Development, 9,* 79–94.

Wuthnow, R. (1998). *After heaven: Spirituality in America since the 1950s.* Berkeley, CA: University of California Press.

Yalom, I. D., & Lieberman, M. A. (1991). Bereavement and heightened existential awareness. *Psychiatry, 54,* 334–345.

Zöllner, T., & Maercker, A. (2006a). Posttraumatic growth in clinical psychology: A critical review and introduction of a two component model. *Clinical Psychology Review, 26,* 626–653.

Zöllner, T., & Maercker, A. (2006b). Posttraumatic growth and psychotherapy. In L. Calhoun & R. Tedeschi (Eds.), *Handbook of posttraumatic growth: Research and practice* (pp. 334–354). New York: Erlbaum.

Zwick, W. R., & Velicer, W. F. (1986). Comparison of five rules for determining the number of components to retain. *Psychological Bulletin, 99,* 432–442.

Chapter 7
Indigenous Healing Practices in India: Shamanism, Spirit Possession, and Healing Shrines

Shubha Ranganathan

Introduction

One of the most striking features of health and medicine in South Asia and South East Asia is the parallel existence of a range of healing systems from different epistemological traditions. With the publication of Leslie's *Asian Medical Systems* (1976), there has been a proliferation of scholarship on the varieties of medical systems in Asia, including India. The availability and deployment of different mechanisms of illness redressal have been variously referred to by phrases like 'medical syncretism' (Addlakha 2008), 'pluralism of genres' (Sujatha 2007) or 'heterogenous cultural model' (Khare 1996). Much of the literature on medical pluralism has focused on two broad systems of medicine, namely, biomedicine/Western medicine/'cosmopolitan medicine' (Dunn 1976) on the one hand, and 'Indian medicine'/'indigenous medicine'/'traditional medicine' on the other hand.[1] Increasingly, however, the boundaries of these binaries are getting blurred. Indigenous medical practices are not impervious to global market forces and therefore it is not uncommon to see the indigenous being recast in a modern *avatar*, whether in the case of herbal medicine (e.g. Mukharji 2009), unani (e.g. Attewell 2007), or ayurveda (e.g. Bode 2008).

[1]The terms 'Indian' and 'indigenous' continue to be retained despite various difficulties. For instance, while unani and homeopathy fall under the rubric of 'Indian Systems of Medicine', unani actually has Greco-Arabic origins and homeopathy originated in Germany. Further, as Mukharji (2009) has pointed out, the ambiguous phrase 'indigenous drugs' does not recognize the plurality of botanical traditions involved; it could refer to drugs available in India, drugs grown in India, or drugs used in indigenous pharmacopoeias.

S. Ranganathan (✉)
Department of Liberal Arts, Indian Institute of Technology Hyderabad,
Kandi, Sangareddy district 502285, Telangana, India
e-mail: shubha@iith.ac.in

G. Misra (ed.), *Psychosocial Interventions for Health and Well-Being*,
https://doi.org/10.1007/978-81-322-3782-2_7

Indigenous healing practices in India can be broadly classified into two categories. The first includes the alternative systems of medicine which have considerable state support and legal backing. Research on Indian systems of medicine or 'Indian medicine' has largely focused on five main classical medical traditions in India, namely ayurveda, yoga and naturopathy, unani, siddha, and homeopathy that are commonly referred to by the acronym AYUSH. As Dalal (2005) points out, in the post-independence period, there was considerable political support for education, research, and practice in ayurveda and unani. These institutionalized medical traditions have now become relatively professionalized and standardized with their own recognized courses, universities, and degrees. In 2014, a separate Ministry for AYUSH was created by the government of India to further focus on these classical medical traditions (Halliburton 2003).

Apart from the Indian systems of medicine which are drawn from classical traditions, large sections of the population in India also resort to practices referred to as 'faith healing' or 'folk healing'. These range from visits to local healers, shamans and *mantravadis* to worship at religious sites purported to have healing properties. Such a pragmatic and pluralistic approach to healing is particularly marked among sufferers of mental illness. Addlakha (2008) found that there was an 'unproblematic reconciliation of different therapeutic systems' (p. 163) for patients—they simultaneously turned to both medical treatment and healing temples without perceiving any contradiction in this. Carstairs and Kapur (1976) found a similar attitude among traditional healers. In their classic study of culture and mental disorder among three communities in a village in Kota (South Canara district or Dakshina Kannada district, Karnataka), it was revealed that traditional healers too accepted the medical model and regarded medical treatment as complementary to their profession.

Observing this widespread pluralism in practice, a number of scholars such as Dalal (2005), Kapur (1979) and Asuni (1979) have called for integrating traditional healing practices within primary care to meet the health needs of the population. They argue that traditional healers are more attuned to the cultural context and beliefs of patients, as they hail from similar socio-economic and cultural backgrounds as patients. Cultural psychologists such as Kakar (1982) and Nandy (1995) have remarked that in India, psychology is generally consumed by a small population comprising the urban elite. Many psychiatrists have embarked on a movement to Indianize the practice of psychiatry, by using language that is more amenable to patients and that reflects the cultural context of their practice (Addlakha 2010; Sébastia 2007). Thus, the intent in collaboration is for professionals to work with healers and healing shrines to meet the health needs of the population.

This chapter reviews the literature on ritual healing, focusing particularly on studies on healing practices in India. Research on religious healing practices has been done from both anthropological and psychological perspectives. Much of this research has attempted to identify what elements of the healing process are important and what factors constitute the efficacy of healing. In trying to delineate the universal factors and processes in healing, research has focused on various aspects of the healing process, such as the symbolic significance of rituals, the relationship between the healer and the patient, the aesthetic aspects of healing, and the psychosocial dimensions of healing. The following sections review this rich body of literature on ritual healing.

Healing as a Symbolic Practice: Studies on Shamanism and Ritual Healing

Research on 'ritual healing' or 'indigenous healing' has been done from different theoretical persuasions. While some researchers have been interested in the performative aspects of healing, others have focussed on the 'cultural therapeutics' of healing. Still, other researchers have looked at the symbolic and socio-political aspects of healing. This section reviews some of the key research on healing done from different theoretical persuasions.

Psychoanalytic Perspectives: Healing as Psychotherapy

Studies on the therapeutic benefits of rituals have been done by psychoanalysts as well as psychoanalytically minded anthropologists. Anthropologists such as Dow (1986) have described healing as involving the transformation of emotions through the use of symbols from a shared mythic world. Others (Scheff 1979) have focussed on the catharsis of repressed emotions in ritual healing. A number of studies have drawn comparisons between psychotherapy and healing (Frank and Frank 1991; Ward 1989).

One of the first psychoanalytic studies of healing traditions in the Indian context was Kakar's (1982) *Shamans, Mystics, and Doctors*. Kakar (1982) proposed that while psychoanalysis and other Western psychotherapies focussed on the individual self through addressing the 'individual myth', indigenous healing addressed the 'collective myth' by reintegrating the self with the community. He added that Western psychoanalysis emphasized the autonomy of the individual and therapeutic growth through insight and understanding. In contrast, Eastern healing traditions emphasized the importance of faith in and surrender to a higher power.

Psychoanalytically-minded anthropologists have also compared psychotherapy with indigenous healing. Notable here is Lévi-Strauss' (1963) explanation of shamanism and psychoanalysis as essentially involving the manipulation of symbols to resolve conflicts. In both cases, the process of abreaction is central, that is, reliving and working through intense emotions and situations during the healing session. He also emphasized the central role of belief in the healing process. According to him, healing was effected through three factors: 'First, the sorcerer's belief in the effectiveness of his techniques; second, the patient's or victim's belief in the sorcerer's power; and, finally, the faith and expectations of the group, which constantly acts as a sort of gravitational field within which the relationship between sorcerer and bewitched is located and defined' (Lévi-Strauss 1963, p. 168).

Obeyesekere's (1977) study of ritual exorcisms in Sri Lanka also drew attention to the cathartic and dramatic aspects of the exorcism. By allowing the possessed woman to act out, he explained, exorcism worked as a 'standard ritual' that tapped the unconscious of the individual and released his/her inhibitions. The dramatic enactment of the establishment of the authority of god over demon was achieved through the performance of the exorcist and patient.

These studies indicate that most scholars have analysed the therapeutic features of rituals in terms of universal processes and mechanisms. The core features of exorcism or ritual healing are regarded as essentially similar to processes in psychotherapy and psychoanalysis. This assumption of universal processes in healing is also seen in phenomenological explanations of the therapeutic benefits of rituals.

Phenomenological Approaches: Culture, Self and Embodiment

Phenomenological studies of ritual healing have also drawn attention to the cultural therapeutics of the healing process. This is seen in the work of Csordas (1983, 1994, 2004) on Pentecostal and Charismatic Movements as well as Navajo healers. Csordas' approach emphasized the role of culture, self and the body in the healing experience. In *The Sacred Self*, Csordas (1994) relied on the phenomenological framework to emphasize charismatic healing as an experience that is personal, cultural as well as grounded in the experience of the body. While focussing on the experience of the patient in the healing process and the transformation of the self that occurred through healing, his work also highlighted the salience of the sacred in the healing process and the embodied nature of healing.

With regard to the efficacy of healing, Csordas and Lewton (1998) identified four factors as relevant: the disposition of supplicants; individuals' experience of the sacred and variations in their capacities for the sacred; the elaboration of alternatives or possibilities in the healing; and actualization of change through the healing process. Csordas (2004) also held that the patient's hopes, desires, and emotional responses were central to the healing process. Csordas' work is an illustration of the psychological anthropology tradition that seeks to draw linkages between culture and self through the theoretical framework of phenomenology.

Symbolic and Interpretive Approaches: Ritual and Social Relations

Most of the approaches to healing discussed so far have been concerned with making broad generalizations about the therapeutic functions of indigenous healing practices. Symbolic and interpretive approaches have been concerned less with the functions of ritual healing, than with understanding the specifics and dynamics of healing in cultural context. Although this category includes a wide range of approaches, all of them focus on healing as cultural practice or text to be interpreted. Some studies make use of symbolic analyses in understanding possession, while others draw on specific theories from the interpretive traditions of anthropology.

Sax (2004) merged various analytic threads in his study of ritual healing, including performative, interpretive and critical traditions. Although he approached healing rituals as performances, he also emphasized the power dynamics involved in these rituals. In his critical approach to the study of ritual, he pointed out that 'social power is constituted not only by relations of material production, but also by relations of ritual production' (Sax 2004, p. 302). Healing rituals reflect and reproduce unequal relations of power by providing and presenting a certain model of society. Sax's (1991, 2009) studies of Himalayan healing practices also emphasized the centrality of family and social relations in shamanism. In *The God of Justice*, Sax (2009) illuminated the important role of shaman in negotiating family relations through possession.

The depiction of ritual healing as an everyday rather than an exotic practice is also reflected in Flueckiger's (2006) *In Amma's Healing Room* about a Muslim woman healer in Hyderabad. Her work was significant in illuminating the variation and flexibility of discourses and practices around illness and healing. She pointed out that such 'vernacular' practices of Islam, such as healing traditions are characterized by considerable fluidity so as to challenge several conventional notions about gender and Islam in South Asia. These works from interpretive anthropology add to the understanding of deity possession and ritual healing as embedded in everyday life and family relations.

Performative Approaches: Healing as Social Drama

Some researchers have emphasized on the performative and expressive aspects of healing rituals. Lee's (1989) dramaturgical perspective of Malaysian healing ceremonies focussed on the social rules of public healing ceremonies and on the relationship between the performer (spirit medium) and the audience. Following Goffman's (1959) approach, he analysed the spirit séance as an interaction based on three rules of role performance: mood changes, status distance and power display. Similarly, Schieffelin (1985) emphasized the dramaturgical and rhetorical aspects of ritual performances. The spirit medium and audience are involved in a 'dialogic mode of constructing reality' where they co-create a new reality through the performance.

Kapferer's (1979) analysis of demonic exorcism in Sri Lanka brought out the performative, expressive, and transformative aspects of rituals. He emphasized that ritual performances are both representative and transformative. They not only represent a certain definition of reality, but also bring about a shift in mood in patients. Kapferer also used symbolic analyses to describe the emotionally expressive behaviour of the patient as constituting a sign/symbol system. The patient's gestures not only reflect their inner experiences; they also work as signs to confirm and prove for the audience the 'actual' internal emotional state of the patient.

Sensorial Approaches: Healing as Aesthetic Experience

Some interpretive approaches have focussed on the embodied and sensory aspects of healing. This is best exemplified in Stoller's (1995) study of the Hauka movement in Nigeria, in which African mediums are possessed by spirits that mimic European figures. Stoller called for a 'sensuous ethnography' that approaches healing trances as bodily experiences involving all the senses. In his study of Hauka spirit mediums, he drew attention to the sentient body and sensory aspects of healing trances—the textures, smells, sights, sounds and tastes. The embodied experience of trance triggers social and colonial memories, thus drawing connections between bodily practices and cultural memories. Stoller's approach emphasizes shamanism as a set of embodied practices involving the sentient body with its textures, smells, sights, sounds and tastes, and as related to cultural memories and practices.

Still, other studies have emphasized the aesthetic aspects of healing. Desjarlais' (1992) study of spirit-related illness and healing in the Nepal Himalayas brought together the sensory grounds of experiences and the 'aesthetics of experience'. In *Body and Emotion* (1992), Desjarlais elaborated on the sensory and cultural grounds of the phenomenon of soul loss among the Yolmo Sherpa in north-central Nepal. Through a "phenomenology of embodied aesthetics", Desjarlais attempted to show 'how ritual performance is grounded within, and governed by, a wider sphere of value and practice: the aesthetics of the everyday' (1992, p. 65). Desjarlais' analysis described experiences of suffering, illness and healing as both culturally constructed and grounded in sensory experience.

This necessarily brief survey gives a glimpse of the wealth of literature on ritual healing. A range of theoretical persuasions and analytic frameworks have been adopted to explore the significance of indigenous healing practices. Each of the different theoretical frameworks is useful in understanding the different dimensions of healing. At the same time, two broad concerns can be discerned in the literature —a focus on the cultural therapeutics of healing and an interest in the symbolic meanings of ritual healing. Apart from shamanistic healing, many individuals also resort to healing practices in religious sites. The next section considers the literature on healing shrines in India.

Healing as Everyday Practice: Studies on Healing Shrines

Several researchers have focussed on the healing aspects of residing in a shrine that is purported to cure one of illness. Many of these studies have been done from psychiatric and psychological perspectives. In general, the psychiatric and psychological literature have been concerned with the effectiveness of healing shrines in curing mental illness. Addlakha (2008) lists the main issues that psychiatric studies on traditional healing have been concerned with: efficacy of traditional healing; characteristics of healers; and collaboration between healing centres and mental health services in order to provide culture-sensitive mental healthcare.

The Pattern of Illness and Cure in Healing Shrines

Stanley (1988) studied a range of healing sites in the state of Maharashtra (Western India) such as *sufi* dargahs, healing churches, local deity shrines, and temples of the Mahanubhav sect. He observed that despite variations in the specific details, there were certain commonalities in the pattern of illness and cure associated with religious sites of healing. Ghost possession typically began with victims having a vague sense of something ‘not right’ with them. Initially, they started to have headaches, backaches and sudden sharp pains. Later, their problems compounded, they had problems at work and in their relationships. Finally, when the problem became severe, they became depressed, unresponsive and unable to work. At this point, they visited doctors. When they obtained no relief from doctors, they approached the healing centre.

Halder’s (2009) study of the Balaji temple in Mehndipur (in the state of Rajasthan in north India) found that most afflicted people suffered from bodily pains, insomnia, and loss of appetite. They initially sought medical treatment but when this did not cure them, they came to the temple. Similarly, Deliège (2007) found that possession usually started out with physical symptoms, gradually leading to problems in work and other areas as well. The occurrence of trance at the temple functioned as the sure sign of possession. Thus, it appears that the pattern of falling ill, visiting temples and going into trance is common to various forms of possession in different healing contexts.

Trance and Possession in Healing Shrines

One important part of healing rituals is the trance that afflicted individuals go through. In the case of shamanism, it is the healer who undergoes trance and cures the sick person. On the other hand, in the case of ghost afflictions for which people turn to healing shrines, it is the afflicted person who goes into a trance. Trance is the central aspect of the healing process as it is believed to draw out the affliction from the person.

Some studies have elaborated on practices of trance and possession in healing shrines. Kakar's (1982) extensive survey of healing traditions in India also included healing traditions in temples. His exploration of healing in the Balaji temple in Mehndipur (in the state of Rajasthan in north India) analysed exorcism as enabling repressed and hysterical women to act out their unacceptable sexual and aggressive urges without guilt. In line with the psychoanalytic framework, he interpreted women's possession as reflecting their unresolved unconscious sexual desires and conflicts. These conflicts are manifested in their dramatized and exaggerated behaviour during trance. By projecting their feelings of hostility onto an external demon, women could act out their unconscious hostility towards their loved ones. Although his psychoanalytic explanation is useful in drawing attention to unconscious motivational processes in possession, there is little exploration of what women themselves experience as healing in the temple.

Dwyer's (2003) elaboration of the healing process in the Balaji temple drew on the phenomenological approach to explore the transformation of the self in the healing process. He described the exorcism in the temple as a transformative experience that brought about physical and mental change. However, Dwyer also compared the exorcist rituals in the temple with psychotherapy, and here, he moved away from a purely phenomenological approach. Thus, he argued that in both exorcist rituals and psychotherapy, the patient draws on shared concepts and beliefs to de-identify with pathological states of being and re-identify with positive self-conceptions. At the same time, Dwyer's comparison between healing and psychotherapy does not highlight what individuals themselves think about healing, thus conflicting with his own stated interest in the 'cultural construction of illness and cure' in the temple.

Pfleiderer (1988) studied healing in a Sufi shrine in Gujarat, the Mira Datar dargah. She analysed the ritual process as a 'semiotic enterprise' (p. 423) of interpreting various related signs and symbols. She argued that patients and their families attempted to read and interpret the 'texts' involved in possession, which included the signs of possession such as symptoms and dreams. In *The Red Thread*, Pfleiderer (2006) added that women used trance and possession as deliberate and instrumental strategies to deceive men. Pfleiderer's explanation of trance and possession as manipulative strategies used by women to gain advantage not only reduces a complex and multifaceted phenomenon but also fails to elaborate women's own perspective of trance, possession and healing.

The Effectiveness of Healing Shrines

A number of scholars have attempted to explain the therapeutic effectiveness of shrines. Asuni (1979) attributed the effectiveness of traditional healing to the fact that healing takes place in a familiar environment and patients had faith in healers, who came from backgrounds similar to those of patients. Padmavati, Thara and Corin (2005) held that shared cultural explanations and belief systems regarding illness played a central role in the effectiveness of healing. Halliburton (2003) found that the aesthetic aspects of healing, such as living in the soothing, pleasant, and spiritual environment of the healing temples, were crucial in the healing process. Raguram et al. (2002) attributed the effectiveness of healing to the benefits of staying in a supportive and non-threatening environment.

Other researchers have found that healing shrines do not just provide a pacifying environment for ill persons, but may even become places of refuge for those in distress. Skultans' (1987a, b, 1991) research on a Mahanubhav temple in the state of Maharashtra (western India) found that the temple sometimes became a permanent shelter for mentally ill women who did not receive care from the family. Similarly, Davar and Lohokare (2009) found that Sufi dargahs often worked as safe spaces for women during times of vulnerability and crisis.

Comparisons between healing shrines and psychotherapy have also been drawn in several studies. Satija et al. (1982) maintained that traditional healing worked through mechanisms of suggestibility, identification, role-playing and catharsis. Dalal (2011) also drew parallels between folk healing and psychotherapy, emphasizing the role of the sacred and holistic nature of healing, which addressed psychological, social, cultural and spiritual dimensions and involved the entire community in the healing of an individual. He added that the healing process itself used mechanisms of suggestion, symbolism, institutionalized catharsis and corrective emotional experiences to redress the problem at the core psychological level. Thus, Dalal (2011) regarded traditional healing as analogous to a culturally specific form of psychotherapy. Dalal and Misra (2011) have argued powerfully for inclusion of the spiritual component in psychotherapy and health psychology, in order to make modern therapies more effective.

This approach of drawing comparisons between indigenous healing shrines and mental health centres is also seen in Sébastia's (2007, 2009a, b) studies. She regarded the shrine of Saint Anthony of Padua in Puliyampatti (Tuticorin district, Tamil Nadu) as analogous to a 'medical care centre' with 'diagnostic', 'casualty', and 'medical care units' (Sébastia 2007, p. 72). Patients were first taken to a space near the church which she referred to as the 'casualty department', and then moved to a "diagnostic centre", where they drew on the power of Saint Anthony to force the possessing spirits to manifest themselves. Finally, they were taken to the 'medical care unit', namely, the shrine of the Virgin Mary where exorcist practices were carried out to expel the spirits.

While many studies, including some of the ones discussed above, regard shrines through the lens of mental health, Bellamy's (2011) analysis of 'everyday healing' practices seeks to understand shrines in their own context. She found that healing in the Husain Tekri dargah (in the north Indian state of Madhya Pradesh) was characterized by the absence of structured healing rituals. Pilgrims did not passively 'receive' healing from a designated healer but instead crafted their own experience of healing, drawing on other pilgrims' narratives and the stories and legends surrounding the Husain Tekri dargah. Her research is significant for bringing out the importance of understanding healing as an active process of becoming familiar with everyday shrine culture and practices. Her work marks an important shift from the study of healing as ritual process to the analysis of healing as everyday practice.

Healing Shrines as Sites of Mental Health Interventions

The above review illustrates that there is considerable interest in the therapeutic functions of healing shrines. In recent times, there has also been interest in looking at healing shrines as potential sites for the delivery of mental health services. In fact, in some dargahs, like the Mira Datar dargah in Gujarat and the Erwadi dargah in Tamil Nadu, psychiatric clinics have also been opened with the within the Dargah precincts.[2] Observing that large numbers of population prefer to access healing shrines when in distress, the state governments of Gujarat and Tamil Nadu have piloted projects that provide psychiatric consultations and medicine to pilgrims residing within the shrines. These moves, largely stemming from pressure on the state to improve the dismal state of public mental healthcare in the country, are based on a biomedical logic of suffering and healing, where distress is equated with disease and healing is substituted with biomedical cure. Such a reductionist model reframes pilgrims' suffering into a psychiatric problem that can be treated with medicines. Yet, as Bellamy's research illustrates, perhaps the most important aspect of healing shrines is the flexibility of the healing narratives that circulate, thereby allowing for pilgrims to experience healing in unique but shared ways.

Further, mental health interventions within shrines primarily rely on medication as the sole line of treatment for pilgrims. In doing so, they ignore the relevance of the social space of the shrine in the healing process. The above review brings out the differences between shamanistic practices and healing shrines. While shamanism is characterized by a dyadic patient–healer relationship, in healing shrines, the bonds that pilgrims form with the shrine community is significant. Given that pilgrims generally stay within the shrine for extended periods of time, they often develop lifelong associations with the shrine and its community. These social and communal aspects of healing are ignored in the biomedical logic of psychiatric treatment.

---

[2]See Ranganathan (2014) for a more elaborate discussion of these initiatives and the controversies surrounding them.

Conclusion: From *Ritual Healing* to *Everyday Healing*

This chapter has described the literature on indigenous healing within anthropology and psychology. Much of the early work in this area has focussed on the practices of healing cults and indigenous healers and shamans. These studies reflect a fascination with the exotic flavour of rituals and a motivation to unravel the symbols and meanings underlying indigenous healing. Traditionally, anthropology has focused more on deity possession or shamanistic practices. There has been much less attention paid to healing in mundane and everyday contexts.

More recent research in India has concentrated on religious shrines where healing is not limited to specific ritual periods or festivals but is integrated into everyday life and practices. These studies—many of which have been done on Muslim healing shrines—have moved focusing on the place of such healing shrines in contemporary religious practices in India. In moving towards the mundane and the routine, these studies have been a useful departure from the conventional anthropological gaze on the exotic.

Along with a shift in focus from 'ritual healing' to 'everyday healing', the literature also shows a parallel shift from an emphasis on the symbolic significance of rituals to the social space of the shrine. The study of everyday healing practices has provided new ways of understanding healing not only in terms of *what* rituals are carried out, but in terms of *where* these healing practices are conducted. Thus, the social space of the healing shrine emerges as a significant part of the healing process. Much of the traditional concern with questions of efficacy has located efficacy in the symbolic significance of the rituals. More recently, however, there has been renewed interest in locating efficacy in the *place* of healing (e.g. Bellamy 2008). In many cases, individuals develop a lifelong association with the shrine and its community. They form strong links with the 'distress community' (Sébastia 2007: 70) or the 'dargah culture' (Bellamy 2011, p. 7) and often frequently return to the shrine at regular intervals to experience trance. These findings indicate that what is important for sufferers is the continued association with the healing site. It is the overall experience of becoming familiar with the shrine and its community that is perhaps at the heart of healing, rather than the performance of specific 'healing rituals'.

References

Addlakha, R. (2008). *Deconstructing mental illness: An ethnography of psychiatry, women and the family*. New Delhi: Zubaan.

Addlakha, R. (2010). 'Indigenisation' not 'Indianisation' of psychiatry: An anthropological perspective. *Sociological Bulletin, 59*(1), 46–68.

Asuni, T. (1979). The dilemma of traditional healing with special reference to Nigeria. *Social Science and Medicine, 13*(B), 27–31.

Attewell, G. (2007). *Refiguring unani tibb: Plural healing in late colonial India*. Hyderabad: Orient Longman.

Bellamy, C. (2008). Person in place: Possession and power at an Indian Islamic saint shrine. *Journal of Feminist Studies in Religion, 24*(1), 31–44.

Bellamy, C. (2011). *The powerful ephemeral: Everyday healing in an ambiguously Islamic place*. Berkeley: University of California Press.

Bode, M. (2008). *Taking traditional knowledge to the market: The modern image of the ayurvedic and unani industry 1980–2000*. Hyderabad: Orient Longman.

Carstairs, G. M. & Kapur, R. L. (1976). *The great universe of Kota: Stress, change and mental disorder in an Indian village*. London: The Hogarth Press.

Csordas, T. J. (1983). The rhetoric of transformation in ritual healing. *Culture, Medicine and Psychiatry, 7,* 333–375.

Csordas, T. J. (1994). *Embodiment and experience: The existential ground of culture and self*. Cambridge: Cambridge University Press.

Csordas, T. J. (2004). Healing and the human condition: Scenes from the present moment in Navajoland. *Culture, Medicine and Psychiatry, 28,* 1–4.

Csordas, T., & Lewton, E. (1998). Practice, performance and experience in a ritual healing. *Transcultural Psychiatry, 35*(4), 435–512.

Dalal, A. K. (2005). Integrating traditional services within primary health care. *Journal of Health Management, 7*(2), 249–262.

Dalal, A. K. (2011). Folk wisdom and traditional healing practices: Some lessons for modern psychotherapies. In M. Cornelissen, G. Misra, & S. Verma (Eds.), *Foundations of Indian psychology* (pp. 21–35). New Delhi: Pearson.

Dalal, A. K., & Misra, G. (Eds.). (2011). *New directions in health psychology*. New Delhi: Sage.

Davar, B., & Lohokare, M. (2009). Recovering from psychological traumas: the place of Dargahs in Maharashtra. *Economic and Political Weekly, 44*(16), 60–67.

Deliège, R. (2007). Demonic possession in Catholic South India. *Indian Anthropologist, 37*(1), 49–66.

Desjarlais, R. R. (1992). *Body and emotion: The aesthetics of illness and healing in the Nepal Himalayas*. Philadelphia: University of Pennsylvania Press.

Dow, J. (1986). Universal aspects of symbolic healing: A theoretical synthesis. *American Anthropologist, 88,* 56–69.

Dunn, F. L. (1976). Traditional Asian medicine and cosmopolitan medicine as adaptive systems. In C. Leslie (Ed.), *Asian medical systems: A comparative study* (pp. 133–158). Berkeley: University of California Press.

Dwyer, G. (2003). *The divine and the demonic: Supernatural affliction and its treatment in North India*. London: Routledge.

Flueckiger, J. (2006). *In Amma's healing room: Gender and vernacular Islam in south India*. Bloomington, Indiana: Indiana University Press.

Frank, J. D., & Frank, J. B. (1991). *Persuasion and healing: A comparative study of psychotherapy* (3rd ed.). Baltimore: John Hopkins University Press.

Goffman, E. (1959). *The presentation of self in everyday life*. New York: Anchor Books.

Halder, F. (2009). Mythologizing distress: Possession and therapy in Balaji Mehendipur (Rajasthan). In B. Sébastia (Ed.), *Restoring mental health in India: Pluralistic therapies and concepts* (pp. 155–183). New Delhi: Oxford University Press.

Halliburton, M. (2003). The importance of a pleasant process of treatment: Lessons on healing from South India. *Culture, Medicine and Psychiatry, 27,* 161–186.

Kakar, S. (1982). *Shamans, mystics and doctors*. London: Unwin Paperbacks.

Kapferer, B. (1979). Emotion and feeling in Sinhalese healing rites. *Social Analysis, 1,* 153–176.

Kapur, R. L. (1979). The role of traditional healers in health care in rural India. *Social Science and Medicine, 13*(B), 27–31.

Khare, S. R. (1996). Dava, daktar and dua: Anthropology of Practiced Medicine in India. *Social Science and Medicine, 43*(5), 837–848.

Lee, R. L. M. (1989). Self-presentation in Malaysian spirit séances: A dramaturgical perspective on altered states of consciousness in healing ceremonies. In C. A. Ward (Ed.), *Altered states of consciousness and mental health: A cross-cultural perspective* (pp. 251–266). New Delhi: Sage Publications.

Lévi-Strauss, C. (1963). *Structural anthropology*. New York: Basic Books.

Mukharji, P. B. (2009). Pharmacology, 'indigenous knowledge', nationalism: A few words from the epitaph of subaltern science. In B. Pati & M. Harrison (Eds.), *The social history of health and medicine in colonial India* (pp. 195–212). Delhi: Primus Books.

Nandy, A. (1995). *The savage Freud and other essays on possible and retrievable selves*. Princeton, NJ: Princeton University Press.

Obeyesekere, G. (1977). Psychocultural exegesis of a case of spirit possession in Sri Lanka. In V. Crapanzano & V. Garrison (Eds.), *Case studies in spirit possession* (pp. 235–294). New York: Wiley.

Padmavati, R., Thara, R., & Corin, E. (2005). A qualitative study of religious practices by chronic mentally ill and their caregivers in South India. *International Journal of Social Psychiatry, 51* (2), 139–149.

Pfleiderer, B. (1988). The semiotics of ritual healing in a north Indian Muslim shrine. *Social Science and Medicine, 27*(5), 417–424.

Pfleiderer, B. (2006). *The red thread: Healing possession at a Muslim shrine in north India*. Delhi: Aakar Books.

Raguram, R., Venkateswaran, A., Ramakrishna, J., & Weiss, M. G. (2002). Traditional community resources for mental health: A report of temple healing from India. *British Medical Journal, 6* (325), 38–40.

Ranganathan, S. (2014). Healing temples, the anti-superstition discourse and global mental health: Some questions from Mahanubhav temples in India. *South Asia: Journal of South Asian Studies, 37*(4), 625–639.

Satija, D. C., Nathawat, S. S., Singh, D., & Sharma, A. (1982). A study of patients attending Mehandipur Balaji temple: Psychiatric and psychodynamic aspects. *Indian Journal of Psychiatry, 24*(4), 375–379.

Sax, W. (1991). *Mountain goddess: Gender and politics in a Himalayan pilgrimage*. New York: Oxford University Press.

Sax, W. S. (2004). Healing rituals: A critical performative approach. *Anthropology & Medicine, 11* (3), 293–306.

Sax, W. (2009). *The God of justice: Ritual healing and social justice in the central Himalayas*. New York: Oxford University Press.

Scheff, T. J. (1979). *Catharsis in healing, ritual, and drama*. Berkeley: University of California Press.

Schieffelin, E. L. (1985). Performance and the cultural construction of reality. *American Ethnologist, 12*(4), 707–724.

Sébastia, B. (2007). A protective fortress: Psychic disorders and therapy at the Catholic shrine of Puliyampatti (South India). *Indian Anthropologist, 37*(1), 67–92.

Sébastia, B. (2009a). The last resort: Why patients with severe mental disorders go to therapeutic shrines in India. In B. Sébastia (Ed.), *Restoring mental health in India: Pluralistic therapies and concepts* (pp. 184–209). New Delhi: Oxford University Press.

Sébastia, B. (Ed.). (2009b). *Restoring mental health in India: Pluralistic therapies and concepts*. New Delhi: Oxford University Press.

Skultans, V. (1987a). The management of mental illness among Maharashtrian families: A case study of a Mahanubhav healing temple. *Man, 22*(4), 661–679.

Skultans, V. (1987b). Trance and the management of mental illness: Among Maharashtrian families. *Anthropology Today, 3*(1), 2–4.

Skultans, V. (1991). Women and affliction in Maharashtra: A hydraulic model of health and illness. *Culture, Medicine and Psychiatry, 15*, 321–359.

Stanley, J. M. (1988). Gods, ghosts and possession. In E. Zelliot & M. Berntsen (Eds.), *The experience of Hinduism: Essays on religion in Maharashtra* (pp. 26–59). Albany: State University of New York Press.

Stoller, P. (1995). *Embodying colonial memories: Spirit possession, power, and the Hauka in West Africa*. New York: Routledge.

Sujatha, V. (2007). Pluralism in Indian medicine: Medical lore as a genre in medical knowledge. *Contributions to Indian Sociology(new series) 41*(2), 169–202.

Ward, C. A. (Ed.). (1989). *Altered states of consciousness and mental health: A cross-cultural perspective*. New Delhi: Sage Publications.

Part II
Interventions Across the Life Span

Chapter 8
Childcare in the Indigenous Health Systems in India from the Perspectives of Developmental and Health Psychology

Malavika Kapur

Concept of Health in the Indigenous Medical Systems

The social context of health and healing is deeply embedded in the indigenous medical systems. The four indigenous systems practised in India and South East Asia are ayurveda, unani, siddha and tibetan medicine. Surprisingly, the core constructs in the four systems are the same, while the language in which they are documented and the practices that emerged according to the geographic regions and diverse cultural influences make them different. The core constructs are based on body and mind unity, man being a part of the universe. The five prime elements are *prithvi* (earth), *Ap* (water), *tejas* (fire), *vayu* (wind) and *akasha* (sky), which is also termed as ether/air. These are prevalent in the unani, siddha and tibetan medicine as well. The three humours too are common, namely, *vata, pitta* and *kapha.* The exception is unani where there are four elements and four humours.

In unani, akasha (sky) is not included. The humours are four in number. Vayu and phlegm remain while pitta (bile) is spilt into black and yellow bile. The *Tridosha* are vata, pitta and kapha are the physical triad or *prakrithi* and the *Triguna* are their psychological counterparts. These are *satva, rajas* and *tamas.* In the unani system, there are eight temperaments. The siddha system is more or less similar to ayurveda with regard to the elements, tridosha and triguna (Mishra 2001; Rahaman 2001; Subbarayappa 2001).

The content is drawn from *Psychological Perspectives on Childcare in Indian. Indigenous Health Systems* (Kapur, M., Springer July 2015).

Kapur and Mukundan (2003)

M. Kapur (✉)
National Institute of Advanced Studies, Indian Institute of Science Campus,
Bangalore 560012, India
e-mail: malavikakapu@ryahoo.co.in

G. Misra (ed.), *Psychosocial Interventions for Health and Well-Being*,
https://doi.org/10.1007/978-81-322-3782-2_8

All the systems follow a holistic approach of correcting the imbalances in the body. The indigenous health practices based on the key constructs in *Charaka Samhita*. In the Tibetan medicine, the same constructs as described in the *Astanga Hridaya* are adopted. However, one finds some differences in the actual treatment methods depending on the regions and the cultures they are rooted in. Being anchored to the social context that these concepts predate modern health psychology by several centuries.

It is in the childcare components of the indigenous systems that one finds marked differences. These appeared to have been due to the melding of folk and medical healing practices. It is in the childcare in the four systems that one finds the component of developmental psychology. The child healthcare practices of the four systems offer fascinating insights. For example in ayurveda, the emphasis in childcare is on the seamless blending of *samskaras* (rites of passage) through healthy practices. In the unani system, the focus is on how to take physical care of children, infants and maternal care. In the siddha system early child development is analysed in detail (Krishnamurthy 1983; Thottam 1983). The developmental phases are termed *paruvams* and these are poetic descriptions of babbling, taking the first steps, viewing the moon with the mother and the mother's communication with the moon on behalf of the child. The paruvams are linked with disorders typical at each stage (Table 8.1).

This merging of developmental stages with disorders is the earliest documented record of developmental psychology and health psychology is uniquely a contribution of siddha medicine. In the Tibetan system, despite the saliency of the original *Bon* religion of Tibet, Buddhist philosophy and Indian ayurveda are effectively combined in Tibetan medicine. The rituals are mostly protective, warding off rituals, referring to the evil spirits of Bon and Indian folk lores. The Hindu deities, demons, *grahas* in particular and the high Lamas and the Buddha offer protection. The childcare systems highlight the importance of the social contexts. Embryology or foetal development is a significant contribution to Tibetan medicine, Buddhist philosophy and Tibetan astrology.

Table 8.1 Developmental phases in the siddha system

Development according to age	Disorders
Kappu Paruvam: Birth to three months	*Grandhi* (two types: black and red)
Mutha Paruvam: Third month to first year	*Thodam*
Thala Paruvam *Sappani Paruvam* *Varugai Paruvam*	*Mandham* and *Karappam*
Third to seventh year	*Ganam* and *Akkaram*
From early infancy to late childhood develop either by themselves or with other diseases	*Suram, Sanni, Kazhical* and *Valippu*

Health Psychology

There are three emerging trends in Western psychology that try to adopt a holistic approach to health and disease. These are positive psychology, developmental psychology and health psychology.

The first theme is positive psychology, a relatively new concept in Western psychology emerging within humanistic psychology through the works of Maslow, Rogers and Fromm. Seligman and Csiszentmihalyi (2000) gave shape to it focusing on four aspects—positive experiences, enduring psychological traits, positive relationships and positive institutions.

However, it needs to be highlighted that ayurveda and other indigenous medical systems place equal emphasis on good health—both mental and physical—while dealing pathology. The Tridosa triad deals with constitutional physical traits. The concept of Triguna deals with constitutionally endowed psychological traits. Of the three *gunas,* the predominance of *rajasik* and *tamasik* denotes psychopathology, while *satvic* represents well-being, a desirable trait. One may be born with this trait. Yet it is not a deterministic notion. It can be cultivated by good lifestyle, diet, good company, etc. Satva renders a person invulnerable to stress and promote resilience (Kapur 2013).

The second theme is developmental psychology. It is relevant in contemporary context to examine childcare practices in ancient India from the perspective of health psychology. In the present chapter, the author proposes to examine childcare practices in ancient India as described in the ancient medical system of ayurveda which deals with health and disease. The paediatric branch of ayurveda is Kaumarabhratya. The works of Charaka, Sushruta and the Vaghbatas, the elder, and the younger, formed the basis for sound clinical practice. The compilations or the Samhitas date back to 1500 in second BC and William Harvey in 1628 had appreciated the holistic approach to health (Kazdin 2000). However, over the years in the West the Cartesian dualism gained a stronghold on the medical practices. In India, the ayurvedic approach has always been holistic and continues to remain so. Two perspectives are at the core of health psychology, accordingly, childcare is examined from two angles—whether it is developmental or holistic.

Developmental psychology is crucial to our understanding of human beings and the basis of child development. It highlights the developmental phases since infancy, the interactions at the bio-psycho-social and cultural stages, as well as the continuities and discontinuities in development. The observations are reinforced by naturalistic observations and empirical studies on infant and children and less on theoretical speculation as in the case of psychology of adults.

The third theme and the most relevant to this chapter is health psychology. It emerged in 1978 as pioneered by Logan Wright (Kazdin 2001), highlighting the importance of bio-psycho-social interactions. Western medicine is borrowed from the Cartesian dualism of the body and the mind. Health psychology in contrast deals with relationship between behavioural, cognitive, psychophysiology, social and environmental factors in establishment, maintenance and detriment of health.

In childhood and adolescence, health psychology was termed as paediatric psychology by Logan Wright in 1967 (Kazdin 2001). It is an interdisciplinary field addressing the interaction of physical, behavioural and emotional development in health and illness issues affecting children, adolescents and the families, within the larger field of health psychology. The focus is not only on children and adolescents but also on the contexts of the child within the family, the school and the medical settings. The emphasis is on the normative development of adaptation to stress resulting from physical conditions, medical treatment and psychosocial interactions with the family, the peers rather than the psychopathological view of children in adjustment and disease.

Three groups of conditions have received attention from the perspective of health psychology.

(i) Interventions for enuresis, encopresis, vomiting, food refusal, chronic abdominal pain, failure to thrive, anorexia and attention deficit disorders.
(ii) Appreciation of psychological principles to understand and intervene with behavioural and psychological constraints of disease, disabilities and medical procedures.
(iii) The focus is on healthy development in conditions such as cancer, AIDS, diabetes and asthma.

The strength of health psychology lies in its holistic approach and the emphasis is on empirical validation.

The domains of development described as discrete chapters in the Western books on child development is an artefact. The physical, intellectual, language, emotional, social, moral and sexual development occurs simultaneously. These are dynamic, interacting and interwoven systems.

Studying children through their developmental phases gives insights to the study of adults. In the Ayurveda, an example of study of temperament is a case in point (Kapur et al. 1997). Triguna is present at birth and gets modified as one grows into an adult. In the study of personality in adults, there are separate tests for children and adults instead of seeing the obvious continuities/discontinuities in the developmental context.

It is of relevance in the contemporary context to examine childcare practices in ancient India from the perspective of health psychology. In the present chapter the author proposes to examine childcare practices in ancient India as described in ancient medical systems that deal with health and disease. However, over the years, as in the West, the Cartesian dualism gained a stronghold on the current medical practices even in India. The Indian indigenous approaches have always been holistic and continue to remain so. These are recognized as medical systems which are embedded in the cultural ethos of the country even today. Childcare in ancient India will be examined from two angles i.e., whether it is **developmental and holistic** in perspective, as these two are at the core of Health Psychology.

Eight Emerging Themes from Childcare in Four Indigenous Health Systems

The four systems of childcare have some common themes amongst them. These are considered essential for the development and care of children. These strongly support the notion that biological, psychological, social and cultural contexts are important for the development of children and caretaking styles are equally essential for the healthy overall development of the child. The themes are as follows:

Qualities of the Physician

In the four systems, the physician's characteristics are of great importance and have been dealt extensively, in terms of training, professional competence, ideal characteristics, spirituality, compassion and many others. In ayurveda, there are four pillars of treatment, namely, the patient, the attendant, the medicine and the physician; and the physician is one amongst the four. The physician's characteristic is hardly mentioned as a key variable even in health psychology.

Care of the Expectant and the Nursing Mother

In ayurvedic texts, the care of the baby begins even before conception. Prospective parents are instructed about the right diet, rituals, prescribed behaviour and psychological attitudes along with prescriptive sexual practices conducive for the birth of healthy infant. The Hindu rite of *Garbhadharana* is described with a complex set of instructions. Gender preference for the male offspring is indicated in a general set of instructions and a specific rite named *pumsavana* is conducted in the third or fourth month of pregnancy. *Jatakarma* is a rite involving medical, psychological and cultural practices associated with birth. The instructions specified for cleaning and feeding the baby and other neonatal care practices are similar to paediatric advice given by medical practitioners. As the new born is exhausted from the birth trauma the anointment of *bala* oil is recommended.

The Mother and the Child as a Symbiotic Unit

The physical and psychological care of the mother and infant are carried out under the assumption that the two form a symbiotic unit. There are a number of do's and don'ts for the expectant and the nursing mother. These range from right diet, sleep, psychological states, behaviour and social interactions. The expectant and the nursing mother are warned about dire outcomes on the physical and the psychological status of the infant if these strictures are disobeyed. An interesting aspect of these ayurvedic texts is the detailed description of the characteristics (physical and psychological) of the mother or the wet nurse (as it was a common practice to hire a wet nurse if mother is not available to breast feed). There are extensive descriptions of different types of breast milk, healthy or otherwise. The above kind of descriptions are absent in current paediatric practice. Currently, there has been empirical evidence to support that exposure of the mother to pollution, drugs, alcohol and nicotine cause adverse effects on the child. The relationship between the quality and quantity of milk and the health of the infant and the mother needs to be examined empirically.

Evolution of the Mind

According to Charaka in the third month of pregnancy, the formation of the head takes place along with the perception of pleasure and pain. Consciousness emerges in the fourth month. It is believed that the foetus is endowed with a mind (*manas*) and wakes up from sleep or subconscious state in the fifth month. The dawn of cognition occurs in the sixth month. The eighth month is considered critical as the total energy (*ojas*) is in a flux for both the mother and the child which causes oscillation between joy and sorrow. The speculation that the foetus has emotions, intelligence and consciousness predates a very contemporary notion of the development of the brain. Currently, it has been discovered by developmental psychologists (Gopnik et al. 2001) that the infant arrives into the world prewired to acquire cognitive and language skills and a temperament underlying emotional predisposition. However, even a few decades back the infant's brain was characterized by 'booming buzzing confusion' according to William James. The development of various faculties may not be scientifically valid but Charaka's assumption that these occurred in foetal stage is indeed remarkable.

The above three sections highlight the interaction between the physical, psychological and environmental and cultural factors in the context of the infant–mother relationship and the impact it has on the development of the infant in health or disease. This indicates that the perspective indeed was developmental and holistic.

Inheritance of Physical and Psychological Predispositions

The concepts of Tridosha and Triguna are central to the ayurvedic practice. These are the physical and psychological predispositions, which are present at birth and even beyond it. The Tridoshas consist of vata, pitta and kapha and are physical predispositions. Of the Trigunas, the rajas and tamas are the psychological traits which contribute to illness while satva is a predisposition to well-being. An individual is seen as a product of various inherited components—*gunas and doshas*. These are the endogenous factors but they interact with various physical and psychological factors in the environment. The ayurvedic system upholds the notion that drugs and other treatments interact differently amongst people with different doshas and gunas. The diseases are caused by varying combination of doshas and gunas, hence the treatment too needs to be varied accordingly. In contemporary medical practice, apart from body weight and age, other individual differences are seen only as side-effects. There is a need to empirically examine individual differences to the responses to treatments according to predispositions as understood by gunas and doshas.

The concepts of Triguna and Tridosha apply equally to children. The interaction or 'match' or 'mismatch' between the mother's and infant's Triguna and Tridosha is recognized as important by the ancient physicians. Once again, the holistic approach is central and the bio-psycho-social interactions are embedded in the constructs of Triguna and Tridosha.

Promotion of Physical and Psychological Health (Samskaras)

The samskaras or rites of passage are cultural practices which promote the achievement of development tasks. While the gunas and doshas reflect on inherited predispositions, samskaras are socially sanctioned rituals carried out at the developmentally appropriate stages. Gunas and doshas represent the nature and samskaras nurture components.

There are 16 samskaras in the life span of an individual; 10 samskaras belong to childhood. The first three—Garvadharana, Pumsavana and *Simanatonnayana*—are carried out before birth. These rituals are essentially related to prospective parents and conducted before the birth of the infant. The remaining seven childhood samskaras are milestones the development of the child (Kumar, p. 91) (Table 8.2).

The above samskaras are socially sanctioned and have medical, psychological and sociocultural significance. These are instituted in a time sequence for the optimal physical and psychological development in each of the developmental phases in the life cycle of a child. While Garvadharana and Pumsavana are steeped in myths, the social connotation is that a healthy child especially a male child is most desired. Simantonnayana is a ritual which gives a special status to the woman who bears the foetus successfully till the risks of abortion or miscarriage has receded, at the seventh month of pregnancy. The rituals aim at protecting her, keeping her safe and happy in order to promote the healthy development of the foetus. This is a special time in the life cycle when the woman is offered the special care and comfort of the maternal home following the ceremony. The ritual highlights the need to promote emotional stability in the expectant mother for the

Table 8.2 Childhood samskaras in Ayurveda (Kumar 1999)

S. No.	Samskara	Period	Assessment
1	*Jatakarma* (birth)	After birth	Rooting and sucking reflex
2	*Namakarana* (naming)	10th day or 12th day or 100th day	Appropriate period for general examination of infants
3	*Niskramana* (outing)	4th Month	(a) Macular fixation and papillary adjustment (b) Reaction to sound (c) Head control
4	*Annaprasana* (feeding cereals)	6th month 10th month	(a) Appearance of first tooth (b) Functioning of digestive system (c) Proper time for weaning
5	*Chudakarana* (tonsure)	1–3 years	Examination and care of anterior fontanelle
6	*Karnavedhana* (ear piercing)	6–8 months	A type of active immunization (*Yukti Krtabala*) initiated with external trauma
7	*Upanayana* (thread ceremony)	6–8 years	(a) Fit for education (b)Assessment of intellect

healthy development of the child. This perhaps needs to be examined empirically in contemporary context.

The seven samskaras after the birth of the infant as seen in Table 8.2, have specific significance to the life stages of the infant. Each of these could be examined empirically from medical, psychological (cognitive, memory, emotional, social development) or sociocultural or anthropological perspective. The samskaras vary according to age, gender and caste, representing the very essence of contemporary developmental approach.

Minor and Major Disorders of Childhood

The disorders of childhood are commonly divided into two categories: minor and major disorders *(balagraha roga)*. Health or disease is a product of inherited physical and psychological predispositions (Tridosha and Triguna), age, gender, caste, diet, lifestyle, season and drugs along with the influence of *grahas* (supernatural elements).

The minor disorders are described with great attention. *Kashyapa Samhita* (Tewari 2002) mentions 46 disorders including headache, ear ache, eye disorders, drooling, pain in the throat, breathing problems, abdominal pain, constipation, and so on. The clinical descriptions are accurate, while the classifications are haphazard. Aetiological explanations are generally multi-factorial, so are the treatments. The treatment ranges from dietary and lifestyle changes to herbal and other remedies.

The pharmacopeia is extensive and calibrated to suit the child's age and the predispositions (Trigunas and Tridoshas).

Serious disorders in childhood, like facial palsy, Koh's abdomen, polio, encephalitis, dehydration, vitamin deficiency, skin disorders and epilepsy, are however, attributed to supernatural forces in addition to the other causes mentioned earlier. These disorders call for the propitiation of grahas who 'seize' the child and cause the diseases (Kumar 1999).

Ayurveda emphasizes on prevention of ailments and promotion of healthy habits. Amongst children, the traditional practice of light oil massage of the baby's body and bathing it has well-established health benefits. Diet appropriate for weaning, the importance of play in childhood are some examples of the promotion of development in children.

To sum up, in ayurveda, treatment and prevention received equal importance in health and disease and the approach is developmental and multifactorial. In the prevention of serious disorders (graha or balagraha) suggestions also abound in the physical and psychological care of the infant such as not to frighten the child, safe places for laying the baby and physical protection of the baby. Once the child is 'seized' by the grahas, in addition to other treatments, magical treatments are called for. The important notion is that of indivisibility of body and mind, the man and the universe. These concepts pre-date the core concepts of health psychology by several centuries. To sum up, child healthcare in ancient India emerged out of the social contexts of the time, and seamlessly blended with social and religious rituals, leading to an ideal way of childcare and healing with safe plant medicines.

Scientific Methodology and the Indigenous Health Practices

Having examined childcare practices in ancient India from the perspective of health psychology, one finds a major lacuna. Relying on *Nyaya* methodology, empirical validation includes:

(i) *Prathyaksha* (seen with one's own eyes)
(ii) *Anumana* (inference)
(iii) *Shabda* (oral knowledge based on experience of sages)
(iv) *Yukti* (experimentation)

Health psychology demands that the interventions or the constructs in order to be accepted need to be empirically validated using only western scientific methodology. Perhaps there needs to be a paradigm shift in health psychology to empirically examine holistic approaches using both quantitative and qualitative methods. Western scientific methodology holds prediction or prognosis as crucial based on scientific evidence. In contrast, in the indigenous health systems these appear somewhat vague and far fetched and are not examined thoroughly.

The construct of temperament in ancient Indian thought was examined empirically by Kapur et al. (1997) on the basis of Trigunas from the Sankhya tradition. The temperamental profile from 17 items was used to provide a theoretical model based on the ancient Indian thought of satva, rajas and tamas, and this construct was validated empirically with a study of normal and disturbed children. Experience of the author and her colleagues revealed that the Western models of temperament as per Thomas and Chess model was difficult for Indian mothers to understand. For the sake of scientific parsimony, Western workers have used narrow band of traits. While the Western models include only biological disposition, the dimensions measured in the Triguna models are: manageability, trust, dependence, sleep, appetite, activity level, morality, emotionality, sociability and aggression. These dimensions go beyond the Western conceptualization of temperament. The study demonstrates that some of the major constructs proposed in ancient Indian literature lend themselves to empirical enquiry as seen below.

The sample consisted of 50 normal nursery school children screened for behaviour problems and handicaps and 30 children with psychiatric disturbance in the age range of four to six years. Both groups were administered the temperament section of Developmental Psychopathology Check List (DPCL) by Kapur (2012). The checklist was orally administered to the mothers who had to say whether the child 'mostly', 'somewhat' or 'not at all' exhibited the particular item of the behaviour. The results showed that 26 of 50 of the normal preschoolers had satvik (good natured and well adjusted) temperament, 14 were predominantly rajasik (high-strung/active), five were tamasik (torpid/dull), and the rest five had no predominance of any particular predisposition. The clinic population of 30 children had three sub groups: one with emotion/learning disorders, one with hyperkinesis/conduct disorders and one with autistic disorders. The three groups, despite the small size of the sub samples, showed distinct profiles. The autistic group had the highest degree of disturbance, with hyperkinesis/conduct disorder in the middle, and the learning/emotion group showing the least degree of disturbance. The groups did not differ on the dimensions of sleep and appetite. The group with emotion/learning disorder had high sociability in the family context and low verbal aggression. Activity level and physical aggression was high in the conduct disorder group. Comparison of the 50 normal and 30 disturbed children revealed that normal group was easily manageable, dependable and trustworthy while the disordered group had higher activity level, emotionality (angry/irritable than cheerful/happy) and sensitivity only towards the self.

Differentiating normal temperament from those typical of psychiatric disorders is of crucial importance not only to the assessment but also to the management. The findings of the present study however need to be examined in larger samples, across time (stability), age, gender, disorder and cultural contexts. The present assessment tool may be used for such studies. The relationship between temperamental traits and psychopathological conditions needs to be examined. Questions whether certain temperamental traits predispose a child to a specific disorder, whether the temperament is an early manifestation of a full-blown disorder at a later date, whether temperament and psychopathology share a common root, remain unanswered. Yet another question is whether satvik temperament is a protective factor against psychopathology as claimed in ayurveda. The above empirical study of temperament based on the Triguna model holds promise for research in the Indian context, not only in the study of psychopathology but possibly to study temperament as a mediating factor in the interaction between child rearing practices and psychosocial development. The holistic models developed in childcare can be adopted for adults and evaluated empirically through ancient Indian constructs to study positive psychology.

Holistic Approach to Phenomenology, Aetiology and Treatment

Some of the key themes of childcare in the indigenous systems are care of the mother and the child as a symbiotic unit, salience of breast milk, rites of passage, childcare systems, scientific methodology and attempts at prognosis or predictions. These themes reveal the extent to which the healing practices are anchored holistic practices.

Multiple causation at the bio-psycho-social level offers a contrast to the scientific parsimony of Western science. However, the study of complex systems has been attempted in the 'general systems theory' and in 'health psychology' and 'chaos' theory. It does not necessarily mean that what cannot be broken into smaller units, cannot be studied. Whatever has been found effective, needs to be studied using appropriate and innovative methods. For example, psychoanalysis has not lent itself for empirical validation but has provided insights of great merit in clinical practice. If one holds what is useful and effective, it is necessary to understand it and study the phenomenology. Perhaps there is a need to develop suitable methodologies along the lines of that employed in examining the 'chaos' theory. These methods should be based on nonlinear theories.

The ancient Indian healthcare systems especially childcare when examined from the perspective of health psychology offer some deep insights. The childcare practices in ancient India predate the core concepts in developmental and health psychology by centuries. However, the major lacuna has been the lack of empirical validation. Such validation is needed to guide us to preferred health practices. Contemporary health psychology could benefit a great deal if it were to introduce the physician characteristics into the equation of effective intervention strategies. There are several possibilities for empirical research in the indigenous systems that may introduce new insights into psychology in general and health psychology in particular.

References

Gopnik, A., Meltzoff, A. N., & Kuhl, P. K. (2001). *The scientist in the crib*. New York: Harper Collins Perennial Edition.

Kapur, M., Hirisave, U., Reddy, M. V., Barnabas. J. P., & Singhal, D. (1997). Study of infant temperament. An Indian perspective. *Indian Journal of Clinical Psychology, 2a*(2), 171–177.

Kapur, M., & Mukundan, H. (2003). *Childcare in Ancient India from the perspective of developmental psychology and pediatrics*. Delhi: Sri Satguru Publications, Indian Book Centre.

Kapur, M. (2012). Health psychology and childcare in ancient India. *Indian Journal of Psychology* (Special Issue), 17–22.

Kapur, M. (2013). Resilience and competence in childhood. In G. Misra (Ed.), *Psychology and psychoanalysis* (pp. 255–298).Vol. XIII Part 3 of History of social science, philosophy and culture in Indian civilization. Gen. Ed. D.P. Chattopadhyaya, New Delhi.

Kazdin, A. E. (Ed.). (2000). Health psychology. In *Encyclopedia of psychology* (Vol. A). New York: Oxford University Press.

Kazdin, A. E. (Ed.). (2001). Pediatric psychology. In *Encyclopedia of psychology* (Vol. 6). New York: Oxford University Press.

Krishnamurthy, J. R. (1983). Paediatrics. In *Siddha medicine* (pp. 382–384). In S. V. Subramanian & V. R. Madhavan (Eds.), *Heritage of the Tamils: Siddha Medicine*. Madras: International Institute of Family.

Kumar A. (1999). *Child health care in Ancient India*. Delhi: Sri Satguru Publications, Indian Medical Sciences Series, Indian Book Centre.

Mishra, S. K. (2001). Ayurveda, unani and siddha systems: An overview and their present status. In *Medicine and life sciences in India* (Vol. IV, Part II, Chap. 15, pp. 479–516). New Delhi. PHISPC Series.

Rahaman, S. Z. (2001). Unani medicine in India. Its origin and fundamental concepts. In B. V. Subbarayappa (Ed.), *Medicine and life sciences in India* (Vol. IV, Part 2, Chap. 10, pp. 292–325).

Seligman, M. E. P., & Csiszentmihalyi, M. (2000). Positive psychology—An introduction. *American Psychologist, 55*(1), 5–14.

Subbarayappa, B. V. (2001). Siddha medicine. In *Medicine and life sciences in India* (Vol. IV, Part II, Chap. 15, pp. 482–451). New Delhi. PHISPC Series.

Tewari, P. V. (2002). Kashyapa Samhita or Vraddhajivikiya Tantra, Varanasi Chaukhambha.

Thottam, B. P. (1983). Childcare and siddha medicine. In S. V. Subramanian & V. R. Madhavan (Eds.), *Heritage of the tamils: Siddha medicine*. Madras: International Institute of Family.

Chapter 9
Lifestyle Intervention at School: A Review of Effectiveness, Barriers, Facilitators, and Strategies

Arun Pratap Singh

Introduction

In contemporary society, proliferation in the number of choices is making adolescent health and well-being increasingly vulnerable. While involvement in risk behaviours (i.e., smoking, drug abuse, violence, unsafe sexual behaviours etc.), sedentary leisure, fast food consumption is increasing, the intake of fruits and vegetables, involvement in physical activity, participation in sports and games is steadily decreasing amongst youngsters (Sidoti et al. 2010; Singh and Misra 2012). According to an updated data on global adolescent health risks by WHO (2014), fewer than one in every four adolescents meet the recommended guidelines for physical activity, i.e., 60 min of moderate to vigorous physical activity daily. An estimated 180 adolescents die each day due to interpersonal violence and one in 10 younger adolescents use tobacco. An estimated 1.3 million premature but preventable mortality is related with a cluster of lifestyle behaviours (i.e., smoking, alcohol, physical activity, inappropriate diet, interpersonal violence, etc.) initiated at a young age (WHO 2014). Prevalence of obesity among Indian adolescents has increased from 9.9 in 2001 to 19.9 in 2012; higher in both boys (3–15.1%) and girls (5.3–13.3%) indicating the early onset of obesity (Sunitha and Gururaj 2014). Increase in irregular sleep may have linkages with relational problems, difficulties in school learning, low academic performance, suicidal ideation, anxiety and mood disorders (Singh 2013). Earlier participation in sexual intercourse may place adolescents at higher risks for a variety of undesirable physiological outcomes, including unintended pregnancy, sexually transmitted diseases, and HIV/AIDS, obstetric fistulae and psychosocial effects, leading to problem behaviour and substance use, and poor school performance (Sunitha and Gururaj 2014). Substance

A. P. Singh (✉)
Department of Psychology, Mahatma Gandhi Antarrashtriya Hindi Viswavidyalaya, Wardha 442005, India
e-mail: jyotiarun13@gmail.com

G. Misra (ed.), *Psychosocial Interventions for Health and Well-Being*,
https://doi.org/10.1007/978-81-322-3782-2_9

abuse may lead to several health complications short term (i.e., respiratory tract infections, decline in physical fitness, low psychological well-being, depressive symptoms etc.) and long term (i.e., increased risk of Coronary Heart Diseases or CHD, cancers of lung, larynx, oesophagus, mouth, bladder and cervix, stroke) in adulthood (Dalal and Misra 2006).

However, despite several assertions, prioritization by governments and arguments for its need in younger age, and establishment of many unhealthy lifestyle habits, multiple chronic concerns and conditions in adulthood (Thirlaway and Upton 2009), LSI has been less attempted and used in schools to cater to the needs of adolescent health due to several difficulties and challenges (Singh and Misra 2012). In particular, health researchers and professionals often get intrigued with critical questions in any attempt for LSI in a school: they become anxious to know about the adolescent health and well-being-associated relevant outcomes of LSI in schools; the barriers and facilitators need to be known for intervention in adolescent lifestyle; how to overcome these barriers and facilitate positive change in adolescent lifestyle; and the theoretical frameworks that can be envisaged to achieve goals for lifestyle change.

Against this backdrop, this chapter aims at providing evidence-based knowledge to health professionals and researchers to enable, motivate, assist and help adolescents to adopt healthier lifestyle. This chapter is divided into three sections. First section elaborates on the effectiveness of LSI in school; second section explicates barriers and facilitators of change in lifestyle; and third section discusses the key theoretical models to address difficulties encountered by lifestyle researchers.

Effectiveness of LSI

Lifestyle is a broad construct which comprises enormous categories of living including fashion, customs, transportation, etc. Present review, in consonance with existing conceptual dynamics of lifestyle in mainstream health psychology and Indian notions contained in the wisdom of yoga and ayurveda, has considered lifestyle as a constellation of diet, sleep, physical activity, daily routine, risk behaviours and religiosity; therefore, LSI as that intervention which manipulated a cluster of living styles related to diet, sleep, activity and risk behaviours. Therefore, effectiveness of LSI in this chapter is limited only to those studies which have involved any two or more than two components of lifestyle.

LSI is effective for promoting functionality, reducing mental health problems and addressing many adolescent health concerns. Walsh (2011) has argued for utilizing lifestyle modifications in therapeutic settings for treating several psychological disorders and promoting health and well-being. A vast research is available for managing lifestyle-related ailments (i.e., diabetes, CVDs, etc.) and reducing ageing-related complications through LSI, but we get minimal research on the effectiveness of LSI for promoting adolescent health and well-being (Singh 2013). However, available review indicated a majority of research work for obesity-related outcomes among school adolescents. Evidences for positive effects of LSI for obesity in school adolescents have been substantially accumulating in the past few years. In addition, a recent review has reported mixed evidences for improvement in anxiety, depression, self-esteem, quality of life and well-being among those overweight adolescents who were exposed to positive change in dietary habits, physical activity and use of leisure time (Hoare et al. 2015). LSI may have potential for increasing mental health within one week (Melnyk et al. 2013).

With the spirit to fill this lacuna, the present researcher has made a small endeavour. He has conducted a one-month field experiment among normal adolescents (n = 100) at a residential school to evaluate the effect of LSI on multiple measures of adolescent health and well-being. Findings revealed that participants reported benefit, who undertook positive change in their dietary habits (avoiding tea, coffee, fast food and maintaining temporal distance between any two meal) sleep (sleeping before 10 O'clock and getting up before sunrise), daily routine (practising yoga and relaxation), and religious behaviours, reported improvement not only in physical health (illness, insomnia and physical fitness) but also in psychological health (body image, self-esteem, depression and anxiety), social functioning (adjustment, empathy, alienation), academic competence and positive health (hope, optimism and quality of life). In school adolescents from disadvantaged sections, LSI may increase physical self-worth, perceived physical condition and self-efficacy in adolescents from disadvantaged schools (Singh 2013).

Barriers and Facilitators for Lifestyle Change

Any LSI cannot be an isolated activity. It requires concerted efforts on the part of all stakeholders. The failure of several LSI programmes reflects critical need for cognizing multiple aspects in its design and conduct (Verhaeghe et al. 2012). For instance, the researchers of a school-based obesity prevention study in New Zealand realized that due to insufficient consideration of several key factors like role of school staff, lack of intensity, their efforts failed to yield any improvement in obesity-related lifestyle behaviours. Henceforth, holistic understanding of barriers and facilitators of LSI is essential to maximize intended effects and improve its design. A variety of barriers on the path of lifestyle change stem from psycho-contextual characteristics of school adolescence. Cultural beliefs, values, socio-economic status, personality, age, and many other ecological factors contribute in initiating and maintaining positive change in adolescent lifestyle (Singh and Misra 2012; Thirlaway and Upton 2009). A summarized caricature of influences and issues related with adherence to lifestyle change is presented herewith.

3.1 First of all, let us discuss those obstructive factors and facilitators which lie in the developmental features of adolescence. Due to 'experimentation' as a feature of this stage of life, adolescents have greater propensity for risk behaviours but less motivation for pursuance of healthy lifestyle. Fragility of self-efficacy often may render them to avoid healthy lifestyle communications. The role of low self-esteem in continuance of many risk behaviours (sexual behaviours, pornography, substance abuse, violence and suicide) and discontinuance of positive living choices has been well-substantiated. Also, sometimes multiple demands of several life tasks may create dysfunctional coping styles and helplessness which in turn result into unhealthy lifestyle choices. For example, adolescents, while coping with developmental stresses created by formation of identity, peer pressure, choice of career goals confirming parental aspirations, may be vulnerable to unhealthy leisure choices and eating habits. In particular, adolescents suffering from mental disorders may not be capable of adhering to positive lifestyle changes (Verhaeghe et al. 2012).

3.2 Family is an important setting for development during adolescence. It plays crucial role in behavioural, cognitive and social development of adolescents. Multiple aspects of family including living arrangements, closeness in relationships, communication patterns, monitoring, support and supervision determine positive or negative orientation of lifestyle choices (Youngblade et al. 2007). Whether parents practice healthy behaviour or demonstrate aggression, their effects accordingly may influence their son/daughter (Youngblade et al. 2007). Non-response or dropping out of LSI is considerably predicted by maternal depression and avoidant attachment attitude (Pott et al. 2009). In low socioeconomic sections, adolescents may get deprived of family support and encouragement in adopting healthy living choices due to principal focus of family on livelihood. Some patriarchal norms and values exhibited and encouraged by family members may induce aberrations in their attempts to inculcate positive lifestyle behaviours. For example, certain aspects of 'sex' as taboo may prevent affirmative, open and dynamic explorations. Ensuring adequate and appropriate acknowledgment, supervision and support by family members can reinforce positive behaviours but also contribute critically in avoiding unhealthy lifestyle behaviours. Therefore, in any attempt of LSI, ensuring family support can augment positive change in lifestyle.

3.3 After the family, any adolescent has to spend most of his time in school. School not only provides academic instruction but also plays a critical role in acquisition and maintenance of health behaviours. Adolescents tend to heed advice of their teachers. Therefore, if teachers are involved in any LSI, then possibility of its success goes up. Second important facilitative/obstructive agency can be company of students. A review has revealed that certain behavioural choices can be easily maintained during adolescence if they get positive peer support and are empowered enough through inculcation of skills and abilities to avoid unhealthy influences of peer pressure (Thirlaway and Upton 2009). Third important pathway is curriculum which is delivered in classroom. By inculcating/delivering information about the relevance of positive lifestyle in textbooks/classroom lectures, school adolescents' mental makeup can be easily prepared for orienting towards participation in LSI.

3.4 Media is a mainstay of sociocultural context of adolescent lives. In current times, when social networking sites are increasingly gaining attention of the younger generation, exposure to particular type of information through tweets and sharing of posts influences adolescent mood and builds up his/her preference or negligence for particular behavioural choices (Singh and Misra 2012). Television and Twitter like social networking sites can be used as mainstay for social marketing to facilitate positive change in school adolescent lives.

Key Theoretical Frameworks and Strategies

Adolescent lifestyle is a complex phenomenon. Several individual, ecological and contextual factors contribute in opting particular lifestyle choices, its patterning with other lifestyle practices and determining related modalities (Dalal and Misra 2006; Singh 2013). Therefore, any one specific theoretical framework cannot explain or resolve all the hassles related with lifestyle changes. Only eclectic strategies derived from several perspectives can offer adequate insights for dealing with challenges related to different domains (i.e., person, ecology and context). Henceforth, this section presents a detailed view of particular psychological techniques related with different psychological perspectives. Table 9.1 presents a summarized view of the key theoretical frameworks and their corresponding strategies.

4.1 Behavioural assertion for manipulating antecedents and consequences has emerged as prominent approach in LSI studies (Singh 2013). In particular, stimulus control, self-management and reinforcement are being used widely. Several attributes of reinforcement including schedule, mode, duration, background scenario have been attended in attempts for changing lifestyle. In a recent analysis of secondary data derived from 14 published randomized treatment-control intervention trials for 2–18 years aged overweight younger generation, significant benefits associated with teaching youth stimulus-control and teaching parents reinforcement has been demonstrated to shape lifestyle practices (Dalton and Kitzmann 2012).

4.2 Cognitive factors including perceptions, beliefs and attitudes are relevant for initiating and sustaining change in lifestyle choices (Singh 2013; Marquez et al. 2009). Many interventions fail because of their failure in addressing attitudes and perceptions (Singh 2013). In paragraphs given below, several cognitive processes and corresponding strategies for changing lifestyle behaviours are elaborated.

According to social cognitive theory, lifestyle habits get ingrained through observation of corresponding behaviours and associated positive outcomes in family members and different sources of mass media (Natale et al. 2014). Self-efficacy is focal determinant in changing any lifestyle practice (Bandura 2004; Dalton and Kitzmann 2012); in particular when adolescents are ready for changing lifestyle (Singh 2013). Individual adolescents high in self-efficacy are less likely to give up when confronted with barriers in attempts for change in lifestyle. It can be enhanced through self-control and management of records of realistic and achievable goals in pursuance of lifestyle change (Bandura 2004). Since the last decade, use of personalized computer-tailored interventions is emerging as promising health-education strategy to accomplish effective self-management and control of behavioural choices in school adolescents (Haeren et al. 2007).

Table 9.1 Basic processes and strategies for lifestyle intervention at a school

Model/theory	Basic assumptions/ processes	Suggested strategies
Classical conditioning	Reflex, stimulus control	Comfortable physical environment
Instrumental conditioning	Reinforcement and punishment	Physical restraint, deprivation and satiation, appreciation, incentives
Social cognitive theory	Reciprocal determinism, vicarious reinforcement self-efficacy	Self-monitoring, computer-tailored LSI, presentations of role models (i.e., actors, sport persons) through the films and power point
Cognitive dissonance theory	Creating dissonance between cognitions	Zero-prize advocacy speech competition in favour of healthy lifestyle
Health belief model	Perception	Risk and benefits assessment
Theory of planned behaviour	Attitude, social influence	recognition by peers and school staff
Self-regulation	Autonomy	Presenting meaningful rational for persuading to change lifestyle goal setting by oneself
Motivational interviewing	Empathy	Empathetic listening, raising awareness, encouragement, confrontation, being receptive to adolescent's point of views and explanation
Ecological model	Interactive influence	Combination of strategies including supportive environment, attractive set up, mass media campaign
Trans-theoretical model	Awareness and motivation	Personalized scrutiny of healthy lifestyle, encourage to make specific concrete plan, setting gradual goals, feedback, reminders

Health Belief Model and theories of reasoning and planning models emphasize on delivery of risk information related to unhealthy lifestyle. Based on these theories, health education programmes have been providing information on potential harmful effects of specific habituations (e.g., cigarette smoking, alcohol abuse, etc.). These programmes are beneficial especially when participating adolescents are motivated by themselves to seek help and information (Singh 2013).

According to self-regulation, autonomy support is an important key to change lifestyle practices (Singh 2013). Therefore, a practitioner needs to acknowledge the perspective a person holds, present choices within the limits of context and meaningful rationale for not providing certain choices. Taking cues from self-regulation theory and humanistic perspective, Motivational interviewing engages adolescents in a non-confrontational and empathic interaction with efforts in highlighting discrepancies between their goals and effects of particular lifestyle behaviours on their health and well-being. It emphasizes not to coerce adolescents but to help them to make their own decisions for altering behavioural choices. Motivational interviewing is useful when adolescents are not motivated to change their lifestyle. In particular, it envisages the following skills/strategies for change in lifestyle: empathy, encouragement, being receptive to adolescent's point of views and explanation. Motivational interviewing has been effective in addressing many risk behaviours and changing diet/exercise favourably (Singh 2013).

4.3 Ecological model is increasingly being utilized for promoting particular aspects of lifestyle. In a multi-level physical activity intervention programme, several ecological strategies (i.e., organizing debates, ensuring access to attractive activities during breaks and after-school hours, supportive environmental conditions) were utilized to promote daily life and recreational physical activity among school adolescents (Simon et al. 2006).

4.4 A recent theoretical innovation-trans-theoretical model proposes that persons are at different stages of readiness to adopt health behaviours. According to this model, LSI can be successful only if action-oriented efforts are undertaken only after acknowledgement of need to change on the part of participant. Many times, persons may relapse from later to earlier stages but stage-wise attempts are repeated until change in lifestyle is successful. Prochaska et al. (1992) enlist the following 10 underlying processes for behavioural change: consciousness-raising, self re-evaluation, self-liberation, counter-conditioning, stimulus-control, reinforcement management, helping relationships, dramatic relief, environmental re-evaluation and social liberation. It is effective in changing dietary habits, physical activity and risk behaviours.

Conclusion

This chapter has summarized comprehensive effects, barriers and facilitators of change and relevant theoretical frameworks and strategies for changing adolescent lifestyle. It has provided evidence-based knowledge for helping adolescents to realize their potentials and fulfil their aspirations to live a healthy, productive and meaningful life. Several potential barriers and facilitators related with LSI and theoretical frameworks are yet to be empirically evaluated. Now, we need to evolve evidence-based knowledge of counselling strategies to help people to accommodate and comply with positive changes in lifestyle.

References

Bandura, A. (2004). Health promotion by social cognitive means. *Health Education & Behavior, 31*(2), 143–164.

Dalal, A. K., & Misra, G. (2006). Psychology of health and well-being: Some emerging perspectives. *Psychological Studies, 51,* 91–104.

Dalton, W. T., & Kitzmann, K. M. (2012). A preliminary investigation of stimulus control, self-monitoring and reinforcement in lifestyle interventions for pediatric overweight. *American Journal of Lifestyle Medicine, 6*(1), 75–89. https://doi.org/10.1177/1559827611402582.

Haeren, S. L., Deforche, B., Vandelanotte, C., Maes, I., & Bourdeaudhuij, I. D. (2007). Acceptability, feasibility and effectiveness of a computer-tailored physical activity intervention in adolescents. *Patient Education and Counseling, 66*(3), 303–310. https://doi.org/10.1016/j.pec.2007.01.003.

Hoare, E., Fuller-Tyszkiewicz, M., Skouteris, H., Millar, L., & Allender, S. (2015). Systematic review of mental health and well-being outcomes following community-based obesity prevention interventions among adolescents. *British Medical Journal Open, 5*(e006586), 1–14.

Lloyd, C. B., & Mensch, B. S. (2008). Marriage and childbirth as factors in dropping out from school: an analysis of DHS data from Sub-Saharan Africa. *Population Studies, 62*(1), 1–13.

Marquez, D. X., Bustamante, E. E., Blissmer, B. J., & Prohaska, T. R. (2009). Health promotion for successful aging. *American Journal of Lifestyle Medicine, 3*(1), 12–19.

Melnyk, B. M., Jacobson, D., Kelly, S., Belyea, M., Shaibi, G., Small, L., O'Haver, J., et al. (2013). Promoting healthy lifestyles in high school adolescents: A randomized controlled trial. *American Journal of Preventive Medicine, 45*(4), 407–415.

Natale, R. A., Messiah, S. F., Asfour, L., Uhlhorn, S. B., Delamater, A., & Arheart, K. L. (2014). Role of modelling as an early childhood obesity prevention strategy: Effect of parents and teachers on preschool children's healthy lifestyle habits. *Journal of Developmental and Behavioral Pediatrics, 35*(6), 378–387.

Pott, W., Albayrak, O., Hebebrand, J., & Pauli-Pott, U. (2009). Treating childhood obesity: Family background variables and the child's success in a weight-control intervention. *International Journal of Eating Disorder, 42,* 284–289. https://doi.org/10.1002/eat.20655.

Prochaska, J. O., DiClemente, C. C., & Norcross, J. C. (1992). In search of how people change: Applications to addictive behaviors. *American Psychologist, 47,* 1102–1114.

Sidoti, E., Paolini, G., & Tringali, G. (2010). A survey on lifestyle and attitudes on fruit and vegetable consumption and participation in physical activity in a sample of secondary school and university students from Palermo, Western Sicily. *Italian Journal of Public Health, 7*(2), 85–93.

Simon, C., Wagner, A., Platata, C., Arveilera, D., Schweitzer, D., Schliengera, J. L., et al. (2006). ICAPS: A multilevel program to improve physical activity in adolescents. *Diabetese and Metabolism, 32*(1), 41–49. https://doi.org/10.1016/S1262-3636(07)70245-8.

Singh, A. P. (2013). Life style counseling: Emerging challenges, missing opportunities and future directions for research. *Asia Pacific Journal of Counseling and Psychotherapy*. Downloadable from http://dx.doi.org/10.1080/21507686.2013.812972.

Singh, A. P., & Misra, G. (2012). Adolescent life style in India: Prevalence of risk and health-promoting factors. *Psychology & Developing Societies, 24*(2), 145–160. https://doi.org/10.1177/097133361202400203.

Sunitha, S., & Gururaj, G. (2014). Health behaviours & problems among young people in India: Cause for concern & call for action. *Indian Journal of Medical Research, 140,* 185–208.

Thirlaway, K., & Upton, D. (2009). *Psychology of life style: Promoting healthy behavior.* New York: Routledge.

Verhaeghe, N., Maeseneer, J. D., Maes, L., Heeringen, C. V., Bogaert, V., Clayes, E., et al. (2012). Health promotion intervention in mental health care: Design and baseline findings of a cluster preference randomized controlled trial. *BMC Public Health, 12*(431), 1–11.

Walsh, R. (2011, January 17). *Lifestyle and mental health.* American Psychologist. Advanceonline Publication. https://doi.org/10.1037/a0021769.

World Health Organization. (2014). Adolescent health risks and solutions. Fact sheet no. 345, updated May, 2014. http://www.who.int/mediacentre/factsheets/fs345/en/. Retrieved on May 24, 2015.

Youngblade, L. M., Theokas, C., Schulenberg, J., Curry, L., Huang, I., & Novak, M. (2007). Risk and promotive factors in families, schools, and communities: A contextual model of positive youth development in adolescence. *Pediatrics, 119*(1), 547–553. https://doi.org/10.1542/peds.2006-2089H.

Chapter 10
Neurofeedback as an Effective Intervention for Academic Performance in Children with Problems in Attention and Concentration

Meena Hariharan, Gadiraju Padmaja and Suvashisa Rana

Attention, Concentration and Academic Performance

Right to education occupies one of the top priorities of developing countries like India. The sanctity of this rests not so much in enrolling all the children in school, but on ensuring that learning takes place in these children in a progressive way that equips them with cognitive skills to match with their developmental stage. Learning calls need to be optimized for developing suitable curriculum and methods on the one hand and proper training and remedial programmes to cater to the deficits in developmental needs on the other. Attention and concentration are the two essential prerequisites for learning, memory and academic performance. Attention refers to the active processing of specific information present in our environment. It is a cognitive process of directing and maintaining awareness of stimuli identified by the senses toward response choice and decision-making. Concentration, on the other hand, refers to the cognitive process of selectively paying attention to one thing and to sustain it for a period of time.

In school, every class is likely to have children who suffer academic failure or underachievement. It is reported that around 20% school children have scholastic backwardness (Karande and Kulkarni 2005). These children's inability to recall learned information is often misjudged and criticized as their disinterest, stubbornness, indifference, non-cooperation or callous attitude. While these reasons cannot be totally ruled out, it could also be because of problems in functioning of pre-frontal cortex caused by trauma (Hariharan et al. 2014). The causes for underperformance may be many ranging from sheer lack of interest to attention deficit or structural changes in the brain. However, as pointed out by Hariharan et al. (2014), demands of schools on children are based on the broad averages of expected abilities of children based on developmental stages. Not much consideration is given to individual

M. Hariharan · G. Padmaja (✉) · S. Rana
Centre for Health Psychology, University of Hyderabad, Hyderabad 500046, India
e-mail: gpadmaja2008@gmail.com

G. Misra (ed.), *Psychosocial Interventions for Health and Well-Being*,
https://doi.org/10.1007/978-81-322-3782-2_10

differences in the pace of development. Barring major causes such as problems with pre-frontal lobe functioning and autism in most cases, problems related to academic performance in school children can be traced back to deficiency or insufficiency of attention. Attention and concentration are the essential ingredients in learning. Academic achievement, which is more often than not a testimony of memory and recall abilities, demand attention and concentration of the learners both in the classroom and during practice sessions of homework. Hence, often the 'non-performers and under-performers' are put on remedial coaching that places higher demand on attention in practice sessions and rote learning. In such cases, exposure to the type of remedial coaching mentioned above may prove counter-productive as they demand longer span of attention. This explains why interventions not based on need assessment often meet with failures. In order to avoid that if interventions are preceded by appropriate screening and need-based planning, the probability of positive and desirable outcomes is increased. For example, in cases where underperformance is attributed to low attention and concentration, if measures are taken to address the attention factor, their memory and performance will automatically show an improvement.

By not targeting to enhance the attention and concentration, children tend to be stuck with persistent non-learning, resulting in repeated under performance. This not only leads to cumulative cognitive deficiency but also impacts the self-esteem and self-efficacy of children. Research studies have demonstrated that having short attention span becomes a block for individuals from effectively or selectively acquiring information. This subsequently results in a lack in competitiveness and the ability to adapt socially. Problems in attention not only affect the academic and cognitive performance, but also manifest in behaviour problems (Ahmed et al. 2007).

The relationship between attention problem and performance has gained the priority of research in the field of developmental psychology and educational psychology for the past several decades. Studies have shown that certain areas of attention dysfunction are correlated with learning problems since attention skills are necessary for accurate perception, storage and retrieval of information. For example, in a study by Accardo et al. (1990), it was seen that in a group of 422 children with attention dysfunction, evidence of learning problems was seen in 73% of them. Another research finding revealed the association between attention problems such as distractibility, low persistence and high activity with grades in reading and also achievement scores in reading and mathematics (Martin and Holbrook 1985).

With the emphasis and insistence on inclusive education, schools are obliged to enroll special children. It is very likely to observe problems indicating suboptimal cognitive functioning among them. Right from the 1960s till late 1990s, even before the policy of inclusive education came into vogue, studies did identify low performance and underachievement among school children that was attributed to problems in attention.

Research shows the prevalence of clinically identifiable attention deficit problems among schoolgoing children which may be categorized under disorders related to cognitive faculties. Research findings indicated that 2–14% children belonging to school age suffer from Attention Deficit Hyperactive Disorder (ADHD) (Swanson et al. 1998). In a study by Gade (1987) using a sample of 321 schoolgoing children between 5 and 10 years, the prevalence of ADHD was found to be 7.17% when a rating scale was used and 0.94% when clinical interview was used, with an overall prevalence percentage of 8.10. One recent study shows the prevalence to be 11.32% with a higher prevalence among boys than girls. The prevalence was highest in the age group 9 and 10 years (Venkata and Panicker 2013).

Nevertheless, percentage of school children who have problem in attention and concentration that is moderate, and can be rectified with proper intervention, could not be located in the literature. Handling the problem of attention at this level is more productive and cost effective than targeting intervention for a cumulative cognitive deficiency at a later stage. Hence, cognitive intervention at primary school must target children who show symptoms of non-clinical (comparatively low) attention and concentration problems.

Neurofeedback and Its Function

Scientifically, neurofeedback is related to biofeedback, which involves recording and providing feedback on data pertaining to biological functions like heart rate, respiration or skin conduction, to a trainee. But instead of working with these peripheral data, neurofeedback works with data from the brain, whereby it can facilitate changes in the brain wave patterns and regional cerebral blood flow (Demos 2005). When the brain operates in a comparatively efficient pattern, feedback is given via auditory or graphic signals or both. Neurofeedback is supposed to strengthen neural pathways while increasing mental endurance and flexibility, which makes it similar to a comprehensive exercise programme.

This helps the people including children to learn and understand through the feedback what happens in their own brains with a change in their state of mind or awareness. During neurofeedback training, the trainees are provided with the feedback when their cycle of brain waves moves into a more desirable pattern. This feedback enables the persons to learn how to re-regulate their distracted thinking and gain control progressively over their activities and tasks with improved and sustained concentration and attention.

The processes involved in this kind of feedback can be traced back to the late 1960s, when Barry Sterman first described operant conditioning (Gunkelman and Johnstone 2005). In the process of neurofeedback training, when there are desirable brain activity changes, a feedback that is rewarding to the individual is given. If the brain activity changes are in the unintended direction, then the given positive feedback is inhibited or a different feedback is provided. These rewards which provide the required reinforcement can range from a simple change in pitch of a tone to a complex type of movement in a video game. Such reinforcement methods are used to teach the brain how to continue and maintain healthy brain wave patterns. Within a few sessions trainees often gain greater awareness of mental drifting and insight into their own mental functioning. Gradually, most of the people who are trained learn to sustain attention for greater periods of time, apparently even during boring tasks in the classroom or at work (Demos 2005).

The process of neurofeedback training involves attaching electrodes to the specific regions on the child's head with a conductive gel. These electrodes transmit the electrical information to an instrument which analyses the brainwaves and feeds the information into a computer. These brainwaves are displayed on a computer screen very swiftly after their actual occurrence within a few thousandths of a second. The child watches the monitor of the computer which displays a picture like a moving object or a graph that indicates the extent to which the child produces the brainwave activity in the intended pattern. Reinforcement is given through a visual or auditory signal whenever the desired brain wave frequencies are produced by the child with the help of the software designed for the purpose. Operant conditioning helps in reducing the brain wave frequencies that are in excess, and increasing those with a deficit. The goal for the child throughout this process is to learn to produce the type of brainwaves associated with a more focused and attentive state. Thus the dysfunctional brain patterns are corrected and the desired patterns are improved.

For the perception of children, neurofeedback is like a video game where they can bring movement and sound in the picture that appears initially static on the computer screen. This movement happens only when the attention and concentration level reaches a set target. The movement of the picture works as a positive reinforcement for the child to enhance the attention span. Thus, the technique, in a way is like taking advantage of children's attraction for video games and utilizing it to enhance their attention and concentration.

Behavioural Principle in Operation

Five brain wave patterns are discussed with respect to performance tasks associated with concentration or focus. Among these, beta wave is associated with an engaged mind state and its subtype Sensory Motor Rhythm (SMR) waves are associated with concentration or focus. The alpha waves are associated with relaxation activity, theta waves with day dreaming state, and the delta waves with deep sleep experience. Neurofeedback therapy aims to train the subjects to maintain the brain waves associated with the desired mental states displaying calmness, relaxation, alertness, and focus during cognitive tasks. Over the past few decades, such techniques have been developed and described in several research reports (Lubar 1991; Lubar and Lubar 1984; Tansey 1991). Kamiya (1969) popularized neurofeedback in the 1960s by publishing his experiments on alpha brain waves. The classic work of researchers such as Sterman, Lubar and others indicated an enhanced efficacy as a result of beta training which also involved sensorimotor rhythmic Electroencephalogram (EEG) activity (Sterman and Clemente 1962).

As has been described in the preceding section, neurofeedback which applies the behavioural principles such as operant conditioning using positive reinforcement has been proved to be efficacious to train the subjects in the ability to monitor their slow and fast brain wave activity. Based on these principles, neurofeedback training programmes are designed for alpha wave or theta wave reduction and for increasing SMR or beta waves thus producing the desired EEG pattern. Studies conducted with such programmes have shown favourable results. For example, in a study done by Loo and Barkley (2005), different programmes of training were used to reduce alpha or theta waves and to increase sensory motor rhythm or beta waves. When the trainee produced the required EEG pattern, the computer was programmed to give a positive response or reward which often was in the form of points earned. Many other studies have also shown learning of different EEG parameters through operant principles both in animals as well as humans (Birbaumer 1977, 1984; Birbaumeret al. 1981; Kamiya 1969; Plotkin 1976; Sterman 1977).

Use of Neurofeedback as a Cognitive Intervention

Around 1970 it was discovered that neurofeedback makes it possible to recondition and retrain brainwave patterns. Neuro-biofeedback, also termed as neurotherapy and EEG biofeedback is a type of biofeedback which illustrates the activity of the brain using real time displays of electroencephalography. This is done usually for the purpose of gaining control over central nervous system activity. The work in this field began with enhancing alpha brainwave activity for simple relaxation (Hardt and Kamiya 1977), with attempts to diminish uncontrolled epilepsy (Lubar and Bahler 1976; Seifert and Lubar 1975) and in treating epilepsy (Sterman 2000; Sterman and Friar 1972). Soon, various researchers began using neurofeedback for handling attention and concentration problems in children with ADHD (Fox et al. 2005; Lévesque et al. 2006; Lubar et al. 1995; Monastra et al. 2002). Thus neurofeedback has been used effectively as a cognitive intervention with disorders involving cognitive deficits as indicated by several researches.

The logical explanation for low attention and concentration in classroom-related activities is that for some children these activities (mostly reading and writing) fail to provide any immediate reward. On the contrary, they have the potential power of receiving punishment for any signal of distraction in attention. Such combination of motivation directed by punishment and negative emotion can have a further undesirable impact on attention and concentration. Going by the principle of classical conditioning this negative association with attention can also have the effect of generalization. One way of helping these children is to reverse this process by creating a simulation which allows the children to experience immediate reward for any marginal increase in attention and concentration. Neurofeedback machine enables the children to bring changes in the animation on the computer screen by enhancing their attention, thus providing an automatic self-reinforcement. Repeated experience of this helps as a training packed with positive reinforcement for progressive improvement in attention and concentration. Thus, negative association with the attention and concentration can be replaced with motivation and self-efficacy which in turn has the power of generalization.

Neurofeedback Intervention for Clinical Sample

Reports of several researches have highlighted the role of neurofeedback in treating Attention Deficit Disorders (ADD) with or without hyperactivity as well as for Learning Disabilities (LD). The EEG biofeedback has been seen to play an important role in improving the attention, cognitive functioning and behaviour as demonstrated by the increase in measures such as IQ scores, grades and educational test scores which is significant (Lubar 1991; Tansey 1990, 1991). It is observed from studies that when neurofeedback training has been used, the conditioned EEG changes that resulted from the training were associated with improvement or normalization of the symptoms of ADHD. It was also reported that the effect of the training has not only been generalized to other facets of life but also sustained thereafter. Studies have shown that these changes have transferred the impact to day-to-day home and school environment even after the treatment is withdrawn (Monastra et al. 2002). Lubar (1991) found that these changes were maintained into adulthood in most treated cases. Researches also pointed to the fact that compared to neurofeedback therapy, no other approach to the treatment of ADHD has been successful in such effects of generalization or maintenance (Pelham et al. 1998; Smith et al. 2006). Multiple advantages of neurofeedback therapy have been reported including improvements in school or work performance, social relationships, self-esteem and plasticity of self-regulatory skills as well as reduction in undesirable patterns of behaviour such as irritability and oppositional behaviour. A review of more than 20 studies using neurofeedback for the treatment of ADHD have shown that 70–80% subjects significantly benefitted which sustained till 10 years after treatment (Lubar 1995). Studies have demonstrated that in addition to IQ scores significant improvements were noticed in classroom performance of children with ADD after neurofeedback training. Distinctly identifiable, EEG differences were noticed after neurofeedback training in children with learning difficulties and attention deficits with or without hyperactivity (Abarbanel 1995; Lubar 1991, 1995; Sterman 1996; Tansey 1990). In a study, a sample of 1089 subjects with attention and behaviour complaints were administered SMR-beta neurofeedback training (Kaiser and Othner 2000). An improvement was reported in areas such as attentiveness, impulse control and response variability after the training, showcasing the importance of neurofeedback training in remediating attentional dysfunction. Mezzacappa and Buckner, (2010) also point to the emerging data suggesting the benefits of interventions designed to improve such skills in both typically developing children and children with impairments. Thus research findings clearly indicate the effectiveness of neurofeedback in bringing positive change in cognitive and behavioural dimensions among children diagnosed with ADHD and LD.

Neurofeedback Intervention for Non-clinical Sample

While the preceding section shows effective results of usage of neurofeedback intervention in children with significant clinical symptoms related to attention, memory and performance, there are also children who have problems with attention, concentration and memory in lower degrees which do not classify them under clinical sample. It is often noticed that children who have problems in sustaining attention and concentration are branded as troublesome or backward in studies and are subjected to methods of rectifying the same either by over-disciplining methods which may be punitive or by neglect. Attention span is related to neurophysiological functioning. Therefore, rather than applying adhoc corrective measures, it is desirable to approach the problem scientifically. For instance, one can contemplate methods of conditioning the neuropsychological functioning of the child.

A careful examination of the research for the past three decades and more shows that several attempts using case study and controlled group studies have been made to examine the effects of EEG biofeedback. Majority of these studies have reported favourable results of this treatment approach. In several studies, quantitative electroencephalographic examination demonstrated improved attention and behavioural control in tests of intelligence and academic achievement (Monastra et al. 2005). Several systematic studies also suggested consistently that neurofeedback training improves attention (Leins et al. 2007), increases IQ scores (Linden et al. 1996) and enhances cognitive performance (Vernon et al. 2003).

Application of Neurofeedback: A Wider Perspective

Contemporary challenges of education and mental health are different from previous decades. With globalization and advanced technology, problems of academic underachievement and attention deficit is not so much due to understimulation as in earlier decades, but because of overstimulation leading to distraction and deviation. Thus the problems are significantly different from what children of 1970s and 80s faced. Hence, the approach to intervention has to be more in line of training to filter attention on selective stimuli, focus and sustain the attention rather than just remedial teaching.

Neurofeedback can be an effective tool for two purposes, i.e., in screening children with problems in attention and concentration as well as in their cognitive training and retraining. Neurofeedback equipment can be used to develop age norms and grade norms of attention and concentration for non-clinical primary school children. Based upon these norms, identification of problems in attention and concentration—the prerequisites for scholastic achievement—may be possible.

The effectiveness of neurofeedback is found in all children with or without developmental psychopathology. Though the studies vary in the methodology in terms of frequency, duration and periodicity, results indicate positive outcome.

Among the healthy children, a single session of neurofeedback training is reported to have resulted in cognitive enhancement (Escolana et al. 2012). Exposure to weekly neurofeedback sessions for seven months is found to be useful in enhancing reading skills and IQ scores in elementary school children having identified learning problems (Orlando and Rivera 2004). Neurofeedback training brings improvement related to symptoms as well as behavioural aspects in children with autism (Jarusiewicz 2002). Significant improvements are also observed in IQ scores following EEG biofeedback in a set of identical twin girls with mild developmental delay and with symptoms suggesting ADHD (Fleischman and Othmer 2006).

The findings of several researches using neurofeedback as an intervention for clinical and non-clinical samples have implications for future educational curricula aiming at improved academic performance. This is possible by identifying the deficits in attention and concentration early enough so that such practical training interventions like neurofeedback are given in addition to educational interventions.

An Empirical Study Using Neurofeedback as an Intervention for Academic Performance in Non-clinical Group of Children with Problems in Attention and Concentration

Considering the vast research which demonstrated that neurofeedback was helpful in children with ADHD and other related clinical problems, the authors conducted a study to measure the effect of neurofeedback as a cognitive intervention in a non-clinical sample. The study attempted to observe if the attention, memory and academic improvement could be brought through neurofeedback intervention in children who were normal. However, their lack of attention and concentration in comparison to other children was often complained by teachers and parents. It was also hypothesized that normal children without any reported attention and concentration problems may also be able to benefit out of this training.

The study adopted a quasi-experimental design, where 50 children studying in Class 3 through 7 having problems with attention and concentration were screened and compared with another group of 26 children who were academically bright with no problems in attention and concentration. The Students' Attention Behavior Rating Scale for Teachers and Children's Attention Behavior Rating Scale for Parents, specifically designed for this study were used as screening instruments to identify the above two groups of children. For the purpose of measuring attention, concentration and memory, PGI Memory Scale (Pershad and Wig 1976) was used, and the examination marks in the pre- and post-intervention phases were taken as measures of academic performance. The intervention consisted of one trial exposure session and ten intervention sessions with a frequency of one session in a week. On termination of intervention, the children were administered a post-test with PGI memory scale and scholastic skills test. The results showed that neurofeedback intervention for ten weeks could bring significant improvement in the academic performance of children. However, this significant improvement did not equate the academic performance of the children with attention and concentration problem with that of bright children who constituted the comparison group. When it came to directly impact attention and concentration, it was found to be very encouraging because the post intervention scores of children with attention and concentration problems was found to be almost at the same level of comparison group. This could be because the training provided in the intervention that required children to sustain their attention on video pictures providing instant reinforcement (movement of the car in the video screen) helped in strengthening the behaviour of sustaining the focused attention. On the other hand, the significant but limited impact in academic performance may be attributed to the factor related to delayed reinforcement associated with academic performance. Perhaps, a direct positive reinforcement for enhanced academic performance would be helpful in improving their performance, which is comparable with their counterparts in the comparison group.

While the desirable outcome in case of children with problems in attention and memory is considered to be a significant contribution to knowledge, equally or more important is the finding that the intervention did not prove as effective in case of children without problems in attention. In fact, a decline in performance was noticed among them after they crossed the half-way mark. This finding suggests the caution to be exercised in prescribing neurofeedback for children. There may be a number of enthusiastic parents who aspire further excellence in their already ‘brilliant’ children. They may ‘seek’ neurofeedback intervention for their children. Similarly, a practitioner who is equipped with the device may feel tempted to use it on children with complaints of performance deficit. Here is where utmost caution needs to be exercised based on the second finding that the intervention proved not effective for the comparison group. Why it was not equally effective on the children without attention problem demands further investigation. It is possible that these children already put their neurocognitive functions to the optimal action, hence the intervention was unable to bring any further improvement that is significant. In such cases, attempts to stretch their attention further should not result in undesirable outcomes. In view of this, screening must be taken up as an essential prerequisite before advocating neurofeedback intervention for any child.

Acknowledgements The study by authors discussed in this article was a part of the project funded by ICSSR.

References

Abarbanel, A. (1995). Gates, states, rhythms and resonances: The scientific basis of neurofeedback training. *Journal of Neurotherapy, 1,* 15–38.

Accardo, P. J., Blondis, T. A., & Whitman, B. Y. (1990). Disorders of attention and activity levels in a referral population. *Pediatrics, 85*(2), 426–431.

Ahmed, A., Khalique, N., Khan, Z., & Amir, A. (2007). Prevalence of psychosocial problems among school going male adolescents. *Indian Journal of Community Medicine, 32*(3), 219–221.

Birbaumer, N. (1977). Operant enhancement of EEG-theta activity. In J. Beatty & H. Legewie (Eds.), *Biofeedback and behavior* (pp. 135–145). New York, London: Plenum Press.
Birbaumer, N. (1984). Operant control of slow brain potentials: A tool in the investigation of the potentials meaning and its relation to attentional dysfunction. In T. Elbert, B. Rockstroh, W. Lutzenberger, & N. Birbaumer (Eds.), *Self-regulation of the brain and behavior* (pp. 227–239). Berlin: Springer.
Birbaumer, N., Elbert, T., Rockstroh, B., & Lutzenberger, W. (1981). Biofeedback of event-related potentials of the brain. *International Journal of Psychology, 16,* 389–415.
Demos, J. N. (2005). Getting started with neurofeedback. In *Diagnosing, and treating AD/HD in children and adolescents* (pp. 235–297). New York: W. W. Norton & Company, Inc.
Escolano, C., Olivan, B., Lopez-del-Hoyo, Y., Garcia-Campayo, J., & Minguez, J. (2012, August 28–September 1). *Double-blind single-session neurofeedback training in upper-alpha for cognitive enhancement of healthy subjects.* Paper presented at IEEE Engineering in Medicine and Biology Society (EMBS): 2012 Annual International Conference of the IEEE, San Diego, CA, USA. https://doi.org/10.1109/embc.2012.6347002.
Fleischman, M. J., & Othmer, S. (2006). Case study: Improvements in IQ score and maintenance of gains following EEG biofeedback with mildly developmentally delayed twins. *Journal of Neurotherapy, 9*(4), 35–46.
Fox, D. J., Tharp, D. F., & Fox, L. C. (2005). Neurofeedback: An alternative and efficacious treatment for attention deficit hyperactivity disorder. *Applied Psychophysiology and Biofeedback, 30*(4), 365–373.
Gade, N. (1987). A study of prevalence and pattern of attention deficit disorder in primary school children. *Indian Journal of Psychiatry, 29,* 113–118.
Gunkelman, J. D., & Johnstone, J. (2005). Neurofeedback and the brain. *Journal of Adult Development, 12*(2–3), 93–98.
Hardt, J. V., & Kamiya, J. (1977). Anxiety change through electroencephalographic alpha feedback seen only in high anxiety subjects. *Science, 201,* 79–81.
Hariharan, M., Chivukula, U., & Swain, S. (2014). Childhood stress and its impact on learning and academic performance. In A. J. Holliman (Ed.), *Educational psychology.* Routledge: London, New York.
Jarusiewicz, B. (2002). Efficacy of neurofeedback for children in the autistic spectrum: A pilot study. *Journal of Neurotherapy, 6*(4), 39–49.
Kaiser, D. A., & Othner, S. (2000). Effect of neurofeedback on variable of attention in a large multi-center trial. *Journal of Neurotherapy, 4*(1), 5–15.
Kamiya, J. (1969). Operant control of the EEG alpha rhythm and some of its reported effects on consciousness. In C. T. Tart (Ed.), *Altered states of consciousness.* New York: Wiley.
Karande, S., & Kulkarni, M. (2005). Poor school performance. *Indian Journal of Pediatrics, 72,* 961–967.
Leins, U., Goth, G., Hinterberger, T., Klinger, C., Rumpf, N., & Strehl, U. (2007). Neurofeedback for children with ADHD: A comparison of SCP and Theta/Beta protocols. *AppliedPsychophysiology and Biofeedback, 32*(2), 73–88.
Lévesque, J., Beauregard, M., & Mensour, B. (2006). Effect of neurofeedback training on the neural substrates of selective attention in children with attention-deficit/hyperactivity disorder: A functional magnetic resonance imaging study. *Neuroscience Letters, 394*(3), 216–221.
Linden, M., Habib, T., & Radojevic, V. (1996). A controlled study of the effects of EEG biofeedback on cognition and behavior of children with attention deficit disorder and learning disabilities. *Biofeedback and Self- Regulation, 21*(1), 35–49.
Loo, S. K., & Barkley, R. A. (2005). Clinical utility of EEG in attention deficit hyperactivity disorder. *Applied Neuropsychology, 12*(2), 64–76.

Lubar, J. F. (1991). Discourse on the development of EEG diagnostics and biofeedback treatment for attention deficit/hyperactivity disorders. *Biofeedback and Self-Regulation, 16,* 202–225.

Lubar, J. F. (1995). Neurofeedback for the management of attention-deficit/hyperactivity disorders. In M. S. Schwartz (Ed.), *Biofeedback: A practitioner's guide* (pp. 493–522). New York: Guilford.

Lubar, J. F., & Bahler, W. W. (1976). Behavioral management of epileptic seizures following EEG biofeedback training of the sensorimotor rhythm. *Biofeedback and Self-Regulation, 1*(1), 77–104.

Lubar, J., & Lubar, J. (1984). Electroencephalographic biofeedback of SMR and beta for treatment of attention deficit disorder in a clinical setting. *Biofeedback and Self Regulation, 9,* 1–23.

Lubar, J. F., Swartwood, M. O., Swartwood, J. N., & O'Donnell, P. H. (1995). Evaluation of the effectiveness of EEG Neurofeedback training for ADHD in a clinical setting as measured by changes in T.O.V.A. scores, behavioral ratings, and WISC-R performance. *Biofeedback & Self-Regulation, 20*(1), 83–99.

Martin, R. P., & Holbrook, J. (1985). Relationship of temperament characteristics to the academic achievement of first-grade children. *Journal of Psychoeducational Assessment, 3,* 377–386.

Mezzacappa, E., & Buckner, J. C. (2010). Working memory training for children with attention problems or hyperactivity: A school-based pilot study. *School Mental Health, 2,* 202–208.

Monastra, V. J., Lynn, S., Linden, M., Lubar, J. F., Gruzelier, J., & LaVaque, T. J. (2005). Electroencephalographic biofeedback in the treatment of attention-deficit/hyperactivity disorder. *Applied Psychophysiological Biofeedback, 30*(2), 95–114.

Monastra, V. J., Monastra, D. M., & George, S. (2002). The effects of stimulant therapy, EEG biofeedback, and parenting style on the primary symptoms of attention-deficit/hyperactivity disorder. *Applied Psychophysiology and Biofeedback, 27*(4), 231–249.

Orlando, P. C., & Rivera, R. O. (2004). Neurofeedback for elementary students with identified learning problems. *Journal of Neurotherapy, 8*(2), 5–19.

Pelham, W. E., Jr., Wheeler, T., & Chronis, A. (1998). Empirically supported psychosocial treatments for attention deficit hyperactivity disorder. *Journal of Clinical Child Psychology, 27* (2), 190–205.

Pershad, D., & Wig, N. N. (1976). A battery of simple tests of memory for use in India. *Neurology India, 24,* 86–89.

Plotkin, W. B. (1976). On the self-regulation of the occipital alpha rhythm: Control strategies, states of consciousness, and the role of physiological feedback. *Journal of Experimental Psychology General, 105,* 66–99.

Seifert, A. R., & Lubar, J. F. (1975). Reduction of epileptic seizures through EEG biofeedback training. *Biological Psychology, 3*(3), 157–184.

Smith, B., Barkley, R. A., & Shapiro, C. (2006). Attention deficit hyperactivity disorder. In E. J. Mash & R. A. Barkley (Eds.), *Treatment of childhood disorders* (3rd ed.). New York: Guilford.

Sterman, M. B. (1977). Sensorimotor EEG operant conditioning: Experimental and clinical effects. *Pavlovian Journal of Biological Science, 12,* 63–92.

Sterman, M. B. (1996). Physiological origins and functional correlates of EEG rhythmic activities: Implications for self regulation. *Biofeedback and Self Regulation, 21,* 3–33.

Sterman, M. B. (2000). Basic concepts and clinical findings in the treatment of seizure disorders with EEG operant conditioning. *Clinical Electroencephalography, 31*(1), 45–55.

Sterman, M. B., & Clemente, C. D. (1962). Forebrain inhibitory mechanisms: Cortical synchronization induced by basal forebrain stimulation. *Experimental Neurology, 6*(2), 91–102.

Sterman, M. B., & Friar, L. (1972). Suppression of seizures in an epileptic following sensorimotor EEG feedback training. *Electroencephalography and Clinical Neuro Physiology, 33*(1), 89–95.

Swanson, J. M., Sergeant, J. A., Taylor, E., Sonuga-Barke, E. J. S., Jensen, P. S., & Cantwell, D. P. (1998). Attention-deficit hyperactivity disorder and hyperkinetic disorder. *Lancet, 351,* 429–433.

Tansey, M. A. (1990). Righting the rhythms of reason: EEG biofeedback training as a therapeutic modality in a clinical office setting. *Medical Psychotherapy, 3,* 57–68.
Tansey, M. A. (1991). Wechsler (WISC-R) changes following treatment of learning. *Australian Journal of Psychology, 43,* 147–153.
Venkata, J. A., & Panicker, A. S. (2013). Prevalence of attention deficit hyperactivity disorder in primary school children. *Indian Journal of Psychiatry, 55,* 338–342.
Vernon, D., Egner, T., Cooper, N., Compton, T., Neilands, C., Sheri, A., et al. (2003). The effect of training distinct neurofeedback protocols on aspects of cognitive performance. *International Journal of Psychophysiology, 47,* 75–85.

Chapter 11
Interventions for Enhancing Health and Well-Being Among Indian Elderly

Nisha Mani Pandey, Indiwar Misra and S. C. Tiwari

Elderly-the Concept

Definition of elderly has been long debated and there is not a single acceptable one. The US and other developed countries consider the age of 65 and above as elderly. Some others classify elderly as: (1) *Young old:* aged 55–65 years; (2) *Old: aged* 66–85 years, and (3) *Oldest old:* aged 85 years and above (Carey 2003). According to Indian studies categorization of the elderly have been done in terms of *young-old:* 60–70 years, *old-old:* 70–80 years and *oldest-old:* 80 years and above (Rao 1993; Rajan 2003). Further, the Census of India provides age-wise data in different age sub-groups, up to 80 years and identifies the elderly with age 60 years and above.

There are bio-medical and philosophical views to define aging and the elderly. Studies suggest that along with chronological age, change in social role (i.e., change in work patterns, adult status of children and menopause) and change in capabilities (i.e., invalid status, senility and change in physical characteristics) are also important components for defining old age or elderly (Glascock and Feinman 1980) In general, the 60th year has been considered as the point of turning old in India. The 'National Policy on Older Persons' (1999) the Government of India defines 'senior citizen' or the 'elderly' as an individual of 60 years or above.

Elderly are often perceived as reservoir of wisdom and intelligence and also perceived as 'deadly desert' with disease, disability and decomposed fraternity. The latter viewpoint is significantly prevailing in society and addressing it is one of the biggest challenges. They have to confront with a number of difficulties including

N. M. Pandey (✉) · S. C. Tiwari
Department of Geriatric Mental Health, King George's Medical University, Lucknow, Uttar Pradesh, India
e-mail: nisha15pandey@yahoo.co.in

I. Misra
Department of Psychology, B.R. Ambedkar College, New Delhi, Delhi, India

G. Misra (ed.), *Psychosocial Interventions for Health and Well-Being*,
https://doi.org/10.1007/978-81-322-3782-2_11

physical, mental, familial, social, environmental, etc. This directly affects their well-being and health. Sense of well-being prevails only in a small proportion of the elderly varying from 20 to 50% (Rao 2001). National Sample Survey Organisation, 2006 also reveal that the elderly experience a greater burden of health morbidity (illness, sickness, injury and poisoning).

There are some physiological/biological causes and a few environmental ones which manipulate the health and well-being of elderly; thus, before finding out ways and strategies to enhance the well-being and health of elderly, one needs to scrutinize the process of age and ageing as well as their status.

Age Related Changes vis à vis State of Mind

The multiple processes of degeneration, which is associated with old age, can be categorized as primary and secondary ageing (Busse 1987). Primary ageing is intrinsic to the organism and is influenced by inherited or hereditary factors, whereas secondary ageing is caused by hostile factors of the environment including trauma and acquired diseases and disabilities in the individual. In human organism, ageing is determined genetically but individual variations are influenced by different environmental factors like nutrition, lifestyle, social and familial environment, illnesses, etc. (Busse 1987).

The objective study of the human ageing is difficult. Many age-related changes often restrict a person in continuing with the normal functions, meet personal needs, maintain dignity and place in family and society as well as fulfil others' demands. The biological, psychological and social problems of human ageing cannot be evaded. These problems are related to physical limitations, occupational redundancy, physical and mental ill health, socio-economic conditions, leisure, retirement as well as maintenance of capacity and performance.

With age the risk for developing certain chronic and incapacitating diseases is significantly high. In the main stages of human life all these factors are closely interwoven; physical and mental declines are added and in the later stage of life. This is the peak year for social and authoritarian achievement, partial/full disengagement from occupational role and community affairs, diminution of sexual function, full or partial dependency because of physical/mental impairment/ handicap or disability. Cognitive changes with ageing are well documented and affect a broad range of functions (Spar and Rue 2009). According to Spar and Rue (2009), effects of ageing on various cognitive functions and ability are explained in subsequent paragraphs.

Intelligence

Vocabulary and knowledge remains stable or increase with age however, in very old age it may decline which is most remarkable for novel tasks. Perceptual motor skills start to decline with chronological age 50–60.

Attention

General attention span may remain the same or there may be minor decline with age but in complex attention, mild decline starts with age and problems with dividing attention, filtering out noise, shift of attention takes place with age.

Language

If there is no sensory deficit, communication ability remains stable at any age. Grammatical and word knowledge which is variable with education, remains the same and stable. Sometimes there is mild decline in verbal fluency or naming and one may often find lapses in occasional word finding. The ability to comprehend also sometimes mildly deteriorates and there may be some worsening in processing of complex messages; however, communication is found to be variable with age and it may be vaguer and repetitive.

Memory

Short-term memory often remains stable or sometimes mild decline occurs. Generally, recall of forward digit span remain intact (7 ± 2 items) but easily disrupted by interference. There is mild to moderate decline in working memory as the ability to manipulate information in short-term memory reduce with age. In general, recent memory also deteriorates moderately though storage remains intact but encoding and retrieval deficits are found to be significantly prevalent with age. Remote memory for major aspects of personal history is found to be variable with age, however, most of the time it remains intact. There is mild to moderate decline on laboratory tasks but the elderly often do better than their younger counterparts on naturalistic prospective memory tasks.

Visio-Spatial Ability

The ability to reproduce drawings (design copying) varies with ageing; however, it is found to be intact for simple designs but not for complex forms/figures. The ability of topographic orientation starts declining with age and it is most noticeable unfamiliar surroundings.

Executive Functions

There is mild to moderate decline in cognitive flexibility. This can be observed in one's thought or action which gets slower and less accurate while shifting from one thought or action with the advancement of age. There is some redundancy and disorganizations in logical problem which also deteriorates with age. The ability of practical reasoning also get affected and mild to moderate decline may be observed in this ability; qualitative practical reasoning remains intact and efficiency on complex and novel tasks worsen with age.

Speed

Slowing of thought and action is the most reliable change of ageing, the velocity to perform different activities also deteriorates with age.

Age-related changes during adult life are less stunning; these changes are generally progressive and cumulative with advancement in age. In later stage of life, biological changes are remarkable and cause progressive, systematic and cumulative adverse changes in physical status and therefore, the psychological and social characteristics also get influenced adversely. Before elaborating on the interventional strategies for enhancing health and well-being various characteristics and environmental aspects need to be discussed clearly.

Socio-Demographic Profile of the Indian Elderly

Reports reveal that in 1901 the proportion of the elderly aged 60 years or above was about 5%, which marginally increased to 5.4% in 1951 (Das et al. 2011). In 2001 there were 7.6% elderly in the country which now has swelled up to 8.6% (Chandramouli 2013). In three decades, the number of older adults has more than doubled, i.e., from 43 million in 1981 to 103 million in 2011 (Chandramouli 2013) and is expected to triple in the next four decades i.e., 316 million (James and Sathyanarayana 2011). Further, there is a steady increase in the expected length of life or life expectancy at birth or life expectancy at the age of 0; it has risen from 49.7 (male = 50.5, female = 49.0) years in 1970–75 to over 63.5 (male = 62.6, female = 64.2) in 2002–06 (Das et al. 2011) and 68.8 in 2017 (https://www.indexmundi.com 2017 accessed on May 7, 2018).

Adding to it, the dependency ratio of elderly is also increasing. Majority of the elderly reported to be dependent and have problem to preserve their lives. According to a recent report (Das et al. 2011) approximately 65% of the elderly have to depend on others for their day-to-day maintenance and the situation of elderly females was reported to be worst than their counterpart males. The analysis further reports that less than 20% of females were financially independent whereas in males majority were found to be economically independent. Feminization of elderly is also on the rise. In the younger population, males outnumber females whereas in the elderly population females outnumber males. According to reports of situation analysis of India (Das et al. 2011), among the elderly 65% individuals are illiterate.

Psycho-Social Profile of Indian Elderly

The Indian society is changing markedly as newer and newer concepts, principles, values and morals are taking place which is eroding our cultural heritage significantly. The traditional Indian societies believe in the concept of '*Vasudhav Kutumkam*' (*the entire world is a family*) and there is a common saying, '*sarve bhavantu sukhinh, sarve santu niramaya; sarve bhadradi pashyantu ma kashchid dukhbhag bhavet*' (*everyone be happy, everyone be healthy; everyone be delighted, no one get any kind of grief/sorrow*). The psycho-social environment was advocated with basic principle of a holistic approach. Generally, collective efforts and responsibilities were being shared. To tackle any situation or problem, the lexicon of 'we' was used. However, with passage of time, the concept of 'we' is being replaced with 'I' in an ever-changing individualistic society. This pattern of ego-centricity in the society is negatively affecting the status of the elderly. Lifestyle issues as well as the changing psycho-social milieu adversely affect the health and well-being of the elderly (Tiwari and Pandey 2014).

In the present scenario, due to influence of the materialistic world and many more transformations in society, newer challenges and problems are taking place (Misra 2010). Verses like '*abhivadansheelasya nitya vriddhopsevinh; chatwari tasya vardhante aayuh, vidya yashbalam* (respecting and serving elderly improves life span, knowledge, fame and strength) (Manusmriti Chapter 2: 121) have became obsolete in today's Indian society. The elderly who previously were respected and revered, now suffer and at times left alone without a single caregiver. Additionally, they have to confront various psycho-social, financial and care-related problems, which directly affect their health and well-being. Such changes adversely affect the social status and relationships with the elderly.

Changes in the family structure, social milieu, technological advancements and transformation in our own values and morals changed the entire psycho-social milieu. As a result, they are not getting adequate care and attention; they have to face an unfriendly, isolated environment and at times feel lonely. Their power of decision making, involvement in family affairs and economic expenditures etc. are gradually declining.

Such familial and social pressures bound the elderly to think themselves as per their own inability and incompetence. Many times they try to cope with the situation and compromise with their desires so that their children or family members do not face any difficulty with them. Sometimes they succeed in developing such changes, especially when they opt for such changes on their own. But if such changes are undertaken due to some compulsion, their well-being get disturbed. Decline in physical health, financial resources, rupture in daily routine, etc., contribute to various social and psychological problems in the elderly and ultimately affect their health and well-being.

Health and Well-Being of the Indian Elderly: An Overview

Health and well-being of the elderly is a challenging issue. Along with physiological, biological, psycho-social issues, they experience health-related problems owing to their high susceptibility to infection, inability to cope with physical and psychological stress, degenerative diseases, cardio-vascular disease, cognitive impairment, etc. Amongst the elderly, certain chronic and incapacitating diseases are significantly high.

Studies report that lifestyle, lack of family support, gender discrimination, socio-economic status, disturbances in families, loneliness and feeling of negligence often lead to psycho-social problems and is clearly associated with increase in psychiatric morbidity among the elderly (Jamuna 1994; Tiwari 2000; Chadha and John 2003; Prakash et al 2004). Low literacy rate and dependency on others also have an adverse effect on health.

It is also reported that majority of elderly suffer with cardiovascular illness, circulatory diseases and cancers (Alam 2000; Ingle and Nath 2008). The prevalence rate of geriatric morbidity because of re-emerging infectious diseases also reported to be high. Recent studies report that rural older people are more susceptible to develop psychiatric morbidity (Tiwari and Pandey 2012; Tiwari et al. 2013) than urban older adults (Tiwari et al. 2014). Studies further reveal that more than 50% of geriatrics are facing physical (Tiwari et al. 2013, 2014) and 20.5% mental morbidity (Tiwari and Pandey 2012).

Co-morbidity may be labelled as a common feature for the elderly as degeneration and deterioration starts in the human organism at the age of 45 or early. However, old age should not be perceived as the age for disease and disability. It is noteworthy that though life expectancy is determined by genes, many of the health hazards may be managed on our own. Environmental factors and lifestyle plays significant role in maintaining and managing the health and well-being of the individual.

Strategies for Enhancing Health and Well-Being of the Elderly

Whenever someone gets ill, some kind of intervention (pharmacological and/non pharmacological) is provided for the improvement and management of the problem. However, the elderly and their caregivers often remain unaware about the available interventional strategies as well as its application. The problem increases, if the healthcare providers do not have clear and proper information regarding available healthcare strategies. One can't refute the significance of pharmacological and non-pharmacological interventions to enhance well-being and health of an elderly. By adopting the following steps carefully and through judicious selection of both type of interventions and their combination as per the need of the subject, problems could be managed more efficiently.

Flowchart-Steps of Interventions
(flowchart near here)

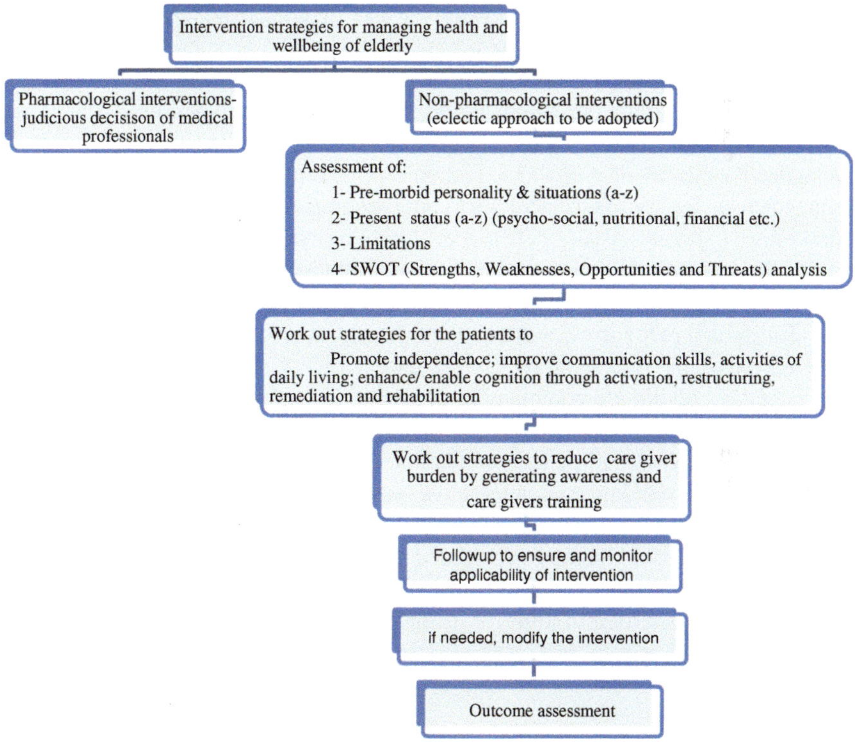

Pharmacological Interventions

The elderly are one of the most vulnerable groups to suffer from drug-induced adverse effects like constipation, urinary retention, delirium, cognitive dysfunction, sedation, postural hypotension, etc. The reasons for such sufferings may be varied (complicated drug regimen, co-morbidity, improper drug selection or dosing, etc.). Careful and conscious therapeutic strategies including non-pharmacological interventions are supposed to be the best option in enhancing elderly health and well-being in today's perspective.

Non-pharmacological Interventions

A number of non-pharmacological interventions are there to enhance well-being and health. It is well recognized that both pharmacological and non-pharmacological type of interventions and treatment strategies are complementary in managing the elderly with multiple morbidity. Studies report that many times non-pharmacological interventions play a significant role in dealing with several common chronic conditions in the elderly (Naci and Ioannidis 2013; Taylor et al. 2014). Individualized and focused interventions are more useful in case of managing the health of elderly. A systemic review provides evidence-based recommendations for non-pharmacological interventions for various common geriatric conditions. (Abraha et al. 2015). For non-pharmacological management one requires proper information regarding patients' illness and his pre-morbid personality as well as habits and lifestyle. In view of overall information the professional may identify and recognize/determine the intensity of problems and then can devise particular steps for interventions. Single interventional strategy is hardly used in most cases as providing a combination of interventions is found to be more useful. Thus, familiarity with various non-pharmacological interventional approaches as well as proper knowledge of its combination use is mandatory.

A number of standard and alternative methods/therapies like-cognitive behaviour therapy, dialectic behaviour therapy, supportive therapies, sensory stimulation therapy, reminiscence therapy, simulated presence therapy, validation therapy, acupuncture, aromatherapy, light therapy, massage or touch therapy, music therapy, yoga therapy etc. are used to improve health and well-being of an individual. These therapies involve certain interventional strategies. The knowledge and understanding about these therapies provides an insight of better management techniques.

Cognitive Behaviour Therapy (CBT)

CBT is a dynamic, systematic, time-bound, structured and investigative method which follows an abstract model of therapeutic interventions. In CBT intervention includes strategies to facilitate learning through repeated presentation of information using different modalities. The elderly are taught to recognize, observe and challenge negative thoughts, behaviour as well as roles and encouraged to develop more adaptive and flexible thoughts, behaviours and roles. As per appropriateness of the strategies, one need to educate and instruct the subject and their caregiver and also monitor the same. This helps in developing pleasant and positive measures. Such interventional sessions consists of 30–45 min sessions following structured guidelines.

CBT aimed to improve cognitive functions and behaviour of the individual. A set of tasks are applied to improve cognitive functions including verbal recall and fluency, concentration, attention, comprehension, reasoning, learning abilities, language and executive functions. At the first step, one needs to recognize the level of deficiency as well as pre-morbid status of the elderly. On the basis of subject's deficiencies one decides frequency, duration, difficulty levels and scope of training sessions. If applied properly, interventions of this therapeutic technique generally helps in improving depressive symptoms, somatization, mild levels of memory deficits, anxiety disorders, etc., as cognitive training helps in improving the 'core' abilities of an individual.

Behavioural Interventions

In behavioural therapies one needs to assess the subject in detail and know the ABC (antecedents, behaviours and consequences) of the particular disorder applying relevant assessment tools. On the basis of findings of the assessment, roots of the particular problems and associated behaviours as well as its impact on the individual should be identified and analysed thoroughly. Behavioural therapies include functional analysis of the particular behaviour. Further, professionals try to find out influences of the stimuli on behaviour, positive reinforcers for behaviours and techniques for strengthening behaviour. In the clinical set-up we found that behavioural interventions not only improve patients' physical and mental health condition but also the well-being and quality of life of the care providers. Generally, behavioural interventions are based on the analysis of these findings. By behavioural interventions the elderly accept their changed roles and get adjusted with their environment in a better way (Ramamurti and Jamuna 2010).

Reality Orientation

Reality orientation aimed to help people by reminding them of facts about themselves and their environment. It is provided in the form of consistent positive reinforcement to correct confused behaviour of the elderly. In this therapy, generally orientation is being provided to the individual specifically regarding their environment using a range of materials and activities. This involves consistent use of orientation devices such as signposts, notices and other memory aids. When an elderly forgets about his/her meal, we often train the caregiver that s/he may provide the meal to the patient and leave the used utensils till the other meal is served so that the patient could recognize that the particular meal is taken by him/her. It is author's own experience during treating patients that reality orientation sessions increase people's verbal orientation and sometimes increase recall.

Validation Therapy

This therapy incorporates a range of specific techniques based on general principles of validation. It can be considered as a kind of philosophy of care. In validation therapy one has to provide a high degree of empathy identifying the subject's entire frame of references. Validation therapy's steps incorporate: classification of particular behaviour/s; stipulation of easy, effortless and practical interventions which facilitate in restoring the dignity; and prevention of worsening conditions of vegetative functions. Further, the therapist should be an emphatic listener as s/he attempts to communicate with individuals by empathizing with the feelings and meanings hidden behind their confused speech and behaviour. It is the emotional content of what is being said that is more important than the person's orientation with the present. Validation therapy promotes contentment, leads to positive affect and behavioural disturbance, produces positive effects and provides the individual with insight into external reality (Hitch 1994).

Reminiscence Therapy

It involves the discussion of past activities, events and experiences with another person or group of people. Revival of past experiences is the core feature of this therapy, especially life's happy events which are intensely there in the memory of the subject like wedding or birth of a child. This therapy can be applied in groups or with individuals. Evidence of significant impact was found to be little in cognitive improvement in one of our study however, after the therapy subject develops feeling of well-being. The application of reminiscence therapy significantly improves the behaviour, well-being, social interaction, self-care (O'Donovan 1993) and motivation (Gibson 1994).

To enhance health and well-being of the elderly there are some alternative non-pharmacological therapies which may play an important role. However, these therapies often lack evidences regarding their impact; thus, they need to be acknowledged and practiced.

Art Therapy

This therapy may be used as a treatment option for those elderly who have some previous (pre-morbid) interests in making drawings or craft. It may provide meaningful stimulation to the subject. A study carried out on patients with dementia (PwD) reports that it improves social interaction and levels of self-esteem (Killick and Allan 1999). Craft-related work as well as drawing and painting stimulates the degenerated brain. If some of the cognitive domains are intact and patients are being involved in such kinds of activities, chances of improvement in cognition will be always there. Such activities provide the patient an opportunity for self-expression and choice for choosing colours and themes for their creations; which also may be analysed further.

Music Therapy

Music therapy involves listening to music or singing. Studies report that people with dementia get benefitted from music therapy (Lord and Garner 1993). Patients get benefits from music, if they get involved in the activity such as singing or playing or listening. Studies report that music therapy helps in increasing the level of well-being; patient may have better social interaction and improvement in autobiographical memory, behaviour as well as agitation (Cohen-Mansfield 2000; Gerdner 2000).

Activity Therapy

Exercises, yoga, meditation, leisure, hobby, etc., related indefinite types of activities may be involved in this therapy. It is a formless group of recreation such as dance, sport and drama. It has been shown that physical exercise can have a number of health benefits for people with dementia.

Aromatherapy

Aromatherapy is one of the fastest growing fields amongst all complementary therapies (Burns et al. 2002). It is advantageous over other treatment options as its application is easy risk of adverse effects is almost negligible. It has a positive image and its use aids interaction while providing a sensory experience. The oil which are usually applied in aromatherapy improve behavioural symptoms; however, supportive studies to establish its significance are minimal.

Spirituality-as Non Pharmacological Intervention

Observing the limitations of the chemical model it is declared that life could be beyond molecules. According to many, including Swami Vivekananda, unselfish love for God as well as for HIS creations—human beings, flora and fauna, environment and all things around in this universe—is the hallmark of a spiritually aroused human being. An individual with spiritual support easily realizes that there are many more important things for long-term happiness and peace of mind than merely taking proper care of one's human form and making adequate provision for material comforts in life. Spiritual care/therapy is usually given in a one-to-one relationship, it is completely personal and makes no assumptions about individual's conviction or life orientation (Singh et al. 2014). Singh et al. (2014) further advocate that comprehensive multidimensional model that combines psychological, social, genetic and neurobiological factors, based on previous research and theory, is needed to guide future research in the area of spirituality. Integrated use of spiritual interventions enhancing individual resilience to stress and the mind–body approaches to stress reduction (e.g., meditation, yoga, mindfulness and Tai Chi) are likely to improve the overall functioning and well-being in older adults.

A study was carried out by the authors in the department on elderly caregivers with adjustment disorders and it was found that spiritual intervention had a positive impact. However, the data is yet to be published. Many individuals with spiritual practices emphasizes that it provides a feeling of contentment as it give calmness, happiness and feeling of emotional balance, peace and love to the elderly and also helps in healing traumatic conditions and gaining health. Again, such experiences need evidence-based documentation, which definitely help in improving the health and well-being of the elderly at large.

All such non-pharmacological therapeutic interventions have positive impact on health and well-being of elderly. Studies reveal that the burden of morbidity among the elderly is enormous; number and proportion of care providers is almost negligible (Tiwari and Pandey 2012). In such a situation, people who are interested in maintaining health and well-being of the elderly need to wake up and join their hands for the betterment of this segment of population. It will be worth mentioning here that there are a number of therapeutic interventions and the application of a combination of these interventions is found to be more result oriented (authors own experience). In managing the health and well-being of the elderly, person-centred approach is more acceptable; however, hardly much study has been conducted in India. Generally, combinations of these therapies are being provided by the professional to get positive, long lasting and significant changes. Few cases involving illiterate elderly with cognitive impairment, who were studied during the authors' post doctoral fellowship in the Department of Geriatric Mental Health (DGMH), are shared here.

Cases and Strategies for Improving Health and Wellbeing of Elderly with Dementia-Evidence Based Interventions

With funding support from Indian Council of Social Sciences Research (ICSSR) during 8 March 2013 to 8 March 2015 authors had an opportunity to carry out a post doctoral fellowship awarded study titled '*Developing Modules for Cognitive Enhancement for Illiterate Older Adults with Cognitive Deficits*'. Some of the case vignettes of this particular project are discussed

Case 1: Smt. DD, 72 years old, widowed mother of three sons and one daughter, living with her middle son and grandchildren since a period of about three years, became more forgetful. Further, she became irritable, agitated and suspicious and also started complaining to others that she didn't get food. She was gradually losing her ability to take care of her day-to-day activities. When she started complaining to everyone that she didn't get food she was brought in the department for consultation and treatment. Specific problems to be addressed, which were pointed out by the caregiver: • Forgetfulness • Irritability • Decrease in complains as it was embarrassing for the care giver and his wife On a detailed assessment by the DGMH team she was diagnosed as case of mild Alzheimer's Dementia (AD) Caregivers were taught to involve Smt. DV in one or other kind of activities of her interest so that she gets engaged They were also taught that the task given by them should be given by accounting her past skills and enjoyments and assist accordingly For remembrance of food intake caregivers were educated that whenever they give them one meal or breakfast keep the utensils there so that she had the remembrance of the same and take away the first meal/BF utensils when the second is to be served They were also taught that the environment of the family should be empathetic for her According to the primary caregiver of the patient DV's irritability and agitation was almost abolished as she was now made engaged with small domestic activities as per her earlier tests and now she was not getting irritated nor was complaining for food. The primary caregiver also shared his view that probably there was no need to provide medication as she was better on non-pharmacological management. However, he advocated that without consultation of the clinician he should not stop medication	**Case 2**: Mr. MB 61 years a married male living with his wife and children came to the department with chief complaints of forgetfulness. MB is a *feriwala* (street vendor) and only earning person in the family. He realized that forgetfulness was his major problem when he was unable to recall prices of the particular items which he sold On detailed assessment he was diagnosed as a case of mild cognitive impairment. The major solution for Mr. MB's problem was to provide some memory aid so that he could be able to perform his occupational duties properly. He was very much disturbed as he was the only earning member of the family and at times due to forgetfulness he became unable to sell his items or give it on less prices. The second problem with him that he was illiterate, therefore, unable to stick a price tag and read the same during his duty hours. A detailed discussion was carried out with him and his major problem was related with his occupation. He was suggested to purchase some rice papers and name them a particular amount and stick its pieces on the items, which are to be sold. Further, he was suggested to purchase a dairy or notepad and stick dummy of rupees and rice papers of different colours accordingly so that if any time he gets confused he may be able to identify the price of a particular colour Practical demonstration was given to him so that he may be able to recall the process This memory facilitation technique along with persistent follow-up enabled Mr. MB to execute his occupational work properly

(continued)

(continued)

Case 3:
Smt. GD living with her husband came with her son-in-law and daughter to the department with complaints of forgetfulness and suspiciousness. She had moderate dementia. Her daughter reported that though she enjoyed receiving friends and relatives, but often became agitated and angry when her father had visitors. The daughter also reported that she often became suspicious and started complaining that her belongings has been stolen by the maid, which often created chaos at home On detailed assessment it was found that initially Smt. GD was an active member of the house and most of the time she used to remain in the kitchen for making some breakfast or edible recipes for family members. Since her daughter-in-law came she took all the responsibilities and gradually she confined herself to her room. Initially nobody noticed, but within a span of three years her cognitive functions declined moderately It is a general principle that for helping anyone one should try to maintain his/her independence as much as possible. Known surroundings, regular and reassuring routine helps the subject in getting well. Unnecessary noise and too many visitors should be avoided. If the subject is embarrassed about his inability to do things, he should be reassured and encouraged. Humour may help in defusing tension. These interventions were provided to caregivers and they were able to manage the subject well For managing illiterate patients suffering from dementia, many other interventions as per patient's/caregiver's needs were provided which have shown beneficial impact. It is well recognized that during the course of illness, patients with dementia lose everyday skills and often become dependent on the care provider. The level of impairment varies from person to person. For maintaining the skills of dementia patients they should remain active. They should be assisted for continuing their previous activities as many as they can. Least required help should be offered to them so that their independence and dignity could be maintained

Some Guidelines for Maintaining Independence and Dignity of the Elderly Patient/Subject

• Daily care routines should be monitored, as these are opportunities for social interaction and physical stimulation
• Provide them with some task to stimulate and get them busy; however, their past skills and enjoyments should be taken into account. For instance, if one enjoys cooking her assistance in kitchen activities may be beneficial for her • One should be sensitive about the energy level of the subject so that s/he should not be burdened unduly. If the person doesn't remember things, rather than asking the person to try and remember, simply give the information. This will help in reducing anxiety and securing cooperation • During providing help the patient should get involved as much as possible. Assistance or help doesn't mean to take over the task from the patient • Support, appreciation and admiration make the patient more confident. Identify what the patient can and actually do and try to de-emphasize the lost skills

(continued)

(continued)

• Many times subject don't remember what they were told as their concentration is poor. Therefore, caregivers should give enough time and trial for performing a task; training is to be given just like a child and s/he should be encouraged and reinforced for positive actions
• Don't criticize the patient
• While providing care one should be mindful of one's own mental state. One should be careful for taking time to rest and relax. Looking after oneself during providing care is a sensitive skill of a caregiver
• If there is strong resistance to get help, the caregiver should take a break and return later
• Caregivers should also take training for skilful management of dementia patients. Study reports that proper understanding of prognosis and complications of interventions helps in avoiding unnecessary aggressive interventions (McCurry et al. 2009) and that reduces caregivers burden and depression as well as delays hospital admission (Brodaty and Donkin 2009).

Along with pharmacological interventions offering dialectic remedies, environmental modifications do wonder. There is a need between synchronization of nutrition (*ahar*), leisure (*vihar*) and thoughts (*vichar*) in proper order (Dalal and Misra 2006).

Some General Interventional Strategies to Improve Health and Well-Being of the Elderly

Maintaining health and well-being of the elderly can be improved only if we are able to provide proper psycho-social environment, economic and social security, and maintain the functional status, well-being and health of elderly. Optimal health is essential at any stage of life and so in old age. Optimal health for the elderly refers to (i) feeling free from disease, (ii) adequate functioning in the particular genetic and environmental condition, (iii) adequate familial and social support, and (iv) ability for continuous personal development. To attain these objectives we need to generate awareness regarding healthy lifestyle and can be achieved if the elderly adopt various healthcare strategies at primary, secondary and tertiary care levels.

Provide Primary, Secondary and Tertiary Care to the Elderly

It can be observed that to address the huge burden of health problems of the elderly, especially mental health, there is an immediate need to identify and involve primary (medical and para medical) and secondary (MD-psychiatry: providing provincial health care services) healthcare providers and give them training to equip geriatric mental health better. With this strategy, the cadre of primary and secondary healthcare providers will be available to make an early diagnosis and initiate treatment in a short period. At the same time, some minimum infrastructures (earmarking some of the existing beds) at least at the district headquarter levels with provisions of medicines to treat and manage the older adults may be made available for geriatric mental healthcare. Basic and elementary healthcare services for elderly in the community itself need to be ensured. Such type of healthcare initiatives and health programmes for the elderly need to be developed according to the ratio of the elderly population in a particular community. For tertiary level care, one full-fledged teaching and training department are to be established in each state to provide superspecialty care for geriatric mental health.

Develop Elderly-Friendly Environment

To maintain emotional state, coping and well-being of the elderly, we need to provide elderly-friendly environment. Their interaction with family and friends develops supportive environment. Engagement of the elderly in their past enjoyable activities may provide physical stimulation. A person who enjoyed cooking or cleaning like activities may be involved in monitoring these activities. Proper arrangements of light, hurdle-free places are to be provided to the elderly to make them more comfortable. If an elderly is not able to handle his/her day-to-day activities, assistance should be given without delay to make them feel relaxed.

Fabricate Better and Strong Individual, Family and Social Relationship

This will help the elderly to remain healthy. Family and society need to understand the emotional and psychological needs of the elderly. Intimate and close relationships are found to be more valuable in old age. Social and family involvement as well as dependency on others is enjoyed by the elderly. It provides a sense of self-efficacy and satisfies a sense of social worth. If the elderly feel himself/herself to be useful for the family, their well-being and mental health will definitely improve.

Provide Economic Protection

Paying capacity of the average Indian elderly is poor; in such a situation, they need a proper policy to maintain their financial status. Healthcare expenditure of the elderly needs to be identified and financial security need to be provided.

Conclusion

It is clearly indicated that the population of the elderly in India is increasing at a fast rate; managing and maintaining their health and well-being from a general perspective to disease level is a prudent issue. Elderly health and well-being may be enhanced by providing peaceful, quiet, composed and conflict-free environment. The government is taking initiatives in this direction by introducing new policies and plans, which will bring more help for the elderly. However, awareness in this population about their needs and rights may also be helpful in upgrading their health and well-being.

References

Abraha, I., Cruz-Jentoft, A., Soiza, R. L., O'Mahony, D., & Cherubini, A. (2015). Evidence of and recommendations for non-pharmacological interventions for common geriatric conditions: The SENATOR-ONTOP systematic review protocol. *BMJ Open,* 5, e007488. https://doi.org/10.1136/bmjopen-2014-007488.

Alam, M. (2000). Ageing in India: A country profile. *Bold, 10,* 5–22.

Brodaty, H., & Donkin, M. (2009). Family caregivers of people with dementia. *Dialogues in Clinical Neuroscience, 11*(2), 217–228.

Burns, A., Byrne, J., Ballard, C., & Holmes, C. (2002). Sensory stimulation in dementia. An effective option for managing behavioural problems. *BMJ, 325,* 1312–1313.

Busse, E. W. (1987). Primary and secondary aging. In G. L. Maddox, G. Roth, R. Atchley, et al. (Eds.), *The encyclopedia of aging* (pp. 5–34). New York: Springer.

Carey, J. R. (2003). Life span: A conceptual review. In J. R. Carey & S. Juljapurkar (Eds.), *Life span evolutionary, ecological and demographic perspectives: Population and development review—a supplement* (Vol. 24, p. 8). New York: Population Council.

Chadha, N. K., & John, V. W. (2003). Social support network among elderly in India. Methodological consideration and implications for rehabilitation. In P. V. Ramamurti & D. Jamuna (Eds.), *Handbook of Indian gerontology.* New Delhi: Serials Publications.

Chandramouli, C. (2013). Census of India 2011 Registrar General & Census Commissioner, India, Ministry of Home Affairs, August, 2013. Retrieved from October 6, 2013. census_2011_age_data-final-12-09-2013.

Cohen-Mansfield, J. (2000). Use of patient characteristics to determine non-pharmacologic interventions for Behavioural and Psychological Symptoms of dementia. *International Psychogeriatrics, 12*(suppl. 1), 373–380.

Dalal, A. K., & Misra, G. (2006). Psychology of health and well-being: Some emerging perspectives. *Psychological Studies, 2*(2–3), 1–33.

Das, S. K., et al. (2011). *Situation analysis of the elderly in India.* Retrieved June, 2011 from http://mospi.nic.in/mospi_new/upload/elderly_in_india.pdf.

Gerdner, L. (2000). Effects of Individualized versus Classical "Relaxation" Music on the Frequency of Agitation in Elderly Persons with Alzheimer's Disease and Related Disorders. *International Psychogeriatrics, 12,* 49–65.

Gibson, F. (1994). What can reminiscence contribute to people with Dementia? In J. Bornat (Ed.), *Reminiscence reviewed: Evaluations, achievements, perspectives* (pp. 46–60). Buckingham: Open University Press.

Glascock, A. P., & Feinman, S. L. (1980). A holocultural analysis of old age. *Comparative Social Research, 3,* 311–332.

Hitch, S. (1994). Cognitive therapy as a tool for the caring elderly confused person. *Journal of Clinical Nursing, 3,* 49–55.

Ingle, G. K., & Nath, A. (2008). Geriatric health in India: Concerns and solutions. *Indian Journal of Community Medicine, 33,* 214–218.

James, K. S., & Sathyanarayana, K. M. (2011). Demographic change, age structure transition and ageing in India: Issues and challenges. *Yojana- A development monthly, 55*, 28–31.

Jamuna, D. (1994). Psychological and social correlates of successful ageing among the Indian elderly women. *Indian Journal of Gerontology, 8*(1&2), 29–36.

Killick, J., & Allan, K. (1999). The arts in dementia care: Tapping a rich resource. *Journal of Dementia Care, 7,* 35–38.

Lord, T. R., & Garner, J. E. (1993). Effects of music on Alzheimer Patients. *Perceptual and Motor Skills, 76*, 451–455.

McCurry, S. M., Gibbons, L. E., Logsdon, R. G., Vitiello, M. V., & Teri, L. (2009). Insomnia in caregivers of persons with dementia: Who is at risk and what can be done about it? *Sleep Medicine Clinics, 4*(4), 519–526.

Misra, G. (2010). Introduction. In G. Misra (Ed.), *Psychology in India: Clinical and health psychology* (Vol. 3). Delhi: ICSSR.

Naci, H., & Ioannidis, J. P. (2013). Comparative effectiveness of exercise and drug interventions on mortality outcomes: Metaepidemiological study. *BMJ, 347,* f5577. https://doi.org/10.1136/bmj.f5577.

O'Donovan, S. (1993). The memory lingers on. *Elderly Care, 5,* 27–31.

Prakash, R., Chaudary, S. K., & Singh, U. (2004). A study of morbidity pattern among geriatric population in the urban area of Udaipur, Rajastan. *Indian Journal of Community Medicine, 119,* 35–40.

Rajan, S. I. (2003). Demography of ageing. In A. B. Dey (Ed.), *Ageing in India: Situation analysis and planning for the future*. Ministry of Health and family Welfare-Government of India & World Health Organization.

Ramamurti, P. V., & Jamuna, D. (2010). Gero psychology in India. In G. Misra (Ed.), *Psychology in India: Clinical and health psychology* (Vol. 3). Delhi: ICSSR.

Rao, V. A. (1993). Psychiatry of old age in India. *International Review of Psychiatry, 5,* 165–170.

Rao, V. A. (2001). The world of the elderlies (preventive geriatrcis). *Annals of the National Academy of Medical Sciences (India), 37*(1&2), 11–17.

Singh, B., Singh, I., & Pandey, N. M. (2014). Spirituality and geriatric mental health. In S. C. Tiwari & N. M. Pandey (Eds.), *Geriatric mental health at a glance*. New Delhi: Ahuja Publishers.

Spar, J. E., & Rue, A. L. (Eds.). (2009). *Clinical manual of geriatric psychiatry*. American Psychological Publications.

Taylor, R. S., Sagar, V. A., Davies, E. J., Davies, E. J., Briscoe, S., Coats, A. J., et al. (2014). Exercise-based rehabilitation for heart failure. *Cochrane Database System Review, 4*, CD003331. https://doi.org/10.1002/14651858.cd003331.

Tiwari, S. C. (2000). Geriatric psychiatric morbidity in rural Northern India: implications for the future. *International Psycho-geriatrics, 12*(1), 35–48.

Tiwari, S. C., & Pandey, N. M. (2014). Geriatric mental health in India. In S. C. Tiwari & N. M. Pandey (Eds.), *Geriatric mental health at a glance*. New Delhi: Ahuja Publishers.

Tiwari, S. C., & Pandey, N. M. (2012). Status and requirements of geriatric mental health in India: An evidence based commentary. *Indian Journal of Psychiatry, 54,* 8–14.

Tiwari, S. C., Srivastava, G., Tripathi, R. K., & Pandey, N. M. (2013). Prevalence of psychiatric morbidity amongst the community dwelling rural older adults in Northern India. *The Indian Journal of Medical Research, 138,* 504–514.

Tiwari, S. C., Tripathi, R. K., Kumar, A., Kar, A. M., Singh, R., Kohli, V. K., et al. (2014). Prevalence of psychiatric morbidity amongst urban elderlies: Lucknow elderly study. *Indian Journal of Psychiatry, 56,* 154–160.

Chapter 12
Alternative Interventions for Fortifying Health of the Indian Elderly

Shyodan Singh and Indiwar Misra

With ever-changing demographic scenario the number and proportion of the elderly is increasing at a fast rate. In the present scenario worldwide life expectancy at birth has increased and professionals related to this field are trying to understand the elderly and the process of ageing. Indeed, the study related to ageing and age-related changes is becoming an area of interest for many namely, health professionals, social scientists, academicians, policymakers, including common man. As an integral process of life, ageing refers to the changes in the individual across the life span, especially during the post maturation phase of development. In a country like India where size of population of the elderly is significantly increasing, the need to find out the opportunities and challenges pertaining to this stage of life is urgently required. With advancing age, people become mature, knowledgeable and experienced but due to increased physical, psychological and social vulnerability, they also require various types of interventions. This age group of population requires fairly good amount of resources to remain healthy. This generates a need to modulate the environment as well as evolve strategic ways to enable them to feel relaxed, comfortable, satisfied and happy. The social scientists, including psychologists are trying hard in this direction by identifying, categorizing and labelling specific problems and then intervening to reduce their impact. Against this backdrop, this chapter draws attention to some alternative interventions which fortify and strengthen the well-being and quality of life of the aged so that they may lead a dignified life.

S. Singh (✉)
Department of Psychology, Zakir Husain College, University of Delhi,
New Delhi, Delhi, India
e-mail: shyodansingh@gmail.com

I. Misra
Department of Psychology, B.R. Ambedkar College, University of Delhi,
New Delhi, Delhi, India

G. Misra (ed.), *Psychosocial Interventions for Health and Well-Being*,
https://doi.org/10.1007/978-81-322-3782-2_12

In Indian culture, there was a noble segregation and demarcation of the stages of life, which was propounded by Manu (Prabhu 1954). According to Manu, 'an individual's life span is divided into four stages or *Asramas* with specific duties and responsibilities for each stage. These were (1) *Brahmacharya asrama* (the celibate educational phase 0–25 years), (2) *Grihastha asrama* (the Family phase 25–50 years), (3) *Vanaprastha asrama* (the disengagement phase 50–75 years) and (4) *Sanyasa asrama* (the renunciation phase, 75+). The Vanaprastha asrama marks the beginnings of old age while the last one, sanyasa, refers to the last stage of life. During vanaprastha asrama one gradually disengages the self from worldly pursuits of life severing one's emotional and possessive bonds to prepare for practicing renunciation and leading the life of an ascetic, ready to give up the physical body. This system was meant to maintain the discipline, peace and harmony in family and society and each of the stages was intended to prepare for the next (Tiwari and Pandey 2012). Vanaprastha and sanyasa were basically related to old age and few of those individuals who were not interested in grihastha activities had opportunity to move from brahmacharya to vanaprastha or sanyasa. The basic training for vanaprastha was to dedicate oneself in intellectual activities and/meditation with a disciplined life including self-control, pursuing altruism for purposes of charity. The elderly persons used to be the key figures in a family set-up. No one denied their presence and they lived a dignified life. However, with many changes in society and environment, this segment of population began to face a number of challenges.

While need for special care of the aged has been recognized the complexity of ageing is often missed out. Ageing is not a singular process. Rather, it consists of at least three distinct aspects i.e. primary, secondary and tertiary ageing (Birren and Cunningham 1985). Primary ageing is normal, disease-free-development during adulthood. Secondary ageing is a series of developmental changes that are related to disease, lifestyle and other environmentally induced changes. Finally, tertiary ageing refers to the rapid losses that occur shortly before death. The ageing process is of course a biological reality which has its own dynamics, largely beyond human control. The cut-off age of 60–65, roughly equivalent to retirement ages in most countries, is said to be the beginning of old age.

With advancing age, people become more susceptible to chronic diseases, physical disabilities and mental incapacities. Due to deteriorating physiological conditions, the body becomes more prone to illness. The illnesses of the elderly are multiple and chronic in nature such as arthritis, rheumatism, high blood pressure and heart problems. Some of the health problems of the elderly can be attributed to the mindset as well. The stereotypical idea that 'old age is an age of ailments and physical infirmities' is deeply rooted in the Indian mind and many of the sufferings and physical troubles which are curable are accepted as natural and inevitable by the elderly.

With regard to the health problems of the elderly of different socioeconomic strata, it has been reported (Siva Raju 2000) that while the elderly from a poor socioeconomic background largely described their health problems on the basis of easily identifiable symptoms such as chest pain, shortness of breath, prolonged cough, breathlessness/asthma, eye problems, difficulty in movements, tiredness and teeth problems, the upper class elderly, in view of their greater knowledge of illnesses, mentioned about ailments like blood pressure, heart attacks and diabetes largely diagnosed through clinical examination. In a study by Mutharayappa and Bhat (2008) NFHS-2 data were analysed to examine the type of lifestyle adopted by the elderly and its effects on their health conditions. The survey revealed that lifestyle adversely affects health and increases morbidity conditions among the elderly. Lifestyle habits such as alcohol consumption, regular smoking and tobacco chewing have adverse effects on one's ability to resist diseases. The needs and problems of the elderly vary significantly according to their age, socioeconomic status, health, living conditions and other background characteristics. As people live longer and into much advanced age (say 80 years and over), they deserve more intensive and long-term care.

With so many convolutions in the familial, societal and cultural milieu old age is emerging as a complex issue that needs immediate attention and care. Because of better health facilities life span has increased and the typical socio-economic conditions like poverty, breaking up of the joint family system and care giving are posing many challenges. Thus, while this increasing number of the elderly is attributed to demographic transition, their deteriorating condition is primarily an outcome of the fast eroding traditional family system in the wake of modernization, migration and urbanization.

The image of ageing has always been overshadowed by negative attitudinal and behavioural characteristics which arouse a sense of fear of growing old. With no exception to India, demographic analyses reveal that the aged population in the world constitutes a significant sub-group within the population. They are becoming one of the important segments of the population pyramid. In spite of the large population with tremendous impact on the nation, research efforts on the aged in India are comparatively insignificant. The Indian research efforts are yet to make their presence felt (Easwaramoorthy and Chadha 1997). It is also observed that only scanty information is available about the situation of the elderly in the different strata of society. Very few studies have been done on the needs and problems of the elderly in rural settings, widowed and widowers, or even about the relatively better off sections of the society (Desai 1988; Dhillon and Singh 2005; Singh 2006). Recently, Singh and Chao (2016) have reported that purpose in life, social support and leisure activities positively contributed to health enhancement of the elderly. This implies that the social class background plays a key role in determining health and well-being.

More efforts need to be undertaken as the existing work is not adequate enough to identify and determine the real picture of the aged. It has been observed (e g., Bose and Gangrade 1988) that there is an urgency to evaluate the needs of the aged for a comprehensive investigation of the elderly people in India. The Census data of India 2011 show that there were 103 million elderly in India, i.e. 8.5% of the total population, up from 77 million in 2001 (see Table 12.1). The number of the elderly in India is expected to increase three-fold to 298 million in 2051, accounting for a little over 17% of the total population. The population aged 70+ has remarkably

Table 12.1 Number and proportion of elderly in India (the estimates and projections)

Age group	1961	2001	2011	2021	2031	2041	2051
Population of elderly (millions)							
60+	25	77	103	132	184	233	298
70+	9	29	39	52	75	104	131
80+	2	8	11	16	20	29	41
Proportion of elderly in the population							
60+	5.6	7.5	8.5	9.7	12.1	14.0	16.6
70+	2.0	2.9	3.2	3.8	4.9	6.3	7.3
80+	0.6	0.8	0.9	1.2	1.3	1.7	2.3
Sex ratio of the elderly population							
60+	103	100	97	102	105	102	
70+	99	108	103	100	108	111	
80+	105	104	114	106	104	115	

Source Censuses of India (+projections), Government of India

increased from 9 million in 1961 to 29 million in 2001 and 43 million in 2011. The share of people aged 70+ in the total population increased from 2% in 1961 to 4% in 2011. The rapid growth in the proportion of the elderly within the total population will continue to grow from 2021 to 2051.

Between 1961 and 2011, the population aged 60+ nearly quadrupled. From 2011 to 2014, it is expected that the share of the population aged 60+ will increase by about 2% every 10 years. The share of the population aged 70+ also increased from 2.0 to 3.6% from 1961 to 2011, and the population share of persons aged 70+ is projected to increase by about 1% by 2031, and then 1% every 10 years up to 2051.

The sex ratio (number of females per 100 males) of the elderly population in India is in favour of females, just as in other parts of the world. Women comprise a majority of this population because female life expectancy is higher. The variation in the sex ratio is small for younger people, but among people aged 70+ and 80+, the sex ratio is expected to continue to increase between 2011 and 2051.

Based on the current rate of change, the 60+ age group is projected to outnumber the age group 0–14 soon after 2050 when the percentage of the child population and the population of the elderly will be the same at about 19%.

The elderly people confront a variety of physical, biological, psychological and social changes which make this stage of life as the most vulnerable stage. The majority of the ageing-related researches focus more on epidemiology, prevalence and the causes of various diseases, disabilities and death. Some of the researchers started working on assessments and evaluation along with strategic interventions to modify and improve the well-being and quality of life of the elderly. Nowadays, a group of professionals are involved in improving and promoting the health of the elderly. This is required for healthy or successful ageing. Recently, research has delivered promising data on the strategies that might alter the course of typical ageing among people with psychiatric disorders, which seem to be associated with accelerated ageing. It is important to note that there is no consensus definition of successful aging. As such, there is no standard outcome upon which the effectiveness of successful aging strategies could be uniformly gauged. The definitions of successful aging vary in its components (e.g. freedom from disability, social engagement), the nature of measurement (e.g. subjective, objective) and the criteria through which 'success' is determined (e.g. normative, impressionistic).

Based on an analysis of diverse views, it seems reasonable that we may focus on 'successful ageing strategy' as a potentially modifiable characteristic or intervention that is intended to enhance the functioning of older adults who could be characterized as aging normally. We shall therefore focus on some of the established interventions, such as physical activity, cognitive training and nutrition/dietary interventions. In addition, we shall also discuss work in emerging interventions, such as complementary and alternative therapies, social interventions, and those focused on enhancing positive psychological traits.

While talking about interventions we need to realize that the growing number of the elderly places increasing demands on the public health system and on medical and social services. The needs of the elderly are distinctive and mostly relate to their health, comfortable and dignified living, psychological well-being (including recreation and social networking), meaningful occupation (with or without economic gains) and security aspects. As Singh (2008) has shown the experienced stress, social support and physical ailments significantly contribute to the enhancement of adjustment of women retirees. These results seem to suggest that social support from colleagues, friends and family enhance both physical and mental health which in turn buffers the effect of experienced stress and thereby promotes better adjustment.

Older persons, therefore, need much more than just medical care, which thus needs an interdisciplinary approach integrating medicine with other functions. These intervention programmes can help the elderly to lead a better life.

Social Support Intervention

Social support is one of the most important intervention programmes which not only enhances the health of the elderly but also can get rid them of several kinds of physical diseases. A social support system is a pattern of continuous or intermittent ties and interchanges of mutual assistance that plays a significant role in maintaining the psychological, social and physical integrity of the individual over time. For it to function, consistency and availability of supporting relationships or resources are required. Both informal and formal activities as well as personal support services that enable older people to remain independent are taken into account. A social support system enables older people to fulfil three needs: socialization, carrying out the task of daily living and personal assistance during time of crisis. Social support is provided by the kin, friends and neighbours. It is precisely these significant others with whom older people have the most frequent interaction, both instrumentally and effectively, and who compose the broad basis of social support system. Yahaya et al. (2013) found that social support especially from non-family member is a significant contributor towards the psychological well-being among older women. There are three distinct key sources of social support, each with a different role to play: children and other relatives, close friends or intimates and neighbours. Most important kind of assistance providers are the children, particularly in situations where there is no spouse at home. Social support motivates the elderly to go on living and not feel being left unattended and unappreciated. Stephens et al. (2011) found that social network reduces loneliness, and consequently enhances mental and physical health of the elderly. Social support provides social security and alleviates stress in crowded residential colonies (Rao 2000; Singh 1993; Sinha 1999). It has implications for formal and informal relations (Kumar 2003; Phillips 1994; Ushasree 2000; Willigen and Chadha 2003) and social networks help in reducing the feeling of well-being and functional competence (Umadevi 1991). Social support interventions could be focused on facilitating long-distance family relationships through newer gadgets of communication technology. This type of intervention is valuable for institutionalized or lonely/isolated elderly who may have very few family contacts. The use of video phones for the family elder was effectively demonstrated in a study by Mickus and Luz (2002) with positive results. The elderly can use mobiles, laptops and computer to talk with family and friends and vice versa. Now, there are different kinds of apps like Skype, Whatsapp, Facebook etc., which can also be used to provide social support for the elderly. Social support intervention can not only reduce loneliness and stress but can enhance the health and well-being of the elderly.

Yoga and Exercise Intervention

Departing from the traditional idea that late adulthood and old age necessarily require disengagement it is found that the elderly need active engagement which is not only about social networking but also about their active connections with the people and surrounding environment. For intellectual and physical fitness of the elderly, Indian cultural context offers many resources. Various types of meditation and yogic practices are available. There is empirical evidence on the effects of transcendental and other kinds of meditation (e.g. Preksha, Vipasana, Sudarshan Kriya) have beneficial effects on mental health and intellectual functioning (Dhar 1997; Ramamurti and Jamuna 1992; Rastogi 1996; Umadevi 2002). In addition, spirituality is also considered as a significant contributor towards mental health and well-being of the elderly. Recent research has shown that yogic meditation and physical activity practices can positively impact the body in many ways, including help to regulate blood glucose levels and keeping the cardiovascular system healthy. It has been shown to have important psychological benefits, as the practice of yoga could help to increase alertness and positive feelings, and decrease negative feelings of aggression, depression and anxiety (Amaranath et al. 2016; DeBruin et al. 2017; Danhauer et al. 2017). The yoga session could include: physical activity, relaxation, regulated breathing exercises and meditation.

Practicing yoga is also a major way to take preventive care of the bone health of the elderly. Bone density naturally decreases with age, but yoga can help to maintain their bones strong and healthy. The pain of arthritis is also managed through yoga. Hypertension can lead to a multitude of health complications if gone untreated, and it is a condition that develops with increasing age. Luckily, yoga helps to control it. Scientists have found that regular yoga practice reduces the diastolic blood pressure. Yoga exercises the body without putting too much pressure on the cardiovascular system, which is exactly what a person with high blood pressure needs. Practicing meditation and *pranayama* can also be highly beneficial. The traditional *asanas* deal with posture and developing self-purification through integration of the functioning of the body and mind. Hatha yoga is an old system that includes the practice of asanas and pranayama (breathing exercise) which help bring peace to the mind and body, preparing the body for deeper spiritual practices such as meditation. Yoga provides strengthening of the body parts of the elderly who may not be keen on exercises like lifting weights. The deep breathing exercises performed in yoga supply more oxygen to the blood, which keeps the body's organs healthy and functioning at an optimal state. Practicing yoga lowers cortisol level in the brain and activates the parasympathetic nervous system. These chemical changes make people less anxious and at ease creating a happier state of mind. The positive and relaxed feelings are also responsible for better sleep quality in the elderly because of the reduced tension in the body as well as relief of pain. The elderly can always benefit from some form of daily movement, but as the age advances, the challenges associated with high impact forms of exercise make things more difficult. Thus, yoga provides a safer way to get moving and stay active. Some form of physical activity like evening and morning walk are important for the elderly to keep them fit and active. Regular physical activity can minimize the physiological effects of ageing and increase active life expectancy by limiting the development and progression of chronic diseases and disabling conditions (Chodzko-Zajko et al. 2009). Dubey and Choyal (2012) also emphasized on the importance of physical activities and highlight its effect on the health of the elderly. Physical activities promote health and well-being and reduce the fear of death. Yoga and physical activity are a means which provide people with a sense of identity and personal autonomy, adds meaning to individual and community life, and encourages personal growth and self-expression (Van der Pas and Koopman-Boyden 2007).

Community Intervention

It is now well accepted that programmes aimed at prevention of illness and promotion of health and well-being of the elderly must be based on an understanding of traditions, belief systems, patterns of family and community interactions and other similar resources. Community interventions need to be planned to improve the psychological conditions of the elderly in India. Community can provide memory interventions which are needed and may be beneficial to the elderly (Lalitha and Jamuna 2004a, b; Verma and Pershad 1996). Culturally relevant activities aiming towards socioeconomic and psychological empowerment of the elderly through senior clubs, forming a volunteer force and development of neighbourhood network groups need to be planned to occupy the elderly meaningfully. Counselling at community centres for the elderly on how to accept and adjust with the concept of growing old and get social support could reduce health and well-being-related problems. Further, this could consist of creating self-awareness, assisting the elderly to set new goals and find a purpose and meaning in life, encouraging them to plan and involve them in physical activities, making a realistic appraisal of themselves and their problems and help them to get rid of their irrational beliefs. Therefore, the important steps in community interventions to improve the health status of the elderly is to promote greater awareness and activities of healthful practices, not only among the elderly but also with respect to the caregivers and the family of the elderly with whom the elderly stay (Jamuna and Ramamurti 2000; Jamuna 2004; Ramamurti 2004; Reddy and Ramamurti 1995; Reddy 1996a, b; Savita and Darshan 1999; Shah 2004; Shah and Prabhakar 1996).

Spirituality and Religious Intervention

Spirituality and religion are important constructs in the lives of elderly (Taylor et al. 2007). For instance, in the study of Newport (2006) 72% elderly had reported that religion is very important in their lives. This represents the highest percentage reported by any of the age groups surveyed by the Gallup organization (Newport 2006). Spiritual beliefs and practices often play a central role in helping older adults to navigate life's challenges (Barusch 1999; Cabassa 2007; Lawrence et al. 2006). Research has associated spirituality with health and wellness (Koenig et al. 2001; Vink et al. 2008), life satisfaction (Yoon and Lee 2007) and self-esteem (Keyes and Reitzes 2007). Similarly, spirituality has been linked with the ability to cope with a variety of issues, including adversity (Barusch 1999), anxiety (Rajagopal et al. 2002), depression (Koenig 2007), fear of falling (Zhang et al. 2006), HIV (Vance 2006), vision loss (Brennan 2002) and lifetime trauma (Krause 2009). In short, empirical research suggests that spirituality typically provides strength to the lives of older adults.

The concern for sacred domains of health and well-being of the elderly however, has been a relatively overlooked topic in gerontology. Some authors, of late, have emphasized that at least some segments of the population are eager for health behaviour change approaches that are based on or are at least consistent with their religious and spiritual beliefs (Smith 2001). Like health, religion and spirituality are complex and multidimensional concepts in gerontology. Religion is viewed as 'denominational, external, cognitive, behavioural, ritualistic and public' while spirituality as 'universal, internal, affective, spontaneous and private' (Richards and Bergin 1997). Viewed in this way, religion is an organized social entity and can be seen primarily as the external manifestation of spiritual experience. Spirituality for some is an attribute of the individual, and pertains to his/her private and affective experiences. Further, various investigators agree that these concepts are probably, but not always, interrelated and often are used in an interchangeable manner. Sharma (2004) examined the efficacy and the complementary nature of certain religious/spiritual interventions (meditation, prayer, and service—volunteering) for health and well-being. Though an essential part of the oriental traditions (various forms of Hinduism, Buddhism, Sufi systems), meditation may exist in religious/ spiritual forms or even in a non-religious form (e.g. Transcendental Meditation: TM). Meditation as a primary intervention variable is observed not only as a relief from suffering, but also as providing power over thinking and emotions not by repressive self-control but by enhanced self-understanding and self-acceptance (e.g., Aruna 1998; Bhawuk 2000; Jain 2003; Kiran Kumar and Raj 1999; Khurana 1996; Sridevi and Krishna Rao 1996; Kapur 2008; Sharma 2004; Taylor et al. 2007).

Healing (recovery) is also seen as a spiritual experience involving an inner sense of well-being, balance, harmony and peace (Anand et al. 2001; Taylor 1997). A healing narrative of middle-aged women, with a major life crisis, was generated by Anand (2004). The process by which those women worked through their emotional pain was identified. It was observed that a progress in healing culminated in self-transformation. Moreover, some practitioners also favour the use of meditation as an adjunct to conventional psychotherapy including psychoanalysis. For example, Kakar (2003) analysed the theory and practice of healing in Eastern (Oriental) spiritual traditions. He observed that the Eastern healing discourse (e.g., meditative practices) goes considerably beyond most traditional psychoanalytic formulation on the nature of empathy in analytic situation. In view of this, Kakar (2003) argues for a place of meditative practice in psychoanalytic education and practice. Prayer is an inherently spiritual or religious activity, and is another self-help health-enhancing activity. Richards and Bergin (1997) cited preliminary evidence suggesting that different forms of prayer (for oneself, others, and for all) are associated with outcome variables like life satisfaction and overall well-being. Anajana and Raju (2002) found that the recitation of Bhagavad Gita (a prayer) contributes positively to personality functioning and quality of life. However, the usefulness of prayer either as an independent intervention or as an adjunct to a therapy remains almost unexplored. Further, service or volunteering can have religious/spiritual or non-religious forms. It can also be an individual or a collective/community volunteerism. Unselfish actions inspired by religion commonly aim to benefit specific individuals, the community as a whole or both (Sinha 1984). Self-less service to others is a way to transcend the egoistic desires promoted by today's consumer-bound culture and can be a predictor of positive health and well-being. Unfortunately, no study has examined service or volunteerism as a significant disease prevention or health promotion variable. Sharma (2004) has argued that meditation, prayer and service have a complementary relationship. Together these interventions can cultivate positive emotions that have undoing effects on negative emotions, and enhance physical and mental health through more adaptive coping (see also Pargament 1997; Smith 2001).

Technological Intervention

Modern scientific and technological advancements have opened up new possibilities for elderly care to support comfortable and dignified living for them. Capabilities of modern technologies coupled with traditional knowledge systems play a vital role in utilizing vast resources for the benefit of the elderly at affordable costs. Many healthcare enterprises are organizing themselves for developing therapeutics by modifying the process of ageing and age-related diseases. The concept of community living is gaining acceptance in India, at least in urban areas where affordability is improving. Technology can play a vital role in such community living spaces. Even existing old age homes, day care centres, etc., can be retrofitted or remodelled with technological equipment. Application of technology to the field of recreation and entertainment is seen as an emerging field which has utility both in urban and rural areas.

Technology Intervention for Elderly (TIE) programme provides technological solutions with a multidisciplinary approach to resolve the problems and improve quality of life of the elderly population. It also aims to provide individual autonomy and independence to persons with disability through holistic development by creating enabling environment for their empowerment through application of science and technology. The department of science and technology (DST) National Policy on Older People (NPOP), DST under its Science and Society Programme has recently launched a new programme on 'Technology Initiative for Disabled and Elderly (TIDE)' to create an enabling environment for the elderly. The TIDE programme has evolved through a series of consultations involving various stakeholders (geriatric specialists, designers, architects, social scientists, senior citizens, etc.). Five thematic workshops were organized to deliberate on specific themes. Under this innovative programme, project proposals are encouraged conceptualization, research and development for finding technological solutions to address the problems faced by the elderly population and to improve their quality of life. Prestigious academic and research institutions (AIIMS, IITs, IISc, SPA, AIIPMR, National Institute of Social Defence) and NGOs (HelpAge India) are actively associated with the TIDE programme.

In TIDE, devices mainly work on the main principle of stimulation to the tactile sense. In this method, individuals are conditioned to perform basic activities in a skill training set-up independently. Same procedure was established for generalization to the home environment. In particular assistive technology is very important. It refers to any equipment or system that assists people who have difficulties, due to age or disability, in carrying out everyday activities. It covers simple items such as walking sticks, bath seats and grab rails, as well as electro-mechanical equipment (e.g. powered wheelchairs), electronic aids (e.g. digital hearing aids and environmental controls), or equipment used by care givers such as lifting aids.

The success of technological applications for the elderly depends on policies and programmes that promote healthy and active ageing. The humane benefits that these technologies promise will certainly be promoted by an elder-care system which accepts new technologies which promote comfort and efficacy for the elderly.

Conclusion

Interventions to promote health and well-being of the elderly are now being widely implemented and recommended to enhance their quality of life. Social support, yoga and physical activity, community and use of technology extend support to the elderly so that they may lead an active life. This can additionally be augmented through elderly participation in physical and social activities like social functions, evening and morning walks, where the elderly can make friends who provide social support when they are in stress, lonely or developing a negative attitude towards death. Engaging in social activities or residence welfare societies provide them self-esteem and love which could enhance resilience and optimism and help the elderly to remain active and healthy. Practice of yoga and regular exercise can reduce cardiovascular and mortality, lower blood pressure and increase metabolism of carbohydrates and fats, as well as provide a range of psychological benefits such as improved self-esteem, positive mood states, reduced life stress, anxiety and depression. The community centre can also play a vital role in counselling and encouraging the elderly to remain alive, active and have a meaningful life. Ageing is an inevitable process and as a person gets old, physical and mental compositions need proper and vigilant attention, care and management. For strengthening and fortifying their health status, participation or involvement in familial and social gathering, religious and spiritual activities and awareness with the surroundings and use of gadgets would be effective. Therefore, the families, caregivers and people involved in the welfare of aging population should develop such intervention plans which can give them a better, safe and secured life.

References

Amaranath, B., Nagendra, H. R., & Deshpande, S. (2016). Effect of integrated Yoga module on positive and negative emotions in Home Guards in Bengaluru: A wait list randomized control trial. *International Journal of Yoga, 9,* 35–43.

Anand, J. (2004). Working through emotional pain: A narrative study of healing process. *Psychological Studies, 49,* 185–192.

Anand, J., Srivastava, A., & Dalal, A. K. (2001). Where suffering ends and healing begins. *Psychological Studies, 46,* 114–126.

Anjana, R., & Raju, S. (2002). Psychological functioning of Bhagavad Gita reciters. *Psychological Studies, 47,* 159–161.

Aruna, G. (1998). Mental health in being-becoming a paradox: JidduKrishnamurthi. *Behavioural Medicine Journal, 1,* 10–13.

Barusch, A. S. (1999). Religion, adversity and age: Religious experiences of low-income elderly women. *Journal of Sociology and Social Welfare, 26,* 125–142.

Bhawuk, D. P. S. (2000). Who attains peace? An Indian model of personal harmony. In J. Prakash & G. Misra (Eds.), *Towards a culturally relevant psychology* (pp. 40–48). Agra: Agra Psychological Research Cell.

Birren, J. E., & Cunningham, W. (1985). Research on the psychology of aging: Principles, concepts and theory. In J. E. Birren & K. W. Schaie (Eds.), *Handbook of the psychology of aging* (pp. 3–34). New York: Van Nostrand.

Bose, A. B., & Gangrade, K. D. (Eds.). (1988). *The aging in India: Problems and potentials.* New Delhi: Abhinav Publications.

Brennan, M. (2002). Spirituality and psychosocial development in middle-age and older adults with vision loss. *Journal of Adult Development, 9,* 31–46.

Cabassa, L. J. (2007). Latino immigrant men's perceptions of depression and attitudes toward help seeking. *Hispanic Journal of Behavioral Sciences, 29,* 492–509.

Chodzko-Zajko, W., Schwingel, A., & Park, C. H. (2009). Successful aging: The role of physical activity. *American Journal of Lifestyle Medicine, 3,* 20–28.

Danhauer, S. C., Addington, E. L., Sohl, S. J., Chaoul, A., & Cohen, L. (2017). Review of yoga therapy during cancer treatment. *Supportive Care in Cancer, 25,* 1357–1372.

DeBruin, E., Formsma, A. R., Frijstein, G., & Bogels, S. M. (2017). Mindful to work: Effects of combined physical exercise, yoga and mindfulness meditation for stress relieve in employees. *Mindfulness, 8,* 204–217.

Desai, K. G. (1988). The aged and the society. In A. B. Bose & K. D. Gangrade (Eds.), *The aged in India: Problems and potentialities.* New Delhi: Abhinav Publication.

Dhar, H. L. (1997). Health and ageing. *Indian Journal of Medical Sciences, 51,* 373–377.

Dhillon, P. K., & Singh, S. (2005). Adjustment of women retirees: Role of health, social support, leisure activities, stress level and demographic variables. *Journal of Personality and Clinical Studies, 21,* 61–70.

Dubey, S., & Choyal, T. (2012). Liesue: Effect on health ageing. *Indian Journal of Gerontology, 26,* 414–423.

Easwaramoorthy, M., & Chadha, N. K. (1997). Quality of life of the elderly in Tamil Nadu. In N. K. Chadha (Ed.), *Aging and the aged: Challenges before Indian gerontology.* New Delhi: Friends Publications.

Jain, S. (2003). Effect of preksha meditation on anxiety and operational efficiency of young convicts. *Psychological Studies, 48,* 82–87.

Jamuna, D. (2004). The statics and dynamics of elder care in the Indian context. In P. V. Ramamurti & D. Jamuna (Eds.), *Handbook on Indian gerontology* (pp. 208–242). New Delhi: Serial Publications.

Jamuna, D., & Ramamurti, P. V. (2000). Burnout among the caregivers of disabled elderly: Effect of intervention. *Psychological Studies, 45,* 150–155.

Kakar, S. (2003). Psychoanalysis and eastern spiritual healing traditions. *Journal of Analytical Psychology, 48,* 659–678.

Kapur, R. L. (2008). *Another way to live.* New Delhi: Penguin.

Keyes, C. L. M., & Reitzes, D. C. (2007). The role of religious identity in the mental health of older working and retired adults. *Aging and Mental Health, 11,* 434–443.

Khurana, A. (1996). *Effect of vipassana meditation on quality of life of undertrials.* Paper presented at national seminar "Quality of life in changing socio-cultural milieu" held at University of Delhi, South Campus, New Delhi, April 12–13.

Kiran Kumar, S. K., & Raj, A. (1999). Ahamkara and ego functions among meditators and normals. *Journal of Indian Psychology, 17,* 46–56.

Koenig, H. G. (2007). Religion and depression in older medical inpatients. *American Journal of Geriatric Psychiatry, 15,* 282–291.

Koenig, H. G., McCullough, M. E., & Larson, D. B. (2001). *Handbook of religion and health.* New York: Oxford University Press.

Krause, N. (2009). Lifetime trauma, prayer, and psychological distress in late life. *International Journal for the Psychology of Religion, 19,* 55–72.

Kumar, S. V. (2003). Economics, health and social networks. In P.S. Liebig & S. I. Rajan (Eds.), *An aging India: Perspectives, prospects and policies.* New York: The Haworth Press.

Lalitha, K., & Jamuna, D. (2004a). Memory status in the Indian elderly. In P. V. Ramamurti & D. Jamuna (Eds.), *Handbook on Indian gerontology* (pp. 328–368). New Delhi: Serial Publications.

Lalitha, K., & Jamuna, D. (2004b). Memory status in the elderly and its correlates: An intervention study. *Indian Journal of Gerontology, 18,* 151–158.

Lawrence, V., Banerjee, S., Bhugra, D., Sangha, K., Turner, S., & Murray, J. (2006). Coping with depression in later life: A qualitative study of help-seeking in three ethnic groups. *Psychological Medicine, 36,* 1375–1383.

Mickus, M. A., & Luz, C. C. (2002). Tele-visits: Sustaining long distance family relationships among institutionalized elders through technology. *Aging & Mental Health, 6,* 387–396.

Mutharayappa, R., & Bhat, T. N. (2008). Is lifestyle influencing morbidity among elderly*? Journal of Health Management, 10,* 203–217.

Newport, F. (2006). Religion most important to blacks, women, and older American. Retrived from http://news.gallup.com/poll/25585/religion-most-important-blacks-women-older-americans.aspx.

Pargament, K. I. (1997). *The psychology of religion and coping: Theory, research and practice.* New York: Guilford.

Phillips, D. R. (1994). Ageing and the implications for services: Formal and informal support systems, accommodation and services. In C. R. Ramachandran & B. Shah (Eds.), *Public health implications of aging in India* (pp. 148–163). New Delhi: ICMR.

Prabhu, P. H. (1954). *Hindu social organisation.* Bombay: Popular Book Depot.

Rajagopal, D., MacKenzie, E., Bailey, C., & Lavizzo-Mourey, R. (2002). The effectiveness of a spiritually-based intervention to alleviate subsyndromal anxiety and minor depression among older adults. *Journal of Religion and Health, 41,* 153–166.

Ramamurti, P. V. (2004). Psychosocial aspects of ageing in India. In P. V. Ramamurti & D. Jamuna (Eds.), *Handbook on Indian gerontology* (pp. 268–327). Delhi: Serials Publications.

Ramamurti, P. V., & Jamuna, D. (1992). Aged in developing India. *Aging and Society: The Indian Journal of Gerontology, 4,* 1–6.

Rao, A. P. (2000). *Kind of supports requires in different kinds of elderly.* Paper presented at the Asia–sub regional seminar for social security for elderly. Social Security Association of India, New Delhi.

Rastogi, A. (1996). Spiritual values to cope with ageing. In V. Kumar (Ed.), *Aging: Indian perspective and global scenario* (pp. 230–237), New Delhi: AIIMS.

Reddy, L. K. (1996a). Health and attitude towards health among elderly. In V. Kumar (Ed.), *Aging: Indian perspective and global scenario* (pp. 231–234), New Delhi.

Reddy, L. K. (1996b). Factors influencing attitude towards health among rural elderly. In I. Chakravarty (Ed.), *Life in twilight years* (pp. 343–349). Calcutta: Kwality Book House.

Reddy, L. K., & Ramamurti, P. V. (1995). Health behaviour among the elderly in India. In *Proceedings of Asia/Oceania Regional Congress of Gerontology*, Hong Kong.

Richards, P. S., & Bergin, A. (1997). *A spiritual strategy for counseling and psychotherapy.* Washington, D.C.: American Psychological Association.

Savita, V., & Darshan, S. (1999). Factors affecting health of aged. *The Indian Journal Gerontology, 9,* 21–37.

Shah, B. (2004). Health care delivery systems of the elderly. In P. V. Ramamurti & D. Jamuna (Eds.), *Handbook on Indian gerontology* (pp. 96–116). Delhi: Serials Publications,

Shah, B., & Prabhakar, A. K. (1996). Healthcare for the elderly. *ICMR Bulletin, 26,* 33–36.
Sharma, S. (2004). Sustaining and enhancing well-being/health of Indian students: The role of certain spiritual or religious oriented interventions. In D. K. Bhattacharjee (Ed.), *Psychology in Indian traditions: Implications for education*. NCERT: New Delhi.
Singh, S. (2006). Perceived health among women retirees. *Psychological studies, 51*, 166–170.
Singh, S. (2008). Psychosocial factors shaping adjustment during widowhood. *Psychological Studies, 53,* 298–302.
Singh, S., & Chao, D. (2016). What makes elderly healthy? An Empirical inquiry into psycho-social dynamics. *Journal of Indian Health Psychology, 10,* 90–99.
Singh, R. R. (1993). Welfare system and psycho-social supports for the aged. In *Proceedings of National Seminar on Ageing Scenario in India by 2001 A.D.* New Delhi: Help Age and Care India.
Sinha, D. (1984). Community as a target: A new perspective to research in prosocial behaviour. In E. Staub, D. Bar-Tal, J. Karylowski, & J. Reykowski (Eds.), *Development and maintenance of prosocial behaviour: International perspective on positive morality* (pp. 445–455). New York: Plenum.
Sinha, S. P. (1999). Role of social supports in alleviating residential crowding stress among elderly. *Indian Journal of Gerontology, 13,* 105–110.
Siva Raju, S. (2000). Ageing in India: An overview. In M. Desai & S. Raju (Eds.), *Gerontological social work in India*. Delhi: B. R. Publishing Company.
Smith, T. S. (2001). Religion and spirituality in the science and practice of health psychology. In T. H. Plante & A. C. Sherman (Eds.), *Faith and health*: *Psychological perspectives* (pp. 335–400). New York: The Guilford Press.
Sridevi, K., & Krishna Rao, P. V. (1996). Yoga practice and menstrual distress. *Journal of the Indian Academy of Applied Psychology, 22,* 47–53.
Stephens, A., Towers, A., & Stevenson, B. (2011). The effects of types of social networks: Perceived social support, and loneliness on the health of older people. *Journal of Aging Health, 23,* 887–911.
Taylor, E. (1997). *A psychology of spiritual healing*. Pennsylvania: Chrysalies Books.
Taylor, R. J., Chatters, L. M., & Jackson, J. S. (2007). Religious and spiritual involvement among older African Americans, Caribbean Blacks, and non-Hispanic Whites: Findings from the National Survey of American Life. *Journal of Gerontology, 62,* 238–250.
Tiwari, S. C., & Pandey, N. M. (2012). The Indian concepts of lifestyle and mental health in old age. *Indian Journal of Psychiatry, 55,* 82–88.
Umadevi, A. (1991). *Study of disability in old age and perception of social support.* Master's Dissertation. S.V. University, Tirupati.
Umadevi, T. (2002). *Psychosocial correlates of disability among the aged.* Unpublished Doctoral Dissertation. S.V. University, Tirupati.
Ushasree, S. (2000). Perceptions of social support among the aged women. *Journal of the Indian Academy of Applied Psychology, 26,* 115–118.
Van der Pas, S., & Koopman-Boyden, P. (2007). Leisure and recreation activities and well-being among older New Zealanders. In P. Koopman-Boyden & C. Waldegrave (Eds.), *Enhancing well-being in an ageing society: 65–84 year old New Zealanders in 2007* (pp. 117–132). Retrieved from University of Waikato Website.
Vance, D. E. (2006). Spirituality and living and aging with HIV: A pilot study. *Journal of Religion, Spirituality and Aging, 19,* 57–74.
Verma, S. K., & Pershad, D. (1996). Self-help groups and cognitive retraining in the elderly. *Research and Development Journal (Help Age India), 3*(1), 28–36.
Vink, D., Aartsen, M. J., & Schoevers, R. A. (2008). Risk factors for anxiety and depression in the elderly: A review. *Journal of Affective Disorders, 106,* 29–44.
Willigen, J. V., & Chadha, N. K. (2003). Social networks of old people in India: Research and policy. In P. S. Liebig & S. Irudaya Rajan (Eds.), *An aging India: Perspectives, prospects and policies* (pp. 109–124). New York: The Haworth Press.

Yahaya, N., Momtaz, Y. A., Hamid, T. A., & Abdullah, S. S. (2013). Social support and psychological well-being among older Malay women in Peninsular Malaysia. *Indian Journal of Gerontology, 27,* 320–332.

Yoon, D. P., & Lee, E.-K. O. (2007). The impact of religiousness, spirituality, and social support on psychological well-being among older adults in rural areas. *Journal of Gerontological Social Work, 48,* 281–298.

Zhang, J.-G., Ishikawa-Takata, K., Yamazaki, H., Morita, T., & Ohta, T. (2006). The effects of Tai Chi Chuan on physiological function and fear of falling in the less robust elderly: An intervention study for preventing falls. *Archives of Gerontology and Geriatrics, 42,* 107–116.

Chapter 13
Yoga as an Intervention for Promoting Subjective Well-Being

Bal Krishna Upadhyay

Subjective Well-Being and Yoga Tradition

Mind is an important part of human psychology wherein many thoughts are buried deep in the unconscious or subconscious. These thoughts reflect on the behaviour of humans and play vital role in promoting well-being and mental health. In today's stress-filled life, more and more people are suffering from stress-borne diseases. This has essentially happened because of mismatched synchronization of mind and body state. It has been established that 'one's body works according to one's mind', and when mind is not healthy it leads to unhealthy body. This ultimately affects the state of well-being experienced by an individual. Yoga as a science is devoted to the integration of mind and body so as to help attaining the highest degree of happiness embodied into a healthy body.

The field of subjective well-being (SWB) has grown substantially in the past three decades, especially with the introduction of positive psychology. There is increasing evidence about the health-enhancing role of SWB (e.g., Cummins 2000; Diener 1984, 2000; Seligman 2002). The concept of SWB as Diener et al. (1997) define refers to people's evaluation of their lives. Haas (1999) has viewed it as a generic term encompassing all aspects of life. Currently, SWB includes life satisfaction, affective experience and subjective responses to the objective conditions. Further, it has also been noted that SWB is a function of the degree of congruence between individual's wishes, needs and environmental demands and opportunities (Jadhav and Havalappanavar 2009). The current view holds that SWB is a function of three variables: life satisfaction, lack of negative mental states and the presence of positive mood and emotion (Thomas 2008).

B. K. Upadhyay (✉)
Faculty of Human Resource Management, Indian Institute of Forest Management, Nehru Nagar, Bhopal 462003, Madhya Pradesh, India
e-mail: bkupadhyay@yahoo.com

G. Misra (ed.), *Psychosocial Interventions for Health and Well-Being*,
https://doi.org/10.1007/978-81-322-3782-2_13

The idea of well-being in the Indian tradition is embedded in the concept of *anand* (bliss) that finds place in the various texts. The Taittiriya Upanishad presents anand as the original state of human consciousness or the atman (the transcendental self. The *panchakosha*[1] (the five sheaths) doctrine draws attention of the varying levels of qualitatively distinct experiences of anand. These five *koshas* are as follows: *annamaya kosha* (related to the satisfaction of sensual pleasures by the acts of satisfying bodily needs of hunger, sleep, sex and fear; *pranmaya kosha* (awareness of duality of atman and body), *manomaya kosha* (related to effective functions of *harsh*, *ullaas*, and *santosh*—excitement, feelings of pleasantness, and being pleased), *vijnaanmaya kosha* (related to wisdom encompassing intuition and intellect) and the *anandmaya kosha* (related to being anandmaya pervaded by bliss) (commentary by Sankara on Taittiriya Upanishad in Sastri (translator) 1923). Each kosha is like a curtain that covers the original state of being. Step by step unfolding of these sheaths leads to the state of anand—the knowledge that 'I am bliss'. Attaining this state of anand is the ultimate state of well-being.

The yogic tradition in India follows the teachings of purifying the self, the atman and the body to attain the ultimate form of well-being, unfolding the anandmaya kosha—the opening of eternal bliss where the person realizes that 'I am bliss'. This implies that a hierarchy of veils has to be lifted and the person has to climb up the ladders one by one to reach the level where ultimate form of well-being is situated.

The first three steps, moving from down to up, in the hierarchy (see Fig. 13.1), that is, annamaya, pranmaya and manomaya koshas is comparatively easier to experience and attain, but the vijnaanmaya and anandmaya koshas are comparatively difficult to attain.

i. ***Annamaya Kosha***: Annamaya kosha is the satiation of the engagements of *indriyas* (sense organs) and assumes that all forms of existence is food to something and forms the base for survival of biological being. All creatures are born out of food and die to become part of food in the 'food chain'. Learning, knowing and removing this sheath of ignorance will lead to the second step up the ladder (from Taittiriya Upanishad with commentary of Sankara, in Sastri (translator) 1923, pp 104–107).
ii. ***Pranmaya kosha***: This second layer relates to the vital life force, which is identified by and is dependent on breathing. The physical manifestation of *prana* (vital life force) is breath and as long as it remains in the person, life exists. By gaining control on the prana, one may remove the sheath surrounding it and move on to the next layer (see Sastri, translator 1923).
iii. ***Manomaya kosha***: The mind sheath is composed of manas (mind, thought, will, wish). The mind along with the five sensory organs is said to constitute the Manomaya kosha. The manas, exists only in individual forms of beings and it is the cause of diversity. Man's bondage as well as liberation is said to

[1]Complete discussion on panchakosha can be found in the verses of Anand Valli's of Taittiriya Upanishad *with* commentary of Sankara.

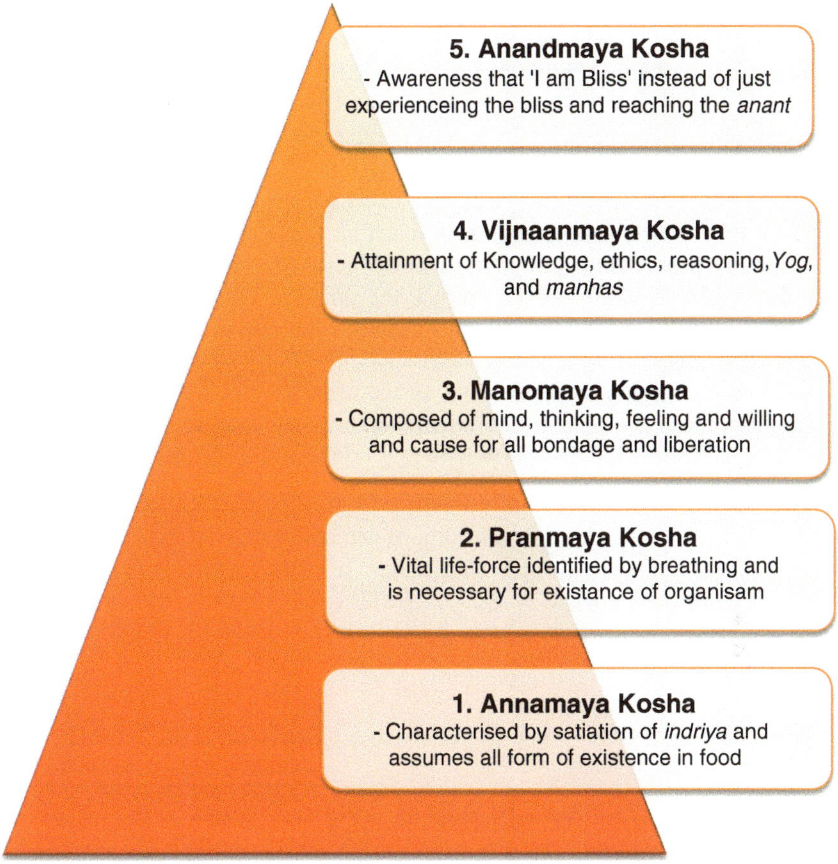

Fig. 13.1 Hierarchy of attaining ultimate well-being or anand by removing the lower sheaths

be caused by the mind, hence, man needs to move beyond this kosha to attain ultimate liberation.

मनएवमनुष्याणांकारणंबन्धमोक्षयोः ।
बन्धायविषयासक्तंमुक्त्यैनिर्विषयंस्मृतम् ॥

*(For man, mind is the cause of bondage and mind is the cause of liberation. Mind absorbed in sense objects is the cause of bondage, and mind detached from the sense objects is the cause of liberation…*Amritabindu Upanishad verse2)

The Manomaya kosha receives its inputs from all the sensory organs and interprets them in various form such as, good, bad and chooses the one most appropriate.

iv. ***Vijnaanmaya kosha***: To reach the Vijnaanmaya kosha or Gyanmaya kosha (the wisdom sheath) one has to detach from the impurity of bondage of all sense organs. This kosha is characterized by knowledge, ethics, reason, yoga, and *manhas* (power to perceive and reason). Nothing is impossible for a man who has removed all the previous sheaths to reach this kosha. The individual at this level is aware and interprets the experience of bliss such as 'I have experienced bliss'. However, the knowledge gained is still not permanent hence the truth has yet not been attained but without entering this state of vijnaanmaya one cannot move towards experiencing the true self or the atman.

v. ***Anandmaya kosha***: Vijnaanmaya kosha envelops the deepest, hidden layer of the realm (unconsciousness) that is the kosha called anandmaya kosha, the ultimate form of well-being. Man reaching the anandmaya kosha gains the capacity to realize the empirical and the spiritual, the conscious and unconscious, the changing and the eternal, the time and the timeless (see Deussen 1980; translation by Bedekarand Palsule). The individual gains self knowledge, realizes the essence and understands that bliss is him and not other. He attains knowledge about elements of the universe and hence attains the ultimate form of well-being, the *satchittaanand,* and liberates from all the sufferings, desires, life and death. Nothing remains but only bliss.

To reach the highest step of liberation or to gain the ultimate understanding of true self (the atman) and become anandmaya one has to remove the sheaths of *dukh* (misery), *klesh* (obstacles), and all barriers of mind, time, body, space and dimensions, which is the part of the four sheaths at the lower levels, as discussed. Thus, understanding the true form of SWB in Indian context is to understand the *panchakoshas* and how to detach from all the lower forms of koshas so as to unveil the anand koshas and become bliss himself attaining the anant (the unlimited).

Yoga as an Intervention to Attain Anand (Subjective Well-Being)

There are many ways apart from contemporary medical advances which have been used very effectively to promote human well-being. Yoga is one such technique considered to be one of the most important, effective and valuable tools available for man to overcome various physical and psychological problems and instill the feeling of happiness. Kuvalyananda and Vinekar (1971) has observed that yoga helps in nurturing positive attitudes and reconditioning neuromuscular systems. Thus, it seems that yoga helps the entire human body to enhance the capacity to withstand greater stress and strain and aims at an integrated and harmonious development of all the potentialities of a person.

Yoga, on the other hand, is also the method of attaining spiritual riches and superiority. The term yoga is made from the word *Yuj*, which means the act of joining. In spiritualism this word is used to explain the unity of the soul and supreme soul. The detachment of soul from the supreme soul results in all sorts of problems and sinful actions, disharmony, crime, immorality, etc. Maharshi Patanjali defines yoga as:

योगःश्चित्तवृत्तिनिरोधः ।2।

(Yoga is restraining the mind-stuff (*chitta*) from taking various forms (*vrittis*)- (*Patanjali Yoga Pradeep, sadhan pad* I:2)

Verma (1994) has operationally defined yoga as a group of techniques and methods consisting of certain exercises e.g., physical and postural exercises, cleansing exercises and breathing exercises, which have a potential to add to our physical and mental health—both positive and negative. Mental health, on the other hand, refers to the physical, psychological, social and spiritual well-being of human beings. It has both negative and positive connotation in terms of mental disease or ill health and the presence of well-being together with yogic exercises contributing to the treatment of mental and medical patients.

It we look at the various definitions provided, it seems that yoga is a group of exercise techniques that strengthen one physically and mentally. But it is not just a group of exercises. Yoga, as a method, is the way of attaining spiritual riches and superiority. This brings good changes in the entire life of a person. Yoga devotion begins with the body and body is the basis for all activities of the world. It is the body that experiences the *sukha* (bliss, happiness), *dukha* (sorrow), *raga* (attachment), *dwesha* (aversions), all forms of *klesha* (afflictions), etc. which has its origin in desires and expectations. These elements of experiences are the various forms of sheaths, which prevent an individual to attain the state of happiness or bliss at large or to simply put it affects the subjective well-being of a person.

Yoga, as a technique, has been known and tested to be important in enhancing cognitive and affective abilities. Thus, yoga may become a vital tool for enhancing the positive evaluation of life.

Yoga and SWB: Some Research and Trends

In contrast to Patanjali's classical yoga, the many schools of post-classical yoga are non-dualistic, that is, they pursue their soteriological programme on the basis of the recognition that 'All is One' (Feuerstein 1998). Various forms of yoga have come up in different ages in form of Vedic yoga, pre-classical yoga, classical yoga and post-classical yoga. However, yogic approaches to health achieved its peak through Hatha Yoga ('Forceful Yoga') and Raj Yoga or Astang Yoga.

It is not the objective of the present work to distinguish between the various forms of yoga, however, understanding of the two most important forms of yoga tradition, Raj Yoga and Hatha Yoga, is felt. While Raj Yoga specializes into leading the practitioner to higher self actualization or realization of the true self, Hatha Yoga specializes in making the body, the home of the atman, healthy and strong. The object of Hatha Yoga is more inclined towards the physical than psychological.[2] Swami Vivekananda (1923) suggested taking advantage of the

[2]See Swami Vivekananda (1923) for more on distinction between Raj Yoga and Hatha Yoga.

techniques of Hatha Yoga, especially the physical purification processes, through which only one can try unveiling the pranmaya kosha and open the manomaya kosha. Thus, practice of Hatha Yoga provides an entry path to the realization of anand kosha. The discussion ahead is based on the combination of Raj Yoga and Hatha Yoga, along with other forms of yogic traditions.

Hatha Yoga specializes in exploring the body's potential for the transformative processes of yogic consciousness technology (Feuerstein 1998). Hatha Yoga is more related to psychosomatic aspect that includes many physical purification techniques supported by a large number of asanas (postures) that exercises the body in various ways providing different benefits, all together. It has always had a close relationship with India's native naturopathic system called Ayurveda, which is profoundly holistic and for this reason has become quite fashionable in the West.

One of the other traditional orientations of yoga is the Viniyoga practiced and propagated by the school of T. Krishnamacharya (1888–1989) and his son Desikachar. Yoga has also been used as a therapy to support traditional Indian medicine for thousands of years. However, yoga therapy in its present form is a new but a growing discipline which has been created by the integration of traditional yoga and contemporary medicine.

Yoga as an Intervention

Contemporary modern society is observing serious changes in the way they live, that is, their lifestyle have changed due to influence of modern electronic gadgets and machines that were not available for the older generation. The American Psychological Association (2012) has reported increase in cases of reported stress in America. However, similar data is not readily available for other countries, but it is assumed that experience of stress has increased the world over. In addition, desire to attain more materialistic pleasures are being observed, in various forms. Working with deadlines and time pressure has made adult population vulnerable to stress which is known to be the major cause of ill health. Rise in stress-induced physical and mental disorders are high, especially virtual dukh and klesh due to overuse of new electronic gadgets. Besides, adults now complain of having no time to exercise that makes them visit medical practitioners on a regular basis so as to get symptomatic relief emerging out in various forms. The recent World Happiness Report 2015 (Helliwell et al. 2015) has also indicated that with increase in age life evaluation decreases. This reveals that SWB among adults, irrespective of gender, is lower than the younger generation.

It has been noted and observed by many scientists and researchers that practice of yoga and meditation brings positive changes in the psychological well-being, overall health and happiness (Malathi et al. 2000). Yoga has been described as a holistic approach to health of which the body, mind and spirit are integral and interdependent part (Bhushan 1998). It has been further noticed that while yoga is still considered as a gentle form of exercise and relaxation, some are drawn towards it for its teachings at a deeper, spiritual level. This change comes from the belief that yoga, when adopted as a spiritual path, can underpin one's entire approach to life (Thomas 2008).

In one of his highly influential article on SWB, Diener (1984) proposed that SWB has three distinct components: life satisfaction (LS), positive affect (PA) and negative affect (NA). Diener et al. (1999) also included satisfaction in specific life domains (e.g., satisfaction with health) in the definition of SWB. When we analyse these components of SWB and the satisfaction in specific life domain, it is found that a positive frame of mind has an inverse effect and reduce health risk and yoga has a mediating effect in enhancing the positives of SWB. In the same line, Upadhyay (2002) proposes certain yogic techniques that help in reducing the symptoms of hypertensions and Coronary Heart Disease (CHD) and enable patients to manage their medical conditions effectively. She has also established that yogic postures can be helpful in reinstating the vital life energy, the prana, while the effects of certain asanas and pranayams may act as a booster to the experiences of positive life evaluations.

The affect component of SWB relates to the positive and negative affect, i.e., emotions, moods and feelings. An emotion is a prime determinant of the sense of subjective well-being and appears to play a central role in many human activities (Santrock 2005). Bhatt (2011) in his study has revealed that there is significant reduction in negative emotions/affect when individuals are exposed to yogic asanas and pranayam. In this regard, it seems that yogic practices allows for greater bonding, better mental or psychological flexibility and working out conflicts with less competition. The findings of Bhatt have also suggested that Yoga reduces the effects of negative affect and is related to improved mental and physical health (Bhatt 2011), hence adding to the feeling of SWB. Besides, Narasimhan et al. (2011) have reviewed and reported that the benefits of reduction in negative emotions improves quality of life in healthy people with increased immunity (Dillon et al. 1985), better pulmonary functions (Kubzansky et al. 2002) and increased lifespan (Danner et al. 2001).

Studies involving short-term Iyengar Yoga (10 h) has shown improvement in self-reported acute mood states of depression trait anxiety, negative mood and fatigue in young adults (e.g., see Woolery et al. 2004). West et al. (2004) have compared African dance and Hatha Yoga and have reported a reduced perceived stress and negative affect with both these practices but higher reduction in cortisol levels in the Hatha Yoga group. Furthermore, the utility of yoga in improving mood and the differential effects has been reported to be related to its positive influence on physiological states of arousal (West et al. 2004) through establishing stable autonomic balance (Vempati and Telles 2002). Thus, yoga induces a positive mind state, that is, it helps in inducing healthy feeling, feeling happier, more content and more at ease and hence, yoga is related to subjective wellbeing positively.

It has thus been established that yogic experiences helps boost the individual's overall subjective well-being. However, it is reminded that practice of yoga is required to be conducted in proper guidance of a trained teacher. Also, the choice of specific technique (*asanas*, and *pranayam*) is very important. to test the hypothesis that yogic practices helps in creating more positive feeling and enhanced experience of physical and mental wellbeing among adult CHD participants, Upadhyay (2002) developed a package for individuals suffering from hypertension and CHD. The yoga package consisted of *Pawan muktaasan* (warming up exercise), pranayam and asanas.

Pawan muktaasan is a series of warming up exercises that has to be done prior to the start of any yogic procedure, as a warming up exercise. It is related to the ayurvedic concept of *tridoshas*, viz., vata (the air), pitta (the fire), kapha (water of life). The wind fans the fire (pitta) and the fire purifies the water of life (kapha) (Frawley 1922). Pawan muktaasan series allows change that leads to renewal and rejuvenation making the practitioner happier and healthy. Similarly, yogasanas are the exercise for the whole body and is the best method to keep the body active, healthy and disease free. The practice of yoga begins with the process of controlling the mind. Patanjali has explained this in one dictum. Yoga controls all the conditions of the mind that forms the greater part of sheaths, which prevents an individual from attaining the ultimate state of happiness. Regular yogasanas help in curing almost all types of diseases and strengthens the nerves and muscles. Where yogasana purifies the mind pranayam purifies the vital life source, the prana. It provides and regulates the additional energy required to work in a positive state of mind. Pranayam controls the playfulness of the mind and its regular practice makes the mind happy preventing any kind of disequilibria in the body.

Using the above package on a sample of 126 adult participants suffering from hypertension and CHD, Upadhyay (2002) concluded that the above yogic postures and techniques are helpful in promoting positive physical and mental well-being leading to enhanced evaluation of life and more positive affect. In the same line, Setterlind (1983) has reported that regular practice of meditation brings a positive change in the well-being of the individual. This entails that yogic meditation may help in increasing of psychological well-being. Besides, Malathi et al. (2000) have observed a significant improvement in 9 of the 11 factors of subjective well-being in healthy volunteers at the end of four months of yoga practice. Kumar (2004) has noticed a remarkable positive shift in a postgraduate student's anxiety and subjective well-being as a result of Yoga Nidra practice on daily basis.

It is now known that yoga has been linked to more advantages than disadvantages. Practices of yoga varies in this contemporary world in terms that it has become a tool for helping people gain better health and most modern meditation techniques aim to train attention and awareness to help bring thoughts under control. Studies show how helpful a regular meditation practice can be for relieving pain, anxiety and stress. In one of the interviews arranged with Dr. Katie Guttenberg for ABC News reports (2013) claims that there are more than 200 schools of yoga taught throughout the world and all of them aim to connect the mind and body through careful breathing and bodily movements. Guttenberg (2013) further reports that studies with meditation find that regularly practice of downward dogs (*adhomukhasvanasan*) and warrior poses (*virabhadrasan*) can help manage stress and anxiety developing out of the various activities that one indulges in one's daily life. There's increasing evidence that yoga can help fight cancer-related fatigue (Blank et al. 2010; Carson et al. 2009), manage high blood pressure (Ross and Thomas 2010; Upadhyay 2002) and ease chronic pain, especially joint pain (Wren et al. 2011).

Comparison of yoga with regular modern form of exercises have revealed that both interventions make subjects feel better, but yoga seems to do better at relieving physical symptoms and perceptions of stress (Oken et al. 2004). It seems that yogic benefits extend not only to physiological and psychological health but is also significant in enhancing the biochemical profile by indicating an anti-stress and antioxidant effect which are important in the prevention of degenerative diseases (Santha et al. 1981; Udupa et al. 1975).

By and by, researches, as discussed, evince that yogasanas and pranayam are useful in worldly life to sustain the health of both physical and vital body. With a healthy body one is better able to undertake spiritual practice leading towards attainment of the purpose of life. Adoption of a yogic lifestyle has been found to be moderately related to measures of SWB (Thomas 2008). Thomas has evinced that people undertaking fulltime yoga studies in colleges and universities reveal higher self-ratings of yogic lifestyle than those attending a weekly yoga class and adoption of a yogic lifestyle is more strongly related to higher levels of life satisfaction in the domains of spirituality, health and community.

By and large, these findings suggest that positive evaluation of life may promote the feeling of subjective well-being and yoga is one such method. The researches further indicate that practice of yoga may impact emotions positively while decreasing the experience of stress and anxiety. Since, yoga is a combination of both physical and mental exercises, it helps in aligning one's mind with the body which helps in creating a better synchronization between the two. Thus, it is clear that yogic practices help not only in building a healthy body but also developing a positive outlook to one's life, hence enhance the experience of SWB in a person. Good physical health and a positive outlook towards life is the first step towards unveiling the veils of ignorance (unveiling of the five sheaths of panchakosha).

Conclusions and Ways Ahead

Yogic exercises are based on the principles of nature and accordingly it helps a person to cure him/herself. Yogic tradition in Indian philosophy is built towards unveiling the panchakoshas so as to experience ultimate liberation or anand. It encourages the practitioner to move towards more simple and easy lifestyle from a complex one. This transition from a complex to simple lifestyle enhances the positive evaluation of subjective well-being in the form of more satisfaction with life, gaining awareness of all elements, developing positive emotions and enhancing the feeling of happiness. Thus, literatures in this field of enquiry seem to indicate that subjective well-being is well related to disciplined yogic lifestyle. A disciplined yogic lifestyle may lead towards uncovering the sheaths of ignorance and move higher up in the steps of panchakosha (annamaya kosha to anandmaya kosha).

Besides, findings available depicts that research on this ancient form of healing (yoga) is being conducted in large numbers, however, they seem to be more confined towards more physiological and or psychological ailments. The related terms like well-being and anand still requires to be integrated in yoga research so that a proper linkage can be drawn between various forms of yogic exercises and dimensions of subjective well-being. Researchers also need to draw their attention to the underpinnings of yoga and its effects on self-esteem. In spite of few researches conducted on how yogic exercises relate to enhancement of positive evaluation of the components of subjective well-being, there still remains a gap. Future researchers may like to undertake studies to indicate how yogic practices can be related to man's happiness and how well it can be used in reducing virtual dukha and klesha so as to increase the individual's subjective well-being.

With the increase in new forms of sufferings like virtual dukha and klesha, the field of yoga and its impact on physiological and psychological well-being are open for the researchers. Whatever, knowledge we have about this system of mental and physical healing is still in infancy. It is not a complete answer to all problems and disorders; however, there may be times when this system is combined with any other healing system to bring the desired results, both in physical as well as psychological domains. The yogic tradition of India has immense potential to lead the understanding on the subject matter of subjective well-being. The only requirement is to prepare to search and learn what is embedded in various ancient texts of one of the world's oldest civilization, India.

अहंनिर्विकल्पोनिराकाररूपो।विभुत्वाच्चसर्वत्रसर्वेंद्रियाणां।

सदामेसमत्वंनमुक्तिर्नबंध।चिदानंदरुपशिवोहंशिवोहं॥ 6 ॥

...I am untouched by the senses, I am neither Mukti nor knowable; I am without form, without limit, beyond space, beyond time; I am in everything; I am the basis of the universe; everywhere am I. I am Existence Absolute, Knowledge Absolute, Bliss Absolute– I am He, I am He (*Shivoham, Shivoham*) (Sri pad Adi Shankaracharya, '*Nirvana Shatakam*').

References

American Psychological Association. (2012). *Stress in America: Our health at risk.* Retrieved May 1, 2015 from https://www.apa.org/news/press/releases/stress/2011/final-2011.pdf.

Bhatt, J. V. (2011). Impact of *yoga* on negative emotions and affects: An organizational based study. *Indian Journal of Applied-Basic Medical Sciences, 13*(13B), 38–44.

Bhushan, L. I. (1998). *Yogic lifestyle and psychological wellbeing*. S.P. East-West psychology national award lecture delivered at Osmania University, Hyderabad on January 4, 1998.

Blank, S. E., Kittel, J., & Haberman, M. R. (2010). Active practice of Iyengar*Yoga* as an intervention for breast cancer survivors. *Journal of the American Association of Nurse Practitioners, 15,* 51–59.

Carson, J. W., Carson, K. M., Porter, L. S., Keefe, F. J., & Seewaldt, V. L. (2009). *Yoga* of Awareness program for menopausal symptoms in breast cancer survivors: Results from a randomized trial. *Supportive Care in Cancer, 17,* 1301–1309.
Cummins, R. A. (2000). Objective and subjective quality of life: An interactive model. *Social Indicators Research, 52*(1), 55–72.
Danner, D. D., Snowdon, D. A., & Friesen, W. V. (2001). Positive emotions in early life and longevity: Findings from the nun study. *Journal of Personality and Social Psychology, 80,* 804–813.
Deussen, P. (1980). *Sixty Upanishads of the Veda—Part I* (V. M. Bedekar, G. B. Palsule, Trans., 1st ed. 2 vols. Vol. 1). Delhi: MotilalBanarsidas (543 p).
Diener, E. (1984). Subjective well-being. *Psychological Bulletin, 95,* 542–575.
Diener, E. (2000). Subjective well-being: The science of happiness and a proposal for a national index. *American Psychologist, 55*(1), 34.
Diener, E., Eunkook, S., & Shigehiro, O. (1997). Recent findings on subjective well-being. *Indian Journal of Clinical Psychology, 24,* 25–41.
Diener, E., Suh, E. M., Lucas, R. E., & Smith, H. L. (1999). Subjective well-being: Three decades of progress. *Psychological Bulletin, 125,* 276–302.
Dillon, K., Minchoff, B., & Baker, K. H. (1985). Positive emotional states and enhancement of the immune system. *International Journal of Psychiatry in Medicine, 15,* 13–18.
Feuerstein, G. (1998). *The Yoga tradition: Its history, literature, philosophy, and practice.* Prescott, Arizona: Hohm Press.
Frawley, D. (1922). *American Institute of Vedic Studies Health Care Professionals Independent Study Course in Ayurveda,* Santa Fe, N.M. Part I.
Guttenberg, K. (2013). *Yoga*, Meditation Benefit Both Brain and Body. *ABC News*, May 22, 2013. http://abcnews.go.com/blogs/health/2013/05/22/yoga-meditation-benefit-both-brain-and-body/. Accessed December 24, 2013.
Haas, B. K. (1999). A multidisciplinary concept analysis of quality of life. *Western Journal of Nursing Research, 21*(6), 728–742.
Helliwell, J. F., Layard, R., & Sachs, J. (Eds.). (2015). *World happiness report 2015.* New York: Sustainable Development Solutions Network.
Jadhav, S. G., & Havalappanavar, N. B. (2009). Effects of *Yoga* interventions on anxiety and subjective well-being. *Journal of Indian Academy of Applied Psychology, 35*(1), 27–31.
Kubzansky, L. D., Wright, R. J., Cohen, S., Weiss, S., Rosner, B., & Sparrow, D. (2002). Breathing easy: A prospective study of optimism and pulmonary function in the normative aging study. *Annals of Behavioral Medicine, 24,* 345–353.
Kumar, K. (2004). *Yoga*nidra and its impact on student's wellbeing. *YogaMimamsha, 36*(1&2), 71–76.
Kuvalyananda, S., & Vinekar, S. L. (1971). *Yogic therapy.* New Delhi: Printed by Ministry of Health, Government of India.
Malathi, A., Damodaran, A., Shah, N., Patil, N., & Maratha, S. (2000). Effect of yogic practices on subjective wellbeing. *Indian Journal of Physiology and Pharmacology, 44*(2), 202–206.
Narasimhan, L., Nagarathna, R., & Nagendra, H. R. (2011). Effect of integrated yogic practices on positive and negative emotions in healthy adults. *International Journal of Yoga, 4*(1), 13–19.
Oken, B. S., Kishiyama, S., Zajdel, D., Bourdette, D., Carlsen, J., Haas, M., ... & Mass, M. (2004). Randomized controlled trial of yoga and exercise in multiple sclerosis. *Neurology,62*(11), 2058–2064.
Ross, A., & Thomas, S. (2010). The health benefits of *yoga* and exercise: A review of comparison studies. *Journal of Alternative and Complementary Medicine, 16,* 3–12.
Santha, J., Shridharan, K., Patil, S. K. B., Kumaria, M. L., Selvamurthy, W., Joseph, N. T., et al. (1981). Study of some physiological and biochemical parameters in subjects undergoing yogic training. *Indian Journal of Medical Research, 74,* 120–124.
Santrock, J. W. (2005). *Psychology essentials* (2nd ed.). New York: Tata McGraw-Hill.
Sastri, S. S. (Translator). (1923). *The Aitereya and Taittiriya Upanishad* (with commentary of Shankara) (pp. 104–112). Madras: The India printing Works.

Seligman, M. E. P. (2002). *Authentic happiness: Using the new positive psychology to realize your potential for lasting fulfillment*. New York: Free Press/Simon and Schuster.

Setterlind, S. (1983). *Relaxation training in school: Review of research and empirical studies*. Goteborg, Sweden: Acta Universities Gothoburgensis.

Thomas, J. (2008). Yogic lifestyle and subjective wellbeing. *Yoga Magazine*.

Udupa, K. N., Singh, R. H., & Shettiwar, R. M. (1975). Physiological and biochemical changes following the practice of some yogic and non-yogic exercises. *Journal of Research in Indian Medicine, 10*(2), 91–93.

Upadhyay, I. B. K. (2002). *Role of* Yogic *Practices in the Treatment of Psychosomatic Disorders*. Unpublished doctoral dissertation, Barkatullah University Bhopal, Bhopal.

Vempati, R. P., & Telles, S. (2002). *Yog*a-based guided relaxation reduces sympathetic activity judged from baseline levels. *Psychological Reports, 90,* 487–494.

Verma, S. K. (1994). Maintaining mental health through *yoga*. *Health for the Millions, 20,* 26–27.

Vivekananda, S. (1923). *Raja yoga: conquering the internal nature*. Calcutta: Advaita Ashrama.

West, J., Otte, C., Geher, K., Johnson, J., & Mohr, D. C. (2004). Effects of Hatha *Yog*a and African dance on affect, perceived stress, and salivary cortisol. *Annals of Behavioral Medicine, 28,* 114–118.

Woolery, A., Myers, H., Sternlieb, B., & Zeltzer, L. (2004). A *yog*a intervention for young adults with elevated symptoms of depression. *Alternative Therapies in Health and Medicine, 10,* 60–63.

Wren, A. A., Wright, M. A., Carson, J. W., & Keefe, F. J. (2011). *Yog*a for persistent pain: New findings and directions for an ancient practice. *Pain, 152*(3), 477–480.

Chapter 14
Religio-Spiritual Interventions for Health and Well-Being

Sagar Sharma and Girishwar Misra

> Spiritual development is the process of growing the intrinsic human capacity for self-transcendence in which the self is embedded in something greater than the self, including the sacred. It is the developmental "engine" that propels search for connectedness, meaning, purpose, and contribution. It is shaped both within and outside of religious traditions, beliefs and practices.
>
> (Roehlkepartain et al. 2006, pp. 5–6).

The contemporary world is characterized by mounting number of chronic psychosocial and other stresses that adversely influence people's health/well-being and quality of life. Increasingly, more and more people are getting fragmented in their personal lives, experiencing alienation and a variety of illnesses. They are less socially connected. Given such a scenario, the current upsurge of interest in understanding the role of spiritual/religious factors in health/well-being and disease is understandable (e.g. Pargament 1997; Thoresen 1998, 1999). In a meta-analytic review of the related literature, Seeman et al. (2003) have provided evidence that spirituality/religiosity is linked with several health-related outcomes, including cardiovascular, neuro-endocrine and immune functioning, although more evidence is desired. Various spiritual interventions also have been reported to be associated with different indicators of health/well-being (Harris et al. 1999; Oman 2013).

In particular, the younger generation is facing serious problems. In view of increasing competition, there is greater emphasis on cognitive performance and far less on optimum emotional development, with resultant high examination stress/anxiety in the younger generation. Parental and peer pressures, along with rising aspirations that far exceed the cognitive capacity and/or available opportunities in life domains, are leading to other negative consequences such as depression, anger/

S. Sharma (✉)
Department of Psychology, Panjab University, Chandigarh, India
e-mail: Sagar1939@gmail.com

G. Misra
Mahatma Gandhi Antarrashtriya Hindi Vishwavidyalaya, Wardha, India

G. Misra (ed.), *Psychosocial Interventions for Health and Well-Being*,
https://doi.org/10.1007/978-81-322-3782-2_14

hostility/aggression/violence, substance abuse and negative school-related behaviours. Spirituality offers opportunity for moral formation, socialization and induction into a sacred worldview, and also provides inner resources to cope with unique life concerns/stresses (Barnes et al. 2000). Against this backdrop, this chapter seeks to address two-fold objectives: (i) clarify the concepts of health/well-being, spirituality and religion, and (ii) examine the relevance and efficacy of meditation, prayer and service-volunteering as spiritual or religious interventions with regard to health/well-being outcomes. The choice of meditation, prayer and service-volunteering is based on traditional, spiritual and religious practices which emphasize a complementary relationship between meditation/prayer and service-volunteering. All of these complementary devotional practices synergize in ways that can sustain and enhance health/well-being through more constructive and adaptive coping with life concerns (Pargament 1997).

Notions of Health/Well-Being and Religion/Spirituality

Health/well-being and religion/spirituality are complex and multidimensional concepts. The similarities and differences depend on the way they are conceptualized. Health/well-being is not a 'default' concept, and is currently defined in positive terms. It also has a range of physical, psychosocial and socio-cultural facets which vary across cultures (see Sundararajan et al. 2013). According to WHO, health is a state of complete mental and social well-being, and is not merely the absence of disease and infirmity. Such an emphasis on harmony/balance or equilibrium is very close to the definition of health in the Indian tradition. Related illustrations include concepts mentioned in Ayurveda (*sama* or balance); *Atisarvatravarjayet* (avoid the extremes); Buddhistic philosophy (*madhyama* or the middle path); Sankhya philosophy (state of *samyavastha* or equilibrium of the three *gunas* or qualities namely, *sattva*—the element of illumination, *rajas*—activity, dynamism; and *tamas*—passivity, inertia darkness). Such a balanced state of human functioning is emphasized in the Bhagvad Gita to be a characteristic of psychological well-being (Misra 2005; Palsane et al. 1986; Sinha 1990).

Religion is viewed as 'denominational, external, cognitive, behavioral, ritualistic and public', and the spiritual as 'universal, internal, affective, spontaneous and private' (Richards and Bergin 1997, p. 13). Thus religion can be seen primarily as the external manifestation of spiritual experience, although people can engage in religious activities independent of having private and affective spiritual experience. It is also possible to consider oneself intensely spiritual while not being religious. While religion is an organized social entity, spirituality for some can be seen as an attribute of the individual. One may also conceptualize spiritual/religious beliefs on an internal/external continuum. Shealy and Myss (1993) refer to religious positions that embrace God as an external being whereas spirituality emphasizes a 'God-Within' reality. They further note that one possible implication of believing one has a God within is that individuals can explore the possibility of being co-creators of their health. Yet another distinction is made in the scientific study of religion: the distinction between believing and belonging. In related research people report aspects of both believing and belonging as they describe their own experiences of religion. Those, identifying themselves as religious, report more of belonging aspects of religion, while their counterparts identifying themselves as spiritual, report more of the believing aspects of religion (Woods and Ironson 1999).

Indeed, human capacity for spiritual and religious belief and engagement appears universal but its exact nature varies across different traditions. They prove to be rich, diverse and illusive phenomena having many connotations. Pargament (1992) defined religion as a 'search for significance in ways related to the sacred' (p. 204) and 'sacred' primarily refers to 'God, divine beings, or a transcendent reality' (Paragmant 2007, p. 33). In contemporary discourse, sacred stands for something consecrated or 'set apart' as well as something that is 'numinous' reflecting divine or supernatural power. Also, it implies an action or ritual that confers sacred status. Of course, what is perceived as sacred depends on the stage of a person's spiritual development. The current thinking is that religion and spirituality are multidimensional constructs characterized by cognitive, affective, behavioural and relational processes. It is observed that the human and spiritual goals are intertwined in the dynamics of everyday life (see Paragament 2013; Sinn 1985). Thus, it is important to understand how religion is used and how the spiritual goals are chosen and pursued. Paragament and Mahoney (2005) observed that spirituality refers to the seeking of something called sacred and religion designates the broader set of ways that sacredness may enter into a search as either the means or as end. The broad explanations for engagement with religion and spirituality put forward include controlling of human impulses and managing anxiety, forming a community of believers, and response to the need for meaning and comprehension.

A brief review of related evidence is provided hereafter that examines the role of meditation, prayer and service (volunteering) in sustaining and enhancing health/well-being. Oman (2013) has indicated that religious/spiritual intervention strategies are diverse and aim at different goals such as (a) supporting an individual in identifying and developing relationships with positive spiritual models, (b) providing individuals with beliefs and tools for learning more effectively from spiritual models and (c) modifying social environments to enhance exposure to positive spiritual models modifying social environments, especially those dismissive of spiritual concerns to project spiritual modelling meta beliefs that are more accurate and supportive (Bandura 1986; Oman and Thoresen 2009). These are not exclusive but complementary intervention strategies.

Meditation-Based Interventions

Although a highly cognitive and sometimes emotional activity, meditation immerses the whole person in a psycho-physiological experience which has been characterized as 'active passivity' (e.g. sitting quietly while being inwardly alert and focused) and 'creative quiescence' (e.g. inwardly calm while being open to expanded awareness) (Shah 1983, pp. 90–91). Meditation is found to have the potential to facilitate self-regulation and may enhance insight and the integration of physiological, emotional, cognitive and behavioural functioning (Kristeller and Hallet 1999; Rubin 1996).

Though an essential part of various forms of Hinduism, Buddhism, Islam, Christianity, Sufi thought, meditation may exist in religious/spiritual forms or even in a non-religious form. Different kinds of meditation serve different purposes and meditation is also associated with transcendental meditation (TM) and its variant for children—Walking Mantra or Word of Wisdom. The TM technique or procedure also has its origin in the ancient Vedic approach to well-being, but it does not require changes in personal beliefs, lifestyle or philosophy. Meditation as a primary intervention variable has been studied on adult groups as a way of reducing their physiological and psychological stress and related illnesses (Benson 1996; Benson et al. 1990; Chopra 1991; Easwaran 1996; Hall 1999; Yogi 1995). Recent research has also focused on the use of meditation as an adjunct to conventional psychotherapy models for alcohol and substance abuse treatment as well as for the alleviation of depression, anxiety, pain and the symptoms of heart disease (Carrington 1998). Koening et al. (2001) have reviewed extensive research in the field. They noted that when people become physically ill, many rely heavily on religious beliefs and practices to relieve stress, have a sense of control, and hope and purpose in life. They argued that religion has multiple roles. It acts as a social support system, reduces the sense of loss of control and helplessness, offers a framework that reduces suffering and enhances self-esteem, brings confidence that one with the help of God could shape the health condition and creates a mindset to relax and allow the body to heal itself. Also, religious involvement helps developing values such as compassion, charity, love and altruism which often help the person to cope successfully with the problems of stress, anxiety and depression.

Yoga is an old indigenous system of knowledge developed in India. Currently, it has gained popularity at a global level. It has been found to be very effective in treating and preventing mental disorders as well as restoring and enhancing physical, psychological and spiritual well-being (Dalal 2011; Dalal and Misra 2006, 2012). The objective of yoga is to develop humans intellectually, morally and spiritually and to prevent their decline. Since majority of health problems are psychogenic, physical treatment does not suffice. The disorders caused by anxiety, frustration, internal conflict, guilt, suppressed desire etc., need that patient's inner attitude be rectified and his reactions transformed.

Among the various forms of meditation, TM (Transcendental Meditation) is worldwide by far the most studied mental relaxation technique. Based on comprehensive statistical meta-analysis of the investigations mainly on samples of adults and the elderly, the TM has been shown as the most effective technique for: (i) reducing anxiety—the most common sign of psychological stress, (ii) increasing self-actualization as reflected in enhanced self-regard, inner-directedness, spontaneity and capacity for few warm interpersonal relations, (iii) reducing alcohol, cigarette and drug abuse, and (iv) for improving psychological health/well-being and maturity (Roth 1994). Though far less in number, some studies on TM have also focused on its efficacy for groups of school children and college students. Such research demonstrates that the practice of TM over a period improves school-related behaviours, basic learning skills, and increases intelligence, creativity and academic performance (Eppley et al. 1989; Galderloos et al. 1991; Nidich and Nidich 1989). Using standardized tests to measure a wide range of cognitive, emotional and perceptual functions, Tim and Orme-Johnson (2001) studied the efficacy of TM on school students in Taiwan. As compared to their control counterparts, TM groups showed significantly greater improvement on all measures such as creative thinking, fluid intelligence field independence and also in the reduction of trait anxiety. Barnes et al. (2003) determined the effect of stress reduction via TM programme on school-related (negative) behaviors in African-American students. They found that four months of TM intervention conducted in school settings significantly reduced absenteeism, suspension rates and rule infractions such as dress violation, excess tardiness, disruptive classroom behaviour like hyperactivity, bullying and fighting. A special strength of this study is the use of documented records rather than typical self-report data. TM is not a rehabilitation programme per se but is a means for self-development. It seems that TM can offer a simple and effective solution to some of the critical problems facing education.

Through meditation, stresses and tensions are released and the nervous system is brought into balance. From balance comes all the benefits such as greater ability to focus on task at hand rather than on self, and this enhances performance. Thus, meditation gives even young children power over their thinking and their emotions, not by repressive self-control, but by enhanced self-understanding and self-acceptance.

Prayer

Like meditation, prayer has been widely used as a self-help health-enhancing intervention. Prayer is an inherently spiritual activity. It is a process of connecting the self, others and the sacred (see Ladd and Spilka 2013). Along with meaning in life, prayer is considered as a significant indicator of appraising spirituality. In the Indian context, prayer relates to Bhakti derived from the root, *bhaj*. Bhakti is a loving attachment to God. It is the devotion to the divine. The divine must be realized to be non-different from 'I'. Bhakti involves unqualified self-surrender to the Supreme God (*Prapatti*) and to try to 'serve' him in every form and in every way. It is called *upasana* which is a ceaseless remembrance of God. Bhakti or prayer makes the person humble and generates a sense of service. It has the capacity to bring the sense of contentment and fulfilment. At the same time it relates to the well-being of others. As Ramanujacharya, a great saint and philosopher, mentioned about *kalyana* which implies service to others by the practice of virtues like *satya* (truthfulness), *arjava* (integrity or purity in thought, word and deed), *daya* (compassion), *dana* (benevolence) and *ahimsa* (non-violence). A bhakta, in his love for

God, directs his love towards the whole creation, and as a result, is free from self-centred love. He is ready to share everything with others as he feels God's presence in all beings.

In the Indian context, several great and little traditions and schools of Bhakti are in vogue (e.g. Shiva, Vaishnava, Shakta, Buddhist, Sufi, Sikh). Therefore, in practice, prayer is not a unitary phenomenon, and as such it can vary by purpose and according to the object and subject of prayer. It can take various forms and modes of expression (e.g., mantra recitation—*japa* or community singing of sacred hymns such as *shabad kirtan*). Further, a prayer can be general or specific for oneself, others or for all to a specific deity or offered more generally.

An ancient Indian invocation that is popular even these days aptly reflects the universal and perennial concern for the well-being of the entire mankind. It runs as:

Sarve Bhavantu Sukhinah
Sarve Santu Niramayah;
Sarve Bhadrani Pashyantu
Ma Kshchidduhkhbhagbhavet.

In English, it means 'let everyone be prosperous and healthy, let no one think of unhappiness of anyone'. Similar invocations of the divine are fully reflected in the prayer of Sikh faith whereby, devotees seek the intervention/blessings of the Eternal Being for complete well-being of all (*sab da bhala*). The Gayatri Mantra is another universal prayer enshrined in the Vedas and considered to be one of Hinduism's most sacred and powerful chants rendered as: '*Aum Bhoor Bhuvah Svaha/Tat Savitur Varenyam/Bhargo Devasya Dheemahi/DhiyoYo Naha Prachodayat*' (Oh God! Thou are the giver of life, remover of pain and sorrow, and bestower of happiness. Oh Creator of the universe, may we receive thy supreme sin-destroying light. May thou guide our intellect in the right direction). The Gayatri may be considered as having three parts—(i) praise, (ii) meditation and (iii) prayer. First, the divine is praised then it is meditated upon in reverence, and lastly an appeal is made to the divine to awaken and strengthen the intellect, the discriminating faculty of persons. It may also be noted that in this invocation the focus is on 'Our', 'We' and not on I. Such prayers along with meaning in life have been described as empirical indicators of appraising spirituality. Meaning in life is an outcome of spirituality, while prayer is an indicator of the defining attribute of connectedness with God (Maraviglia 1999).

In Indian traditions, God is also represented in Mother Form. This is amply reflected in Swami Vivekananda's vision of the Divine Mother at Kanyakumari or his spiritual preceptor Sri Ramakrishna's child-like adoration of the mother or in the grand Indian festivals of Durga Puja or Navratri (nine nights devoted to the worship of Divine Mother). Relating to God as Mother forges a personalized relationship strengthening the bond between Bhakta (devotee) and Bhagvan (God), as between a child and mother. Such a connectivity with God in Mother form through prayer can enhance psychological well-being and personal integration that counters distress, anomie and alienation. Given the ever-existing special bonding in a mother-child relationship, connectivity to God as Mother ought to be natural, easier and faster for school children than the adults including their parents and teachers. The relevance of prayers like Vande Mataram and Saraswati Vandana, as significant aspects of school-related activities, can also be seen from such a perspective.

Richards and Bergin (1997) cited preliminary evidence suggesting that different forms of prayer may have differential associations with outcome variables like effective coping with stressful situations, overall well-being and life satisfaction. Likewise, Sawni-Sikand et al. (2002) report that a high frequency of prayer is associated with more positive mental health/well-being. The usefulness of prayer as an adjunct to child counselling, however, remains almost completely uninvestigated. Further, there are potential ethical and role boundary issues that need to be addressed when considering the use of prayer in students' counselling. These include the danger of imposing certain beliefs or values on students or usurping or conflicting with religious authority. While explaining the relationship of prayer with healing and holistic health, Hughes (1997) argued that the belief of the praying person in the power of prayer itself stimulates healing, and the relaxation response and the sense of personal efficacy gained through act of praying may enhance the immune system. Despite such explanations of the mechanisms through which prayer promotes healing/holistic health, there sometimes exists a facet of prayer and healing that mystifies researchers and defies rational explanation. This seems to suggest the existence of higher power as a potential explanation for healing.

Service-Volunteering (Selfless Service)

Service (*sewa*) also exists both in spiritual or non-spiritual forms. It can also be an individual activity or a collective/community volunteerism (e.g., *kar sewa*). The association between service/volunteering to help others and the world's major faiths is understandable. Unselfish action commonly aims at the benefit of specific individuals, the community as a whole or both (Sinha 1984). Those who are spiritually focused but not active in any organized religion may view serving others as a key dimension of their spiritual life and health/well-being. In fact, for most such persons the very essence of their spirituality lies in service to humanity. Such persons also see service to others as a way to transcend the egoistic desires promoted by today's consumer-oriented culture. Even those persons who initially volunteer their desire for sociability (an extrinsic motivation) may still experience some benefits from lessened self-centered focus on 'me, my and mine' by a gradual transition towards 'thou, thy and thine' (Brake and Thoreson 1996). Such a transformational religious coping could lead a person gradually to internalize core teachings of a spiritual tradition. A person may then volunteer or do service (sewa) for primarily selfless motives, but still experience heightened social and emotional support by volunteering (Pargament 1997).

Only a few studies have dealt with service or volunteerism as a possible health promotion and disease prevention variable. Matthews et al. (1998) compiled evidence to show that volunteerism or service is a predictor of positive physical and mental health outcomes for adults. Similarly, adolescents who volunteered to help community members or in classroom activities report a wide range of positive effects such as a better resolution of multiple problem behaviours that share a common underlying causal agent (Allen et al. 1997; Moore and Allen 1996; Waterman 1997). The work by Allen et al. (1997) also observed that the most successful programme sites for adolescent volunteers offered a second intervention component consisting of classroom activities which helped students to cope with important (psychosocial) developmental tasks. Such studies suggest a complementary relationship between service (volunteerism) to help others and the activities that enhance the skills for coping with urgent life tasks. The reason for enhanced well-being for those who help others may also include greater social networks/integration that can buffer stress effects, distraction from their own troubles, enhanced meaning in life or a more physically active life. Given such benefits, the effort to instill an ethic practice of helping others in need among the young children must be continued since (i) early volunteerism strongly predicts adult volunteerism (Hodgkinson and Weitzman 1996); and (ii) because such a practice supports a moral or spiritual orientation toward giving to others (Sokolowski 1996). Social service in school settings takes the form of mass participation in awareness programmes (e.g. HIV/A1DS, environmental and gender issues) and other voluntary activities involving helping classmates, juniors and the disadvantaged in and outside school systems.

As stated earlier, meditation (and to a lesser extent prayer) is characterized by 'active passivity'. Service or volunteering (especially 'selfless service') is also a kind of prayer that is reflected in a wholesome and meaningful social activity involving body, mind and spirit. It represents a quest for the sacred in life and beyond by serving others. In the process, both societal well-being as well as personal well-being are enhanced. Meditation, prayer and service share a complementary relationship and together facilitate cultivating positive emotions (e.g., joy. contentment) that have undoing effects on negative emotions (e.g., anxiety, depression, anger); and thus enhance physical and mental health through more adaptive coping mechanism (Pargament 1997). Perhaps Saint Francis in his widely used prayer well captured the practical implications of such a complementary relationship: 'For it is in giving that we receive' (quoted in Easwaran 1996, p. 30).

Concluding Comments

Taken together, meditation, prayer and service can form a holistic and effective self-help health package for all people including the youth. Nonetheless, certain research, policy and ethical issues merit attention. There is now ample evidence on the efficacy of various forms of meditation (particularly the TM) even on samples of school students. Thus, some form of meditation can be incorporated at least as an adjunct to counselling. In comparison, the support for the effectiveness of prayer and service is more theoretical than empirical. Notwithstanding the paucity of empirical studies, the significant role of prayer and service has always been acknowledged by educators and planners. This is reflected in the continued presence of these interventions as an integral part of socialization in families and schools. However, the significance of such interventions gets devalued when conducted in 'ritualistic' and 'cosmetic' forms.

The paucity of systematic studies in this area necessitates comprehensive research. Thus, the relative efficacy of such spiritual or religious-oriented interventions needs to be empirically established using various health and other indicators for groups with different religious or spiritual backgrounds as well as for those who do not consider themselves religious or spiritual. Use of qualitative interview studies of students whose intervention has involved some form of meditations/prayer and/or service, could be used to complement the knowledge gained from controlled studies. While the practice of such interventions appears important for all persons, their relative effectiveness may depend on the content, form and frequency of each of these interventions, and the religious denomination or spiritual orientation of the person (Sharma and Misra 2010). Thus, a counsellor or a teacher must also take precautions against the usual lapse called 'uniformity myth' i.e., assuming that all students are same and need the same extent of intervention. Further, additional supportive evidence in favour of certain religious or spiritual interventions can facilitate their implementations not only for groups of students but their immediate role models like parents and teachers.

Given the sensitivity of issues related to spiritual interventions, the educationists, counsellors and planners need to develop comprehensive framework of spirituality and moral education in which issues like the form, content and meaning of meditation, prayer and service and that of other related interventions are addressed gently and appropriately with dignity, respect and integrity. Lastly, the professionals must also guard against: (i) trivializing the numinous or the sacred, (ii) engaging in questionable priestcraft by usurping religious authority, and (iii) imposing their own religious or spiritual values on students.

References

Allen, J. P., Phillibee, S., Herlig, S. S., & Kuperminc, G. P. (1997). Preventing teen pregnancy and academic failure: Experimental evaluation of a developmentally based approach. *Child Development, 68*, 729–742.

Bandura, A. (1986). *Social foundations of thought and action.* Englewood Cliffs, NJ: Prentice Hall.

Barnes, L. L., Plotnikoff, G. A., Fox, K., & Pendleton, S. (2000). Spirituality, religion and pediatrics: Intersecting worlds of healing. *Pediatrics, 106,* 899–908.

Barnes, V. A., Bauza, L. B., & Treiber, F. A. (2003). Impact of stress reduction on negative school behavior in adolescents. *Health and Quality of Life Outcomes, 1,* 1–7.

Benson, H. (1996). *Timeless healing: The power and biology of belief.* New York: Scribner.

Benson, H., Malhotra, M. S., Goldman, R. F., Jacobs, G. D., & Hopkins, P. J. (1990). The case reports of the metabolic and electroencephalographic changes during advanced Buddhist meditation techniques. *Behavioral Medicine, 16,* 90–95.

Brake, R. E., & Thoresen, C. E. (1996). Reducing Type A behavior patterns: A structured group approach. In R. Allan & S. S. Scheidt (Eds.), *Heart and mind: The practice of cardiac psychology* (pp. 255–290). Washington: American Psychological Association.

Carrington, P. (1998). *The book of meditation*. Boston: Element.

Chopra, D. (1991). *Creating health: How to wake up the body's intelligence.* New York: Houghton Miffin.

Dalal, A. K. (2011). Folk wisdom and traditional healing practices: Some lessons for modern psychotherapies. In R. M. M. Cornelisson, G. Misra, & S. Varma (Eds.), *Foundations of Indian psychology* (pp. 21–35). New Delhi: Pearson.

Dalal, A. K., & Misra, G. (2006). Psychology of health and wellbeing: Some emerging perspectives. *Psychological Studies, 51,* 91–104.

Dalal, A. K., & Misra, G. (Eds.). (2012). *New directions in health psychology*. New Delhi: Sage.

Easwaran, E. (1996). *Meditation: A simple eight-point program for translating spiritual ideas into daily life* (2nd ed.). Tomales, CA: Nilgiri Press.

Eppley, R. R., Abrams, A. I., & Shear, J. (1989). Differential effects of relaxation techniques on trait anxiety: A meta analysis. *Journal of Clinical Psychology, 45,* 957–974.

Gelderloos, P., Walton, K. G., Orme-Johnson, D. W., & Alexander, C. N. (1991). Effectiveness of transcendental meditation program in preventing and treating substance misuse: A review. *International Journal of Addiction, 26,* 293–325.

Hall, P. D. (1999). The effect of meditation on the academic performance of African American college students. *Journal of Black Studies, 29,* 408–415.

Harris, A. H. S., Thoresen, C. E., McCullough, M. E., & Larson, D. B. (1999). Spiritually and religiously-oriented interventions. *Journal of Health Psychology, 4,* 413–433.

Hodgkinson, V. A., & Weitzerman, M. S. (1996). *Giving and volunteering in the United States: Findings from a national survey.* Washington, D.C.: Independent Sector.

Hughes, C. E. (1997). Prayer and healing: A case study. *Journal of Holistic Nursing, 15,* 318–324.

Koening, H. G., McCullough, M. E., & Larson, D. (Eds.). (2001). *Handbook of religion and health.* New York: Oxford University Press.

Krsteller, J. L., & Hallett, C. B. (1999). An exploratory study of a meditation-based intervention for binge eating disorder. *Journal of Health Psychology, 4,* 357–363.

Ladd, K. L., & Spilka, B. (2013). Prayer: A review of the empirical literature. In K. L. Pargament (Ed.), *APA handbook of psychology, religion and spirituality context, theory and research* (Vol. 1, pp. 293–310). Washington: American Psychological Association.

Maraviglia, M. G. (1999). Critical analysis of spirituality and its empirical indicators: Prayer and meaning in life. *Journal of Holistic Nursing, 17,* 18–33.

Matthews, D. A., McCullough, M. E., Larson, D. B., Koenig, H. G., Swyers, J. P., & Milano, M. G. (1998). Religious commitment and health status: A review of the research and implications for family medicine. *Archives of Family Medicine, 7,* 118–124.

Misra, G. (2005). From disease to wellbeing perspectives from an indigenous tradition. In R. Singh, A. Yadav, & N. Sharma (Eds.), *Health psychology* (pp. 281–294). New Delhi: Global Visions.

Moore, C. W., & Allen, J. P. (1996). The effect of volunteering on the young volunteer. *Journal of Primary Prevention, 17,* 231–258.

Myss, C., & Shealy, C. N. (1998). *The creation of health: The emotional, psychological, and spiritual responses that promote health and healing*. London: Harmony.

Nidich, S. I., & Nidich, R. J. (1989). Increased academic achievement at Maharishi school of the age of enlightenment: A replication study. *Education, 109,* 302–304.

Oman, D. (2013). Spiritual modeling and the social learning of spirituality and religion. In K. L. Pargament (Ed.), *APA handbook of psychology, religion and spirituality context, theory and research* (Vol. 1, pp. 187–204). Washington: American Psychological Association.

Oman, D., & Thoresen, C. E. (2009). Spiritual modelling: A key to spiritual and religious growth. *The International Journal for the Psychology of Religion, 13,* 149–165.

Palsane, M. N., Bhavsar, S. N., Goswami, R. P., & Evans, G. W. (1986). The concept of stress in the Indian tradition. *Journal of Indian Psychology, 5,* 1–12.

Paragament, K. I. (1992). Of means and ends: Religion and the search for significance. *The International Journal for the Psychology of Religion, 2,* 201–229.

Paragament, K. I. (1997). *The psychology of religion and coping: Theory, research and practice.* New York: Guilford Press.

Pargament, K. J. (2007). *Spiritually integrated psychotherapy.* New York: Guilford Press.

Pargament, K. (Ed.). (2013). *APA handbook of psychology, religion and spirituality,* vol.1. Washington D.C.: American Psychological Association.

Pargament, K. J., & Mahoney, A. (2005). Sacred matters: Sanctification as a vital topic for the psychology of religion. *The International Journal for the Psychology of Religion, 15,* 179–198.

Richards, P. S., & Bergin, A. E. (1997). *A spiritual strategy for counselling and psychotherapy.* Washington, D.C.: American Psychological Association.

Roehlkepartain, E. C., Benson, P. L., King, P. E., & Wagener, L. M. (2006). Spiritual development in childhood and adolescence: Moving to the scientific mainstream. In E. C. Roehlkepartain, P. E. King, L. M. Wagener, & P. L. Benson (Eds.), *The handbook of spiritual development in childhood and adolescence* (pp. 1–15). Thousand Oaks, CA: Sage.

Roth, R. (1994). *Maharishi Mahesh Yogi's transcendental meditation.* Washington, D.C.: Primus.

Rubin, J. B. (1996). *Psychotherapy and Buddhism: Toward an integration.* New York: Plenum Press.

Sawni-Sikand, A., Schubiner, H., & Thomas, R. L. (2002). Use of complementary/alternative therapies among children in primary care pediatrics. *Ambulatory Pediatrics, 2,* 99–103.

Seeman, T. E., Dram, L. F., & Man, M. (2003). Religiosity/spirituality and health: A critical review of the evidence for biological pathways. *American Psychologist, 58,* 53–63.

Shah, I. (1983). *Learning how to learn.* London: Octagon Press.

Sharma, S., & Misra, G. (2010). Health psychology: Progress and challenges. In G. Misra (Ed.), *Psychology in India. Clinical and health psychology* (Vol. 3, pp. 265–316). New Delhi: Pearson.

Shealy, C. N., & Myss, C. M. (1993). *The creation of health: Merging traditional medicine with intutitive diagnosis.* Walpole: Stillpoint Publishing.

Sinha, D. (1984). Community as a target: A new perspective to research on prosocial behaviour. In E. Staub, D. Bar-Tal, J. Karylowski, & J. Reykowski (Eds.), *International perspective on positive morality* (pp. 445–455). New York: Plenum.

Sinha, D. (1990). Concept of psychosocial well-being: Western and Indian perspectives. *NINIHANS Journal, 8,* I–11.

Sinn, M. (1985). *Freedom from self: Sufism, meditation and psychotherapy.* New York: Human Science Press.

Sokolowski, S. W. (1996). Show me the way to the next worthy deed: Toward a micro structural theory of volunteering and giving. *VOLUNTAS: International Journal of Voluntary and Nonprofit Organizations, 7,* 259–278.

Sundararajan, L., Misra, G., & Marsella, A. J. (2013). Indigenous approaches to assessment, diagnosis, and treatment of mental disorders. In F. A. Paniagua & A.-M. Yamada (Eds.), *Handbook of multicultural mental health: Assessment and treatment of diverse populations* (pp. 69–84). New York: Elsevier, Academic Press.

Thoresen, C. F. (1998). Spirituality, health and science: The coming revival? In S. Roth-Roemer, K. Robinson, & C. Carmtn (Eds.), *The emerging role of counseling psychology in health care* (pp. 409–431). New York: Norton.

Thoresen, C. F. (1999). Spirituality and health: Is there a relationship? *Journal of Health Psychology, 4,* 291–300.

Tim, A. K., & Ormi-Johnson, D. W. (2001). Students' intelligence and creativity improved by transcendental meditation technique. *Intelligence, 29,* 419–440.

Waterman, A. S. (1997). *Service-learning: Applications from the research.* New Jersey: Lawrence Erlbaum.

Woods, T. E., & Ironson, G. H. (1999). Religion and spirituality in the face of illness. *Journal of Health Psychology, 4,* 393–412.

Yogi, M. M. (1995). *Maharshi's Vedic approach to health.* Vlodrop, Holland: Maharshi Vedic University.

Chapter 15
Behavioural Intervention Programme for Promoting Healthcare Practices in the Community: An Initiative

Nisha Mani Pandey and S. C. Tiwari

Health is the prime concern for every nation. Behaviour is the key to health. Inter relatedness between health and behaviour is well documented; it is an established fact that many of the illnesses are the result of faulty/unhealthy behavioural patterns (Vaillant and Mukamal 2001; Gary and David 2001; Tiwari et al. 2007; Shukla et al. 2016). The long-term behavioural patterns which is often referred to as 'lifestyle', are responsible for a variety of chronic communicable diseases i.e., diarrhea, dysentery, malaria, tuberculosis, conjunctivitis, AIDS, etc., and non-communicable health problems i.e. hypertension, coronary heart disease, diabetes, cancer, etc. Unhealthy lifestyle, with little exercises, poor diet and smoking may reduce one's lifespan by 23 years (*The Telegraph*, 7 July 2015). Evidences reveal that faulty or maladaptive behavioural patterns are one of the most usual reasons for developing illness/disease/disability including inadequate physical environment, hygienic and dietary practices, lethargic lifestyle, smoking, reckless driving, inappropriate health-seeking behaviour, disregarding preventive aspects etc. (Aggarwal et al. 2015; Assefa and Kumie 2014; Barton et al. 2016; Borg et al. 2017; Rose 1981; Shukla et al. 2016; Tiwari et al. 2007).

The links between behaviour and health had been clearly and widely recognized (Heald et al. 2017; Friis et al. 2017). However, deliberate and purposeful efforts to monitor this interrelatedness has never been studied thoroughly. Medical sciences significantly contributed in reducing and curing most of the illnesses but the burden of morbidity in the community is still widespread. The major aim of medical science is to preserve, reinstate and/promote health by reducing the burden of illnesses and distress as well as to provide proper treatment. A large number of health professionals are working on preventive aspects of health. Trails are being

---

N. M. Pandey (✉) · S. C. Tiwari
Department of Geriatric Mental Health, King George's Medical University,
Lucknow, Uttar Pradesh, India
e-mail: nisha15pandey@yahoo.co.in

G. Misra (ed.), *Psychosocial Interventions for Health and Well-Being*,
https://doi.org/10.1007/978-81-322-3782-2_15

made to prevent risk of disease, injury, disability and death. And most of the preventive measures can be adopted just by accepting one or the other kind of healthy behaviour.

Why is it so? What are the reasons behind it? How should one approach the community to eradicate the burden of illness? The answer is simple but difficult to achieve—modify the ill/unhealthy behavioural pattern and adopt a healthy one. This will help in reducing the burden of illnesses, morbidity and mortality. Assessment of relationships between environmental/behavioural/psychosocial and biological factors of health and disease is very difficult. Unpleasant environment or any psychological stressors has a significant role to play in introducing and aggravating communicable and non-communicable diseases. It is reported that some of the psychosocial complications of physical disorders include marital and financial difficulties, personality changes, affective disturbances, memory impairment and intellectual deterioration; psychotic reactions may also occur in some cases (Abiodun 1994). The article further indicates that psychosocial intervention techniques may be required in the management of psychosocial consequences of physical disorders and for some physical illnesses application of biofeedback and relaxation training etc., are beneficial as these help in the management of hypertension. In developing countries where available resources are limited, attention to the behavioural, psychological and social aspects of medical care particularly, will be beneficial (Abiodun 1994; Meinck et al. 2015).

To remain healthy and to preserve health there are three types of preventive measures i.e.—(1) **Primary prevention**: This level is related to pre-disease status and advocates for protection of health by personal and communal efforts such as enhancing nutritional status, immunization and eliminating environmental risks such as contaminated water supplies; (2) **Secondary prevention**: Basically related with early diagnosis and early treatment of the disease when symptoms occur; and (3) **Tertiary prevention**: At this level diseases take its advance shape and one needs to take steps to minimize disabilities and promote the patient to live a dignified life. Another level of care was also added to these three levels of prevention, i.e., **Primordial prevention** which aims at eradicating, eliminating or minimizing the impact of disability or diseases (John 1995). It will be worth mentioning here that preventions which brings much benefits to the people often offers little to each participating individual (Rose 1981).

It can be clearly observed that ultimate connections of all these levels of preventions are related with the behavioural action of the individual (Kang et al. 2010; Band et al. 2015). However, evidence based research from India in relation to the role, nature, dynamics of behaviour correlates in the causation, perpetuation, treatment and outcome of both communicable and non-communicable diseases, is scant. Nonetheless, legislations advocate for abuses of various kinds of substances, sex, child, immorality etc. and awareness generation through mass media for adopting healthy behavioural practices against unhealthy behavioural practices, viz., regulated life, hygienic practices, physical exercises, yogic exercises, health seeking and health information seeking behaviour etc., is present. But the critical question is that how could it be implemented or how many people would adopt it?

It is an established fact that human behaviour is too complex to be understood and explained by armchair theorizing, not so acquiescent to change without active participation and involvement of the index person or community (Joseph and Jaswal 2014). Verbal and/or visual communications apparently are not enough to bring about the desired changes in illness-breeding behaviours. Communications by modelling and knowledge about dynamics (rationale/modus operandi) of intervention compounds may hold key to the success of behavioural interventional strategies. In view of this, a pilot study was planned, developed and carried out by funding support of World Bank through Uttar Pradesh Health System Development Program by the King George's Medical University, Lucknow, in the state of Uttar Pradesh during 2002–2004. The study was named as 'Impact of Behavioural Interventions on illness breeding behaviors' (Tiwari and Associates 2004). The study was aimed to identify faulty behavioural patterns (illness breeding behaviour) in the areas of daily living, healthcare and health promotion as well as to provide strategic interventions to replace those patterns with healthy behaviours. A detailed and comprehensive assessment had to be attained in the following study objectives in a phase-wise manner:

A. **Short-Term Objectives**:

- **Project Development and Intervention Phase**:

  To survey the community:

  (a) To study the operant behavioural correlates in daily living, healthcare and health promotion suspected to be breeding illnesses.
  (b) To identify, train and engage peripheral health workers and people from the community (community interns) in behavioral intervention programmes.
  (c) To study the perceptions and requirements of the community regarding available health education materials through social marketing.
  (d) To carry out interventions employing I.E.C. strategies with identified behavioural correlates.

- **Project Evaluation Phase**:

  To resurvey the community:

  (a) To study the impact of behavioural intervention.
  (b) To finalize Behavioural Intervention Package for primary and secondary prevention for use in healthcare delivery systems.

B. **Long-Term Objectives**:

(a) To develop skilled human infrastructure (resource) from the community and peripheral health workers at primary care level for capacity building, primary and secondary prevention, healthcare and health promotion through behavioural interventions.

(b) To develop health consciousness and positive health-seeking behaviour in the community to care for their own health.
(c) To develop disease-specific and general Behavioural Intervention Packages (Health Education Materials) for use at primary care level for primary and secondary preventions.

It was a pre-post assessment study. Each study area was mapped with the help of local influential persons and with their help at the local level some community volunteers were also identified for getting help in approaching the families. These community volunteers were named as community interns. They were made aware about the programme and trained to visit and strengthen the behavioural interventions. A qualified research team carried out the entire research activities. The research team was also trained to work out behavioural interventions in specific areas with key informants/indexed subjects and impress upon them the need to adopt these interventions in their day-to-day living, as and when required. The research data was collected on a number of schedules and proforma which were developed to find out familial details, physical/mental health status of the family members and illness breeding behavioural correlates in the family.

The research team members (psychologists, medical officers and social workers) along with community interns visited the included families. During the initial phase, socio-economic status (SES) and other details of the family were recorded by a social worker. The medical officer and psychologist assessed the physical and mental health status of each family member on a pre-coded proforma. Faulty (illness breeding) behavioural profiles operant in the family on different aspects related to their physical environment, cooking practices, dietary and nutritional habits, healthcare, interpersonal relationship, child rearing and elderly care, etc., were assessed individually by each team member on a structured and coded proforma. On the basis of all these information, the psychologist and medical member of the team worked out and provided adoptable and feasible interventions to the key informant/index person. On an average, around two hours were usually needed and therefore spent with each family for the entire activity. Subsequently, community interns of the locality also followed up the families at least once a month to advise them on the implementation of the worked out behavioural interventions.

The senior members of the research team did mid-term evaluation of the families after three months of the initial inclusion to enquire about facilitators/difficulties in the implementation of the worked out interventions. Feasible interventions were worked out again as per the requirement. After six months of initial evaluation, final evaluation was carried out and results were found to be very encouraging. Through perceived outcomes of the impact of community, behavioural intervention may be judged (Table 15.1).

The respondents were asked to give their overall assessment about the impact of behavioural interventions in terms of 'perceived' positive changes (in percentage) with regard to some common physical health problems or difficulties that the families usually used to encounter before behavioural intervention. The figure in NA column of Table 15.1 shows the percentage of families where the index health

Table 15.1 Distribution of perceived positive changes (%) in the overall profile of common problems/difficulties amongst study families following behavioural interventions (visual analogue scale)

Problems/ difficulties	Nature of change				
	Nil to negligible	Some impact (25–50%)	Appreciable impact (50–75%)	Significant impact (75 and more)	N.A.
Fever	18	27	42	13	–
Common cold	9	21	47	23	–
Diarrhoea	7	12	31	39	11
Dysentery	3	13	16	27	41
Sleep problems	6	5	11	19	59
Low moods	11	13	16	8	52
Conflicts and quarrels in family	3	12	17	29	39
General well being	19	38	19	17	7
Substance abuse	23	15	17	8	37
Behavioral problems	13	16	37	13	21
Daily living	11	22	31	16	20
Healthcare	7	11	33	18	31
Health promotion	19	23	18	13	27
Family planning practices	21	26	23	11	19

problems were denied. It would appear from Table 15.1 that fever, common cold, lack of general well-being, diarrohea, problems associated with use of family planning practices, problems of daily living behavioural problems were commonest among families (present in more than 75% of the families). Problems associated with health promotion, healthcare, non-medical use of dependence producing drugs, conflicts and quarrels in the households and dysentery were reported to be the next common (present in 50–75% families), sleep problems, problems associated with low moods were common in 40–50% families. Through behavioural interventions it was possible to negotiate profitably the conflicts and quarrels in the household, dysentery, sleep problems, diarrohea, healthcare and common cold in more than 90% of the families; low moods, daily living, behavioural problems, fever and problems associated with general well-being in 80–90% families; family planning practices, substance abuse in 75–80% families. The most noticeable impact of behavioural intervention was reported in counteracting diarrohea and common cold, an 'appreciable to significant' impact in 70% families. Other common problems/difficulties where the impact of behavioural intervention was from an 'appreciable to significant' extent in 50–55% families were reported to have fever, healthcare and behavioural problems. Behavioural interventions had an 'appreciable to significant' impact on 40–50% families who had problems/difficulties associated with daily living, conflicts and quarrels in the households, dysentery and sleep problems. Behavioural interventions were also reported to have had an 'appreciable to significant' impact on 30–40% families with problems/difficulties in areas of general well being, family planning practices and health promotion. Substance abuse and low moods were reported to be the two problem areas where behavioural interventions could make an 'appreciable to significant' dent in 25 and 24% of families respectively. In majority of the families (38%) only 'some' dent could be made through behavioral interventions with regard to the problems associated with general well-being followed by fever (27%), family planning practices (26%), health promotion (23%), daily living (22%), common cold (21%), behavioral problems (16%), substance abuse (15%), low moods and dysentery (13% each), conflicts and quarrels in the household and diarrhea (12% each), healthcare (11%) and sleep problems (5%).

All those behaviours had been sorted out which had positive impact on the healthcare of family members. On the basis of these interventions, information, education and communication (IEC) materials were prepared in the areas of DL, HC and HP. The behavioural intervention package (BIP) in all the areas incorporated behavioural posters/calendar, songs, flip books. This revealed possibility for devising those research instruments through which one can identify 'illness breeding' and 'health ameliorating' behavioural profiles in the areas of 'daily living', 'healthcare' and 'health promotion'. Some of the studies demonstrated that community participation can be successfully utilized in the development and implementation of healthy behavioural strategies (Sakalidis and Geddes 2016; de Souza-Talarico et al. 2009; van der Meer and van der Weel 1999). The study also revealed that cooperation and participation of the community can easily be enlisted through communication, modelling and modus operandi explanations (Adamchak and Mbizvo 1991; Bhatia et al. 2004). Community awareness on health-related issues can be enhanced without argument and positive health-seeking behaviours can be strengthened (Delfabbro and King 2017; Saaka and Galaa 2011; Siril et al. 2017). This will also be worth mentioning that community participation in their own healthcare-related issues can be increased through the establishment of 'health clubs' manned by enthused, motivated and trained local 'community interns'. Behaviour holds the key to '*health*' and '*morbidity*': healthy behaviours promote wellness, preserve health; protect from illness, and reduce morbidity. A health logo and slogan was also devised:

SWASTH VYAVAHAR

SWASTH PARIWAR

'*Na Koi Kharch, Na Koi Killat; Swasth Vyavhar Hi Kare Jeevan Unnat*', which means *without making any expenditure, without scarcity, healthy behaviour improves life*.

In view of findings of the presented study it may be said that in healthcare services with *least input, maximum output* can be achieved by applying behavioural interventions.

Implications:

- Introduction of new syllabus for 'Behaviour and Health' in 'medical education' and 'general education' courses.
- The need and gains of behavioural changes, and the usual behaviour modification procedures to be popularized.
- Development of field evolved cost-effective, feasible and acceptable Behavioral Intervention Package (IEC materials).
- Integration of physical and mental healthcare services.
- Creation of the positions of 'Behaviour Scientist' at primary health centres, counsellors at sub-centres.
- Use of mass media communication methods at community level to increase health consciousness.
- 'Health promotion' programmes to be given more emphasis along with 'Healthcare' programmes.
- The language, presentation and dissemination of healthcare and health promotion materials should have a mass appeal.
- Health education materials should ensure participant and personalized delivery.
- Introduction of 'least input maximum output' concept at the primary healthcare level.
- Introduction of new paradigm in primary healthcare: community health clubs and community interns for healthcare.
- The behavioural interventions should have three components: (a) audio-visual communications; (b) communications through modelling; (c) rationale/modus operandi.
- Emphasis on human infra-structural development and community capacity building for primary healthcare.
- Integration of like-minded services and programs sponsored by other governmental and non-governmental agencies operant in the community.
- Establishment of training, research and data retrieval cell at every district headquarter.
- Extension and application of Behavioral Intervention Package (I.E.C. materials) to other areas of the state.

References

Abiodun, O. A. (1994). The role of psychosocial factors in the causation, course and outcome of physical disorders: A review. *East African Medical Journal, 71*(1), 55–59.

Adamchak, D. J., & Mbizvo, M. T. (1991). Family planning information sources and media exposure among Zimbabwean men. *Studies in Family Planning, 22*(5), 326–331.

Aggarwal, A., Unger-Saldaña, K., Lewison, G., & Sullivan, R. (2015). The challenge of cancer in middle-income countries with an ageing population: Mexico as a case study. *Ecancermedicalscience, 9,* 536. https://doi.org/10.3332/ecancer.2015.536.

Assefa, M., & Kumie, A. (2014). Assessment of factors influencing hygiene behaviour among school children in Mereb-Leke District, Northern Ethiopia: A cross-sectional study. *BMC Public Health, 14,* 1000. https://doi.org/10.1186/1471-2458-14-1000.

Band, R., Wearden, A., & Barrowclough, C. (2015). Patient outcomes in association with significant other responses to chronic fatigue syndrome: A systematic review of the literature. *Clinical Psychology: Science and Practice, 22*(1), 29–46. https://doi.org/10.1111/cpsp.12093.

Barton, C., Ketelle, R., Merrilees, J., & Miller, B. (2016). Non-pharmacological management of behavioral symptoms in frontotemporal and other dementias. *Current Neurology and Neuroscience Reports, 16*(2), 14. https://doi.org/10.1007/s11910-015-0618-1.

Bhatia, V., Swami, H. M., & Kaur, A. P. (2004). An intervention study to enhance AIDS awareness among underprivileged population in Chandigarh. *Indian Journal of Dermatology, Venereology and Leprology, 70*(2), 87–91.

Borg, S., Öberg, B., Nilsson, L., Söderlund, A., & Bäck, M. (2017). The role of a behavioural medicine intervention in physiotherapy for the effects of rehabilitation outcomes in exercise-based cardiac rehabilitation (ECRA)—the study protocol of a randomised, controlled trial. *BMC Cardiovascular Disorders, 17*(1), 134. https://doi.org/10.1186/s12872-017-0557-7.

de Souza-Talarico, J. N., Chaves, E. C., Nitrini, R., & Caramelli, P. (2009). Stress and coping in older people with Alzheimer's disease. *Journal of Clinical Nursing, 18*(3), 457–465. https://doi.org/10.1111/j.1365-2702.2008.02508.x.

Delfabbro, P., & King, D. (2017). Prevention paradox logic and problem gambling: Does low-risk gambling impose a greater burden of harm than high-risk gambling? *Journal of Behavioral Addictions*, 1–5. https://doi.org/10.1556/2006.6.2017.022.

Friis, R., Skov, L. R., Olsen, A., Appleton, K. M., Saulais, L., Dinnella, C., et al. (2017). Comparison of three nudge interventions (priming, default option, and perceived variety) to promote vegetable consumption in a self-service buffet setting. *PloS One*, *12*(5), e0176028. https://doi.org/10.1371/journal.pone.0176028.

Gary, E. F., & David, J. S. (2001). Ten years of life: Is it a matter of choice? *Archives of Internal Medicine, 161,* 1645–1652.

Heald, A. H., Anderson, S. G., Khan, A., Stocker, J., Davies, S., Bliss, K., et al. (2017). Success rates in a diabetes specialist nurse-led education programme: Re-setting the glucostat. *Experimental and Clinical Endocrinology and Diabetes: Official Journal, German Society of Endocrinology [and] German Diabetes Association*, *125*(5), 297–300. https://doi.org/10.1055/s-0042-108055.

John, M. L. (1995). *A dictionary of epidemiology* (4th ed.). USA: Oxford University Press.

Joseph, J., & Jaswal, S. (2014). Psychosocial framework for understanding psychological distress among survivors of the November 26, 2008 Mumbai terror attack: Beyond traumatic experiences and emergency medical care. *Prehospital and Disaster Medicine, 29*(3), 330–338. https://doi.org/10.1017/S1049023X14000478.

Kang, Y., Yang, I.-S., & Kim, N. (2010). Correlates of health behaviors in patients with coronary artery disease. *Asian Nursing Research, 4*(1), 45–55. https://doi.org/10.1016/S1976-1317(10)60005-9.

Meinck, F., Cluver, L. D., & Boyes, M. E. (2015). Household illness, poverty and physical and emotional child abuse victimisation: Findings from South Africa's first prospective cohort study. *BMC Public Health, 15,* 444. https://doi.org/10.1186/s12889-015-1792-4.

Rose, G. (1981). *Strategy of prevention: Lessons from cardiovascular disease, 282,* 1847–1851.

Saaka, M., & Galaa, S. (2011). Improving the utilization of health and nutrition services: Experience from the Catholic Relief Services supported the Development Assistance Programme in Ghana. *Primary Health Care Research & Development, 12*(2), 145–156. https://doi.org/10.1017/S1463423610000411.

Sakalidis, V. S., & Geddes, D. T. (2016). Suck-swallow-breathe dynamics in breastfed infants. *Journal of Human Lactation: Official Journal of International Lactation Consultant Association, 32*(2), 201–211; quiz 393–395. https://doi.org/10.1177/0890334415601093.

Shukla, D., Pandey, N. M., & Tiwari, S. C. (2016). Impact of behavioral intervention program on overall health of families: A report from Barabanki, Uttar Pradesh. *GJRA—Global Journal for Research Analysis, 5*(2), 214–216.

Siril, H., Fawzi, M. C. S., Todd, J., Wyatt, M., Kilewo, J., Ware, N., et al. (2017). Hopefulness fosters affective and cognitive constructs for actions to cope and enhance quality of life among people living with HIV in Dar Es Salaam, Tanzania. *Journal of the International Association of Providers of AIDS Care, 16*(2), 140–148. https://doi.org/10.1177/2325957414539195.

Tiwari, S. C., Agarwal, G. G., Kumar, A., & Pandey, N. M. (2007). Preventing illnesses: A community based behaviour intervention approach. *Springer, 52*(1), 77–84.

Tiwari, S. C., & Associates. (2004). Impact of behavioural intervention on illness breeding behaviours. Unpublished.

Vaillant, G., & Mukamal, K. (2001). *Successful Aging, 158*(6), 839–847.

van der Meer, A. L., & van der Weel, F. R. (1999). Development of perception in action in healthy and at-risk children. *Acta Paediatrica (Oslo, Norway: 1992). Supplement, 88*(429), 29–36.

Part III
Cultural Perspectives on Intervention

Chapter 16
Illness, Health and Culture: Anthropological Perspectives on Ethno-Medicine in India

P. C. Joshi and Nilisha Vashist

Concept of Ethno Medicine in Anthropology

Anthropology, since its very inception as an academic discipline has dabbled with the aspects of medical systems of the so-called 'primitive' or non-western people; often, these systems came heavily entwined with systems of religion and magic and found their place even in the earliest monologues as dedicated chapters. W. H. R. Rivers and F. Clements, the earliest pioneers, before the officially known sub-discipline of medical anthropology emerged, effectively owe us the initiation of concepts of disease causation and indigenous medicine. Clements (1932, in Foster and Anderson 1978) in the first comparative worldwide survey of beliefs of disease causation and Rivers (1924, ibid) through magico-religious and naturalistic worldviews of health in his book *Medicine, Magic and Religion*, showed the deeply cultural underpinnings of native understanding of disease and health as also the stereotype that magic and religion are always connected to medicine in indigenous societies.

The ever-strengthening field of medical anthropology has documented and argued for the centrality of culture in every aspect of human illness and health in societies around the world, whether it is at the level of conceptualizing and describing illness, functional v/s experiential nature, causation and etiology, symptoms, treatment seeking, sick-role, patient-healer interaction, notions of efficacy, cure, etc. Remaining true to its roots of the physical anthropology, accounts of native medical systems and mental health and the field of public health, medical anthropology has consistently tried to enquire into the biological as well as cultural and preventive as well as curative aspects of various medical systems at a cross-cultural level.

P. C. Joshi (✉) · N. Vashist
Department of Anthropology, University of Delhi, New Delhi, Delhi, India
e-mail: pcjoshi@anthro.du.ac.in

G. Misra (ed.), *Psychosocial Interventions for Health and Well-Being*,
https://doi.org/10.1007/978-81-322-3782-2_16

The sub-field of ethno-medicine articulates with other sub fields on both a theoretical and applied level. So, whereas the universal occurrence of beliefs in illness and healthcare across societies make ethno-medicine an interesting enterprise to collect data on knowledge and practices of different societies related to psychosocial, physical and functional aspects of health and healthcare, it is also utmost necessary on a practical level to apply this knowledge in a better manner in order to contribute towards a more effective and culturally accepted public health in regions with indigenous populations in increasingly multi-cultural nations.

Most medical anthropologists dealing with ethno-medicine take somewhat of a systems approach in their work. Major areas of study among biological medical anthropologists include diet and nutrition, evolutionary adaptation, genetic and epigenetic aspects of populations, etc. while socio-cultural medical anthropologists show mostly an ethnographic interest in health knowledge, beliefs and medical systems along with the paraphernalia firmly embedded within the cultural nuances of people under study. A mid-way ground sees health ecologists, medical geographers and epidemiologists combining these two approaches.

Ethno-medicine today is broadly understood as 'those beliefs and practices relating to disease which are products of indigenous cultural development and are not explicitly derived from the conceptual framework of modern medicine' (Hughes 1968: 99 in Foster and Anderson 1978). However, it has increasingly been accepted in the academic circles that modern or bio-medicine is also a form of ethno-medicine since it is essentially drawn upon western cultural constructs thereby eluding the gold standard of 'scientific objectivism' previously assigned to it (Lock and Schepher-Hughes 1990; Rhodes 1990). But for the sake of avoiding confusion, ethno-medicine in this chapter should be seen as consistent with the aforementioned definition.

Such terminology also creates some conflicting assumptions about different indigenous medical systems. For example, in Indian context where tribal groups practice their native medicine and health and illness beliefs, the mainstream population following great traditions has its own indigenous health systems viz., Ayurveda, Yoga, Unani, Siddha, which as per the definition above and commonly employed stand different from the cosmopolitan western bio-medicine.

Sometimes, these two diverse types of medical systems are also collectively called traditional medical systems. However, the term ethno-medicine should generally be used for native groups which have undocumented orally perpetuated systems of medicine and healthcare unlike the national medical systems which are codified and documented.

A number of perspectives arise when one thinks of ethno-medicine in India. India being an extremely culturally diverse country is marked by changing cultural connotations every few miles. Not only different communities but also different sections of the same community practice differing sets of practices and belief systems. Added to these are the overarching great traditions which permeate these different sets of beliefs and practices. In relation to the conception of health and illness, beliefs of causation and cure, these complex cultural groundings influence the notions of sickness, disease and treatment in a unique manner (Mutatkar 2013).

The modern medical system or bio-medicine has low outreach and majority of it is concentrated in the urban areas serving a minority of population, thus, leaving a wide chiasm to be filled in by effective understanding and application of ethno-medical practices and beliefs of such areas. Even in a few societies, where modern medical system has been introduced, the efficacy remains low due to non-acceptance of such a healthcare system by the natives, compelling the health scientists and planners to come up with insights on a better suited healthcare system to indigenous people.

Various studies done on different aspects dealing with indigenous beliefs on health and illness, etiologies, epidemiology, traditional medical practitioners, healthcare systems as well as interaction between various medical systems, health policy planning, etc. shed some important insights into anthropological understanding in the field of ethno-medicine. Some of these are discussed as:

Conception of Health and Illness in Indigenous Groups

The conception of health varies from culture to culture and so does that of illness. Most medical anthropologists today distinguish between illness and disease, where former relates to the subjective and lived experiences of people articulated through a common cultural understanding; disease is a pathological concept used to technically narrow down the unit of malfunction from a wider experiential illness description in the bio-medical model of health. As such, the concept of health and subsequent illnesses are grounded in a holistic and inclusive cultural frame in all societies.

Different indigenous communities conceive health in their own culturally rooted manners and have a native conception of body organs and functions called as ethno-anatomy and ethno-physiology which influences their beliefs related to health, body processes and illnesses (Khundongbam et al. 2012). Many a times, contradictory versions of health also appear in native beliefs where bio-medical views on germs and diseases clash with native models like the case of Jaunsar-Bawar, where intestinal worms are looked upon as beneficial to health rather than as a disease (Joshi 1986, 1995).

The ethno-physiology of *jenukuruba* tribe of Karnataka places importance on the liver as the chief organ where food is transformed into blood. Thin and red-coloured blood is a sign of agility and health while thick and blackish red blood is a sign of illness and loss of strength. These are manifested in young and old bodies respectively. Also, health and intelligence is attributed to lean and short-statured body type. As such, various causes, natural or personal, may turn blood thicker and discoloured giving rise to many types of illnesses (Vijayendra and Bhat 2004).

The menstrual beliefs of body among the *andro* community of Manipur (Krishnakumari et al. 2013) relate menstrual blood to be flowing out of a lotus shaped sac in the women's womb, which if encounters male semen is conceived as a baby. Also, the ethno-anatomy of womb is seen as having numerous placentas in the womb which determine the sex of the baby; if conceived on the right side of the womb it is a male offspring and to the left is a female. Also, various reproductive illnesses (in press) like vaginal discharge, prolapse, menstrual irregularities, etc. are described in terms of ethno-anatomical perception and beliefs on body processes. For example, it is believed among the *andro* women that wearing pads and intra-uterine devices causes obstruction in expelling impure menstrual blood and leads to illness, highlighting the role of folk anatomical and physiological beliefs in healthcare.

As with many ecologically oriented groups, various indigenous communities describe health in functional rather than medical sense of being. As such, disability to perform usual life functions is seen as illness rather than presence of some ailment per se.

The *kamar* of Chhatisgarh describe their health in terms of ability to maintain levels of energy to perform daily tasks and vigour of blood. So, youth is seen as the healthiest stage of life where one's blood is warm and red while due to weakening of blood in old age, a person becomes susceptible to illness (Khatua 2012). Apart from this, other illnesses may either be caused due to natural or individual factors.

Similarly, the hill *korwa* of Chattisgarh attribute health to proper functioning of the body that permits hard physical work and intake of heavy food. Also, a good pulse rate denotes a healthy body. They differentiate between *kaccha* (young) and *buddha* (old) body through the vigour of blood where fluidic and red blood signifies youth and thick and black blood signifies loss of youth leading to an unhealthy body (Khatua 2012).

For the *baiga* of Madhya Pradesh, health is an ability to do work without feeling tired and have a good appetite while illness almost invariably stems from decrease in amount of blood in the body due to various natural and individual causes (Khatua 2012).

The *mishings* of Assam also view health in functional terms of ability to carry on day-to-day tasks at ease like ability to plough one bigha of land in two days or ability to cover 2 km on foot at a stretch, etc. with an ideal body which meant being tall and strong with healthy white teeth and the ability to laugh loudly with additional features of long, black hair and the potentiality to give birth to 4–5 children in women (Kar 2013).

The native beliefs on the organization of body organs and their functions is an important aspect of their medical systems (Joshi and Khattri 2008) which leads them to deduce the causes of mal-functioning of certain body organs as well as types of explanations used for such mal-functioning. So, one find these societies using various etiological concepts that are derived from and relate to native understandings of their bodies.

Disease Etiologies and Causality Concepts

Foster and Anderson (1978) discuss non-Western disease etiologies in two realms —the personalistic and the naturalistic which lead to different types of causality concepts for the explanation of illness. The naturalistic medical systems explain illness in impersonal, systemic terms of natural factors of climate, humoral mis-balance, etc. As such health is essentially a state of equilibrium when all insensate elements in the body—hot and cold or various humours are in proportion to an individual in her/his physical and social environment (ibid). Contrary to this, personalistic medical systems describe illness to be caused by an active and purposeful intervention of some sensate agent supernatural in origin like a ghost, evil spirit, angry gods or a human being in command of such forces like witch, sorcerer, etc. (ibid). However, no society exhibits a neat delineation or simply one type of causality etiologies and one comes across causality attributes on a spectral level.

In Indian contexts, most of the communities have causality concepts that effectively attribute illness and disease to both types of etiological categories. So, one finds most of the communities including the tribal groups, essentially distinguishing between personalistic and naturalist causes and categories of illnesses.

Joshi (2013) lists the differentiation of *bimari-dos* among the Jaunsari tribe of Uttarakhand where *Dos* includes all kinds of sufferings and misfortunes including an individual's illness as well as calamities affecting a large group but bimari refers to bodily disturbances in the case of an individual (Joshi 2013). Ailments like cold, fever, headache, body ache, bone fracture, snake-bite, skin infections like scabies etc. are treated as natural ailments (Rizvi 2013) occurring due to imbalance of various humours and ecological-environmental hazards. The essentially personalistic *dos* not only explains etiologies in a sensate manner due to various hierarchies of demi gods, spirits and evil entities but also points towards a more holistic nature of indigenous causality factors extending the conception of health not only to the individual bodily processes but to successful integration of individual body into a wider social world. This is also to be seen in several other indigenous communities that offer personalistic etiologies for a variety of illness concepts that may or may not be labelled diseases according to a bio-medical view.

The *chenchus* (Sharma and Srinivasu 2013) and *yerukala of* Andhra Pradesh ascribe natural causes to diseases like jaundice, stomach pain, dysentery, headache, cough, fevers during rainy season, rheumatism, bone-fractures, etc. while other illnesses like small pox, snake/scorpion bite, body-swelling, psychological illnesses, etc. are understood through personalistic causality factors (Reddy et al. 2013).

The *kannikar tribe* of Kerala distinguishes between two broad categories of illnesses—*rogam* and *upadravam* (Menon 2013) where *rogam* are attributed to natural factors and require medication while *upadravam* illnesses are attached to supernatural beings like evil spirits, angry deities, etc.

Similarly, the *irular* people of Tamil Nadu consult medicine men or herbalists *rangamsamiar* for both body ailments requiring only medication and ailments due to sorcery or *kodangi* depending upon the causality logic involved (Saheb 2013).

Also the *mishings* of Assam ascribe certain ailments to natural causes while still invoking the personalistic etiologies for most of the others. So, ailments at personal and community level like epidemics, accidents, sudden onset of fevers, diaorrhoea or diseases like leprosy, paralysis, tuberculosis, etc. are understood to be caused by supernatural personalistic forces while other illnesses like upset stomach, cold-cough, body aches, skin-diseases, etc. are thought to be causes by natural forces under rules of purity and pollution and humoral imbalances (Kar 2013).

The *rathwa* tribe of Gujarat attribute majority of illnesses to supernatural entities or sorcery including small pox, leprosy, severe body aches and other illnesses due to evil eye, high fever as also general misfortune and societal misintegration. Minor ailments like headaches, minor fevers, oils, skin ailments, toothache, constipation, etc. are attributed to imbalance of bodily humours and resorted to medication (Das 2004).

The *gaddis* of Himachal Pradesh (Kaushal 2004; Kaushal and Joshi 2007) attribute the causes of various ailments to factors like punishment from deities or affliction by supernatural entities like *autars*, *kailung*, *gunga* or by magic and witchcraft while many day-to-day ailments like body-aches, minor fevers or bruises, skin infections, etc. are treated through the use of locally available herbs.

Among the *moyons* of Manipur (Moyon 2004), though most of the people resort to allopathy for their illnesses, those ailments that cannot be diagnosed by doctors are taken to visionaries who tackle illnesses caused due to spirit intrusion and other supernatural entities. In addition, various locally available herbs are also used to cure illnesses like cold and cough, joint pains, dysentery, indigestion, jaundice, etc.

The *monpas* of Arunachal Pradesh (Ibata 2004) conform to a highly spiritual *bon* religion in which the mountain spirit *pfu* influences all aspects of health and illnesses in combination with the malefic forces *don* and *grib*; diseases are cured by a *monpa*, the traditional healer, and the spiritualist *bonpo.* However, bonpos distinguish between illnesses occurring due to natural causes and those due to spiritual ones and no rites are performed for natural ailments like fractured bones, aches due to strenuous work, some ailments of blood, diseases like cholera. For these ailments a *bonpa* sends patients to doctors trained in western medicine. For spiritual illnesses like psychological and social maladjustments, chronic and lingering illnesses, etc., a number of rites are performed.

The common thread that binds the disease etiologies and causality attributes in all these and similar indigenous groups are a native understanding of severity of deviation from health in the personalistic illnesses. These illnesses are different from diseases or bodily troubles in being assimilated at a wider level of social and communal well-being in addition to lingering or chronic versions of naturally attributed illnesses. These are to be satiated at the level of social body in terms of Lock and Schepher-Hughes (1990) as well as individual body. This brings in the major role played by religious specialists or diviners or medicine men who perform various rituals and thus, aim at rooting out the causes of hiatus through a sleuth of supernatural entities. These medicine men often perform the role of herbalists also, while in some more hierarchal organized tribes; different roles may be given to different specialists (Joshi 1981a, c, 2013). The herbalists take care of most of the illnesses attributed to natural causes. It is also interesting to note that in most of the indigenous societies, the illnesses belonging to the realm of personalistic causality factors can often also cause other ailments pertaining to the natural causality factors but not vice versa (Joshi 1981b, 1988, 1991, 2004, 2013), hinting at the priority given to social sustenance and group well-being over individual well-being.

Traditional Healers in Ethno Medicine

The centrality of traditional healers is a characteristic of indigenous medicine. Whether these native medical systems are naturalistic or personalistic or combine both, traditional healers that include herbalists, faith-healers, diviners/shamans, etc. are found in all scenarios. These traditional healers are informally trained in their healing practices by virtue of culturally accepted idioms of illnesses and their healing and may get their training from previous healers like herbalists through apprenticeship or over a time with experience or through special abilities that are inborn and refined through elder practitioners like shamanism, etc. The informality of occupation results in their close association with the people as these healers interact with patients in a culturally meaningful therapeutic discourse. Kleinman (1978) calls this form of healing as the folk sector which is largely resorted to by the indigenous communities but is also found in communities with a more established professional sector of health consisting of certified doctors. The cultural orientation in explaining, understanding and reciprocating idioms of distress of the sufferers by these healers lends cultural credibility to their practices.

The role of shaman is central in medical systems of various communities in India. So, one finds regular mention of sacred healers who act as a mediator between patients and mystical powers like *siamphu* among *paite* tribe, *kamyou* among *jangkhul* nagas, *thempu* among *rongmeis*, *ithim* among *thadou* kukis, etc. (Hemlata and Kumari 2004).

These shamans or witch-doctors perform various functions in a community which range from warding off epidemics by following preventive measures of sacrificial offerings to protecting the community and individuals from attacks of evil spirits, ensuring crop production by bringing rains, treating various diseases like small-pox, cholera, etc. In Uttarakhand, among *tharus*, the shaman *bharra* performs functions like tracing out diseases by spelling out the name of responsible spirits, warding off epidemics and protecting villages from evil spirits by invoking goddess *bhawani* and *sayana* of *bhoksa* tribe is consulted for treatment of diseases like chicken pox and cholera (Singh 2004).

Often, different types of traditional healers may be found in one community who perform different functions. For example, Joshi (1981a, 2013) describes the hierarchy of traditional healers consulted for various illnesses by the Jaunsari people of Uttarakhand, where the priest cum astrologer, the *baman*, and the diviner cum shaman, the *mali*, deal exclusively with personalistic attributed *dos* whereas herbalist and pulse specialist *jariyara* and the female specialist deal with naturalistic illnesses called bimari.

Similarly, the *anals* of Manipur (Hemlata and Kumari 2004) differentiate between two types of *athim* (physician)—the *larni* (those who are possessed by spirits) and *patakang* (those who heal without being possessed).

Among the *suskal* of Gujarat (Das 2004), the shaman is known as *bhua* who is consulted for various chronic and other ailments thought to be due to supernatural causes while other types of healers are snake-bite specialists, local herbalist or *vedji* in addition to practitioners of allopathic medicines.

The hill *korwa* of central India depend traditionally upon the services of *ojha* as diviner and shaman, village priest *baiga*, spiritist cum medicine man *panda*, while herbal medicine is taken from herbal specialist called *dewar* (Khatua 2013). Similarly, the Birhors of Chattisgarh also rely on ojhas for ailments related to supernatural causes. The tribal doctor among the *kamars* of Chattisgarh is called *gunia* who performs all types of healing from herbalism to shamanistic. *Gunia* is usually consulted along with the free medical treatment available to them through government health centres (Sinha and Banerjee 2013).

The religious specialist *plathi* among the *kannikars* of Kerala (Menon 2013) are consulted to treat maladies due to *upadravam* or supernatural causes. This is usually done simultaneously to other types of naturalistic treatments and bio-medicine.

The psychosocial aspects of the shamans or other faith healers have been widely discussed in anthropology (Devereux 1961; Lewis 1971; Taussig 1987; Eliade 1961). In the context of shamans in Indian communities, a few studies highlight these psychosocial aspects. Joshi (2010) discusses the processes leading to successful initiation of a shaman among the *jaunsaris* of Uttarakhand. Here a shaman is seen not only as a person who provides family therapy and counselling to psychosocially troubled people but also as a psychosocially rehabilitated person himself who by virtue of effective and culturally valued rehabilitation, has been able to gain better healing for himself which he then perpetuates to others. He, through his therapy, not only mitigates the various illnesses but also acts as an agent of social justice and functioning according to the cultural norms.

Faith-healing is prevalent not only in indigenous tribal groups but also in various rural and urban communities belonging to organized religions. Faith-healing in *dargahs* and temples like Balaji in Rajasthan also contribute to traditional ways of healing of the psychologically affected (Joshi and Vashist forthcoming).

Ecology, Health and Ethno Medicine

Medical anthropology has always been ecological in its orientation which deals with the inter-relationships between humans and their environment, combining the biological and sociocultural dimensions that determine health and illnesses. Though nature provides its own determining limits to the availability of resources and orientation of certain diseases more than other, the sociocultural dimensions of health govern many different factors ranging from social cognizance of 'food' from amongst the available sources of nutrition, various aspects of environment-specific diseases and cultural institutions to deal with them as also the cultural factors that trigger disease and the environment in which the patient gets after-care or treatment (Bhalla 2013; Gadekar et al. 2013). Also, the cultural norms of marriage and mating also play a central role in perpetuation of certain genetic disorders through the effect of inbreeding (Ramachandraiah 2013).

Owing to the pathological and sociopsychological dimensions of illnesses, ecology occupies a central place in determining the health of people occupying a certain niche. Various dimensions become significant of which nutrition is preliminary. Nutrition, as a bio-cultural feature, is determined by availability in the natural environment, however, what becomes available to humans is culturally determined and defined as the edible part of all sources of nutrition, known as 'food' (Foster and Anderson 1978).

Various communities in India classify food according to the prevalent ayurvedic tridosha theory where food is believed to be of *vayu*, *pitta* and *kapha* nature which is further categorized as hot and cold. This classification of food determines the edibility of food according to various beliefs of body-functioning and processes as also environmental concerns like for illnesses caused due to hot elements like sunstroke, it is believed that eating cold nature foods like curd would provide relief.

The *bettakuruba* of Karnataka (Vijayendra 2013) classify food into hot or *churuka*, cold or *thampu* and gaseous or *vaya* substances in accordance to the *pitta*, *kapha* and *vaya* elements in these. Thus, during summer season cold foods like jackfruit, guava, banana, millets as *ragi*, meat of pig and sheep are preferred while during winter and rainy season hot foods like fried vegetables and cereals are preferred. The native beliefs lead them to totally discard egg, chicken, raw papaya consumption by pregnant women. Also, gaseous foods are to be avoided during pregnancy while foods like bottle-gourd and papaya are known as milk-enhancers and encouraged during lactation.

The *savara* women of Andhra Pradesh (Narahari 2013) deny the new-born the first milk or colostrum by squeezing it out and alternatively feed the new-born sugar water or honey or castor oil to clean the digestive tract. The same is also true of other tribes like *gadaba* and *porja*.

Pasuvula Banda of Visakhapatnam (Subramanyam 2004) have a taboo against consumption of their own totemic plants and animals. Extensive dietary restrictions are placed on pregnant and lactating mothers that may or may not be in sync with that of nutritional requirements as per the bio-medical standards. Prohibitions like consuming liquor are beneficial while on the contrary those like prohibition of fish, meat, eggs and vegetables like pumpkins, cause a substantial protein deficit in pregnant and lactating women.

Due to ecological factors, certain diseases caused due to vitamin A and B deficiency are also prevalent, so are those pertaining to skin and urino-genital tract due to constant contact with microbes in their immediate environment. Similarly, infant and child mortality as well as maternal health are important concerns in many of the indigenous groups in the country. Among the *moyons* (Moyon 2004), main diseases among the children are air and water borne like chicken pox, whooping cough, fever, cold diarrhoea, dysentery, jaundice, cholera, typhoid, etc.

Nutritional anaemia has been a consistent factor for low health among most women in indigenous communities (Paliwal 2004). Coupled with factors like malarial environment, genetic abnormalities like thalassemia, G6PD deficiency and sickle cell disease, this constitutes major disease burden among the indigenous population. For example, *Birhors* and hill *Korwas* (Sinha and Banerjee 2013) report a high incidence of nutritional anaemia, more in women due to heavy workload, low dietary intake and burden of multiple pregnancies as well as diseases like cataract, thalassemia, etc. while sickle cell trait is absent unlike most of the tribal groups in India.

Ethno-Medicine in Interaction with ISM and Biomedicine: Current Issues

Owing to the immense ethnic diversity of India, there is a great variation in the nature of health seeking among people across country. In the face of illnesses, different communities seek different types of medicine based on their cultural beliefs and availability of health resources. Though every community possesses its own intrinsic knowledge of various ailments and resources needed to cure these, often pragmatism in healthcare leads them to simultaneously seek other options available. The Indian medical system comprises several locally based and valued ethno-medical systems under an over-arching pan-Indian systems of Indian medicines like ayurveda, unani, siddha, etc., which is further diversified by a hegemonic western or bio-medicine. With the proliferation of Western medicine worldwide, there have been sustained efforts on part of the government to allocate modern health resources and personnel to indigenous areas.

Medically pluralistic societies deal with numerous aspects that are of interest to the medical anthropologist like, decisions influencing selection of available medical systems, role expectations of patients, clientele, patient–healer interaction and patient satisfaction, notions of efficacy, treatment and types of cure, placebo effect, interaction of various medical systems, strengths and weaknesses of indigenous systems vis-à-vis medicine. In context of national medical systems, questions of mainstreaming the ISM, interaction of ISM and ethno-medicine as well as successful incorporation of western medicine, its extent and reach, issues in outreach and acceptance are also of significance. Also, the essential premise that a medical system needs to always be analysed in terms of cultural background and the total social system, makes the issue of interaction between various medical systems a complex one.

Owing to the resource limitation in healthcare sector in highly populated and diverse countries like India, there is a strong need for integration of ethno-medicine and ISM to the mainstream model of healthcare that focuses heavily on western medicine. Of late, attempts have been made to incorporate AYUSH in national policies for health delivery but ethno-medicine still lags far behind due to various reasons. The foremost among such reasons is a lack of documentation of the native systems of medicine, others being lack of 'scientific' evidence, loss of bio-diversity leading to reduction in ethno-medical base of pharmacopeia, informal nature of healing that is difficult to incorporate in a formal nationalized system, hierarchical and distrustful role of professional healers for traditional ones, insufficient cultural sensitivity, etc. (Banerjee et al. 2013; Reddy 2013; Kakar 2013).

Conclusion

Ethno-medicine is a rich field of enquiry in the discipline of medical anthropology. Cross-cultural in nature, it aims at not only documenting the indigenous beliefs about the concepts of health, illness, disease and healthcare but also an applied interest in studying and implementing the trajectories of efficacy, utility, cultural validity and interaction of ethno-medicine with professional medicine for the betterment of healthcare in a multi-cultural world. In India, as also other developing nations, where professional healthcare is heavily affected by limitations in health resources and personnel, an effective health planning needs to incorporate locally available resources for wider health coverage.

As such, medical anthropology with its emic and culturally situated perspectives is of great significance in bridging the gap between healthcare demand and availability with its grass-root oriented and practical interventions through the studies of indigenous medical systems. Various dimensions pertaining to the ethno-medicine in India have been covered in this chapter which deal with issues ranging from conception of health and illness, etiological dimensions, healing beliefs and traditional healers as well as interaction of ethno-medicine with other systems of medicine like the Indian systems, viz., ayurveda, unani, etc., and the Western medicine system or allopathy. Various empirical studies have consistently described the ethno-medical richness of beliefs, cultural settings, ecology in governing the formation and sustenance of native medical beliefs. These medical beliefs may or may not be syncretic to Western notions but nonetheless form the very basis of the social system of indigenous communities. For effective healthcare in India, the anthropological perspectives on these aspects have immense significance for a culturally acceptable, efficacious and pragmatic healthcare that is accessible to all.

References

Banerjee, B. G., Kaur, G., & Sinha, A. K. (2013). An anthropological perspective in medical pluralism: Some observations. In H. K. Bhat, P. C. Joshi & B. R. Vijayendra (Eds.), *Illness, health and culture* (Vol. 1, pp. 94–113). New Delhi: Concept Publishing.

Bhalla, A. K. (2013). Medical anthropology in context of culture, environment, disease and health. In H. K. Bhat, P. C. Joshi & B. R. Vijayendra (Eds.), *Illness, health and culture* (Vol. 1, pp. 55–66). New Delhi: Concept Publishing .

Das, M. (2004). Disease and illness and their ethno-medical treatment among rathwas of Suskal, Gujarat. In A. K. Kalla & P. C Joshi (Eds.), *Tribal health and medicines* (pp. 283–300). New Delhi: Concept publishing.

Devereux, G. (1961). Shamans as neurotics. *American Anthropologist, 63,* 1088–1090.

Eliade, M. (1961). Recent works on Shamanism. *History of Religions, 1*(1), 152–186.

Foster, G., & Anderson, B. G. (1978). *Medical anthropology*. New York: Wiley.

Gadekar, P. H., Apte, H., & Gambhir, R. D. (2013). Environment as a cause and cure: A study among fishermen community. In H. K. Bhat, P. C. Joshi & B. R. Vijayendra (Eds.), *Illness, health and culture* (Vol. 1, pp. 287–295). New Delhi: Concept Publishing .

Hemlata, O., & Kumari, P. K. (2004). Health care practices among tribes of Manipur. In A. K. Kalla & P. C Joshi (Eds.), *Tribal health and medicines* (pp. 276–282). New Delhi: Concept Publishing .

Ibata, A. (2004). Bon medicine among Monpas in Western Arunachal Pradesh. In A. K. Kalla & P. C Joshi (Eds.), *Tribal health and medicines* (pp. 318–340). New Delhi: Concept Publishing.

Joshi, P. C. (1981a). Concept and causation: Ethno-medicine in Jaunsar-Bawar. *Journal of Social Research, 23*(2), 16–26.

Joshi, P. C. (1981b). Perception and classification of illness among the Khasa tribals of Dehradun. *Tribe, 23*(1), 16–26.

Joshi, P. C. (1981c). Illness and social control: A study in ethno-medicine. *Research Proceedings, 8*(1&2), 9–16.

Joshi, P. C. (1986). Health and healing in the Himalayas. *Journal of Himalyan Studies and Regional Development, 10,* 111–117.

Joshi, P. C. (1988). Traditional medical systems in Central Himalayas. *The Eastern Anthropologist, 41*(1), 78–86.

Joshi, P. C. (1991). Culture, health and illness: Aspects of ethno-medicine in Jaunsar-Bawar. In S. K. Biswas (Ed.), *The Central Himalayan panorama* (pp. 253–280). Calcutta: Calcutta Institute of Social Research and Applied Anthropology.

Joshi, P. C. (1995). Don't let me down: Place of worms in culture and reflections on ethno-physiology in a Central Himalayan Tribe. *Journal of Indian Anthropological Society, 30,* 253–258.

Joshi, P. C. (2004). The world of tribal healers. In A. K. Kalla & P. C. Joshi (Eds.), *Tribal health and medicines* (pp. 202–241). New Delhi: Concept Publishing.

Joshi, P. C. (2010). Psychotherapeutic elements in Shamanistic healing in the context of Himalayan traditions. *Delhi Psychiatry Journal, 13*(2), 254–257.

Joshi, P. C. (2013). *Relevance of traditional medicine in global era*. New Delhi: Icon Publications.

Joshi, P. C., & Khattri, P. (2008). Traditional medical system of the Bhils: Characteristics, function and change. In R. K. Pathak, A. K. Sinha, R. N. Vasishat, B. G. Banerjee & C. J. Edwin (Eds.), *Bio-social health issues* (pp. 471–486). New Delhi: Northern Book Centre.

Joshi, P. C., & Vashist, N. (In press). Ritual healing and Shamanism. *The Eastern anthropologist*.

Kakar, D. N. (2013). Problems and prospects of healthcare in India. In H. K. Bhat, P. C. Joshi & B. R. Vijayendra (Eds.), *Illness, health and culture* (Vol. 1, pp. 21–31). New Delhi: Concept Publishing.

Kar, R. K. (2013). Societal dimensions of health; Some rambles on the tribal scenario. In H. K. Bhat, P. C. Joshi & B. R. Vijayendra (Eds.), *Illness, health and culture* (Vol. 1, pp. 229–240). New Delhi: Concept Publishing.

Kaushal, S. (2004). Healing practices among Gaddi Tribe of Himachal Pradesh. In A. K. Kalla & P. C Joshi (Eds.), *Tribal health and medicines* (pp. 301–310). New Delhi: Concept Publishing.

Kaushal, S., & Joshi, P. C. (2007). Ethno medical practices in a high altitude Vashist village in Himachal Pradesh. *South Asian Anthropologist, 7*(1), 37–46.

Khatua, N. (2012). *Health, ecology and culture: An anthropological study among the three tribes of Central India*. Kolkata: Anthropological Survey of India.

Khatua, N. (2013). Problems and prospects of modern healthcare services: A case of hill Korwa Tribe of Chattisgarh. In H. K. Bhat, P. C. Joshi & B. R. Vijayendra (Eds.), *Illness, health and culture* (Vol. 1, pp. 198–208). New Delhi: Concept Publishing.

Khundongbam, G., Joshi, P. C., & Singh, M. M. (2012). Perception of childhood diarrhoea in Langmeidong village, Manipur. *South-Asian Anthropologist, 12*(2), 135–140.

Kleinman, A. (1978). Concepts and a model for comparison of medical systems. *Social Science and Medicine, Bulletin* 85–93.

Krishnakumari, P., Joshi, P. C., Kumar, M. A. & Singh, M. M. (In press). Women's perception of reproductive illness in Manipur, India. *Journal of Anthropology*.

Krishnakumari, P., Joshi, P. C., & Singh, M. M. (2013). Beliefs and practices on reproductive health among Andro of Manipur. *South Asian Anthropologist, 13*(2), 111–119.

Lewis, I. M. (1971). *Ecstatic religions: An anthropological study of spirit possession and Shamanism*. Middlesex, UK: Penguin Books.

Lock, M. & Schepher-Hughes, N. (1990). A critical interpretive approach in medical anthropology: Rituals and routines of discipline and dissent. In T. M. Jhonson & C. F. Sargent (Eds.), *Medical anthropology; contemporary theory and method* (pp. 41–71). New York: Praeger.

Menon, V. (2013). Health-seeking among forest-dwelling Kanikkar in Kerala. In H. K. Bhat, P. C. Joshi & B. R. Vijayendra (Eds.), *Illness, health and culture* (Vol. 1, pp. 144–169). Concept Publishing: New Delhi.

Moyon, L. N. (2004). Women and health among the Moyons. In A. K. Kalla & P. C. Joshi (Eds.), *Tribal health and medicines* (pp. 168–175). New Delhi: Concept Publishing.

Mutatkar, R. K. (2013). Medical anthropology, past, present and Future. In H. K. Bhat, P. C. Joshi & B. R. Vijayendra (Eds.), *Illness, health and culture* (Vol. 1, pp. 47–54). New Delhi: Concept Publishing.

Narahari, S. (2013). Mother child healthcare practices. In H. K. Bhat, P. C. Joshi & B. R. Vijayendra (Eds.), *Illness, health and culture* (Vol. 2, pp. 163–169). New Delhi: Concept Publishing.

Paliwal, M. (2004). Risk factors of HIV/AIDS among tribals in India. In A. K. Kalla & P. C. Joshi (Eds.), *Tribal health and medicines* (pp. 104–111). New Delhi: Concept Publishing.

Ramachandraiah, T. (2013). Bio-anthropological studies and their and their relation to health sciences: Medical anthropology. In H. K. Bhat, P. C. Joshi & B. R. Vijayendra (Eds.), *Illness, health and culture* (Vol. 1, pp. 67–73). New Delhi: Concept Publishing.

Reddy, P. K. (2013). Medical pluralism and mainstreaming AYUSH: An anthropological analysis of health policy. In H. K. Bhat, P. C. Joshi & B. R. Vijayendra (Eds.), *Illness, health and culture* (Vol. 1, pp. 77–93). New Delhi: Concept Publishing.

Reddy, K. V., Gangadhar, J., Manoj, D. K. & Kumar, M. K. (2013). The relevance of ethno-medicine and healthcare practices among the Yerukala and Chenchu tribes of Nallamala forest range of Andhra Pradesh. In H. K. Bhat, P. C. Joshi & B. R. Vijayendra (Eds.), *Illness, health and culture* (Vol. 1, pp. 250–264). New Delhi: Concept Publishing.

Rhodes, L. A. (1990). Studying bio-medicine as a cultural system. In T. M. Johnson & C. F. Sargent (Eds.), *Medical anthropology: Contemporary theory and method* (pp. 165–183). New York: Praeger.

Rizvi, S. N. H. (2013). Indigenous medicine and its practice among the Jaunsari. In H. K. Bhat, P. C. Joshi & B. R. Vijayendra (Eds.), *Illness, health and culture* (Vol. 1, pp. 241–249). New Delhi: Concept Publishing.

Saheb, S. A. A. (2013). Ethno-medicine and traditional treatment: A case study of Irular of Tamil-Nadu. In H. K. Bhat, P. C. Joshi & B. R. Vijayendra (Eds.), *Illness, health and culture* (Vol. 1, pp. 265–273). New Delhi: Concept Publishing.

Sharma, B. V. & Srinivasu, N. (2013). Health status and healthcare among the Chenchus. In H. K. Bhat, P. C. Joshi & B. R. Vijayendra (Eds.), *Illness, health and culture* (Vol. 1, pp. 188–197). New Delhi: Concept Publishing.

Singh, A. P. (2004). Healing practices among the tribes of Uttaranchal. In A. K. Kalla & P. C. Joshi (Eds.), *Tribal health and medicines* (pp. 242–246). New Delhi: Concept Publishing.

Sinha, A. K. & Banerjee, B. G. (2013). Health and health seeking behaviour of 'primitive tribal groups' of Chattisgarh: Some socio-demographic dimensions. In H. K. Bhat, P. C. Joshi & B. R. Vijayendra (Eds.), *Illness, health and culture* (Vol. 1, pp. 114–143). New Delhi: Concept Publishing.

Subramanyam, V. (2004). Ecology, diet and health status among tribes; A study in Pasuvulabanda Village of Visakha agency area, Andhra Pradesh. In A. K. Kalla & P. C. Joshi (Eds.), *Tribal health and medicines* (pp. 115–130). New Delhi: Concept Publishing.

Taussig, M. (1987). *Shamanism, colonialism and the wild man: A study in terror and healing*. Chicago: University of Chicago Press.

Vijayendra, B. R. (2013). Food habits and beliefs among the BettaKuruba of Karnataka. In H. K. Bhat, P. C. Joshi & B. R. Vijayendra (Eds.), *Illness, health and culture* (Vol. 2, pp. 74–84). New Delhi: Concept Publishing.
Vijayendra, B. R., & Bhat, H. K. (2004). Ethnomedicine among the JenuKuruba of Karnataka. In A. K. Kalla & P. C. Joshi (Eds.), *Tribal health and medicines* (pp. 391–407). New Delhi: Concept Publishing.

Chapter 17
Towards a Culturally-Informed Counselling and Psychotherapy

Tissy Mariam Thomas, Baiju Gopal and T. Sasidharan

The methodological shift ensued in the academic sphere of psychology in India since the 1980s witnessed its ripples in the popularization of cultural psychology, indigenous psychology, transpersonal psychology, Indian psychology, Asian healing practices, health psychology, positive psychology and community psychology. Even though these disciplines found their origins in western psychology, they offer a space for cultural debates. Emergence and implementation of qualitative research methods in studying human behaviour opened up a wide range of lines of investigation to make inquiries of cultural imprints. The predominant positivist-empirical approach with its deductive outlook created more obstacles than facilitating context-dependent studies about human behaviour (Misra 2003). Rethinking culture-psychology interface with an inductive research perspective transcended disciplinary boundaries. Examining the Western and non-Western cultural perceptions gave rise to diverse and plural conceptualizations of psychology.

Cultural Construction of Self

Culture as defined by Malinowski (1944) is 'composed of partly autonomous, partly coordinated institutions. It is integrated on a series of principles such as the community of blood through procreation; the contiguity in space related to cooperation;

T. M. Thomas (✉)
Department of Psychology, University of Kerala, Thiruvananthapuram, Kerala, India
e-mail: talk2tissy@gmail.com

B. Gopal
Department of Psychology, CHRIST (Deemed to be University), Bangalore, India

T. Sasidharan
Department of Psychology, University of Calicut, Malappuram, Kerala, India

G. Misra (ed.), *Psychosocial Interventions for Health and Well-Being*,
https://doi.org/10.1007/978-81-322-3782-2_17

the specialization in activities; and last but not the least, the use of power in political organization. Each culture owes its completeness and self-sufficiency to the fact that it satisfies the whole range of basic, instrumental and integrative needs'. Cultural psychology, therefore, holds a semiotic (sign-mediated) direction and an activity orientation. Semiotic mediation is part of the system of organized psychological functions which symbolically capture the intra and inter psychological processes. The idea of folk models, one of the forms of sign mediation fits into the views of cognitive anthropology which views culture as existing knowledge and core conceptual structures (D' Andrade 1984, cited in Valsiner 2007). The activity-theoretic perspective of culture argues that 'humans develop through their changing participation in the socio-cultural activities of their communities, which also change' (Rogoff 2003 cited in Valsiner 2007). Thus an individual doesn't lose own culture in the fusion of structurally divergent cultures rather transforms one's own. By drawing contrasts between mutually interdependent cultural practices, cross-cultural psychologists overcome the 'blinders' of existing tacit assumptions. They believe in the implied properties of qualitative homogeneity and temporal stability of cultures.

Extending the study of cultures, Hofstede (2011) has noted six important dimensions of cultural variation, i.e., power distance, uncertainty avoidance, individualism/collectivism, masculinity/femininity, long/short term orientation and indulgence/restraint. Individualism pertains to societies in which the ties between individuals are loose: everyone is expected to look after himself or herself and his or her immediate family. Collectivism characterizes the societies in which people from birth onwards are integrated into strong, cohesive in-groups, which throughout people's lifetime continue to protect them in exchange for unquestioning loyalty (Hofstede 1991 cited in Kim 1997). The individualistic values are upheld by Western Europe and North American cultures and Asian cultures represent collectivistic values. Cultures emphasize feminine orientation, stress minimum emotional and social differentiation between genders and men and women share a balance between family and work. Masculine cultures are marked with a strong emotional and social role differentiation between genders. France, Portugal, Thailand follow a feminine culture whereas Japan, Germany and Mexico are of masculine cultures. Cultures with a short-term orientation focuses on immediate need gratification and believe that most important events in life have occurred in the past or take place now whereas cultures with a long-term orientation give less importance to need gratification and observe that most significant events in life are yet to come in future. Cultural accounts of mental health/illness, therefore, typify an individual's religion, caste, language, family structure and relationships in their community.

Construction of self through socialization of one's own culture has its implication for the development of a personal culture. Sigmund Freud's classical psychoanalysis linked it with the development of personality and psychopathology. Mead held that self-concept is mediated through language. The self which passes through preparatory, play and game stages finally stabilizes by taking into account the social forces of the culture (Mead and Strauss 1964 cited in Fraser and Burchell 2001, pp. 29–30). Selfhood depends on the socialization of a child into one's social world and through this the acquisition of relevant materials for knowing the self is acquired. The making of a personal and social self find their raw materials from the language, values, norms, beliefs, roles and social collectives. The degree of harmony or integration a person experiences within the various elements of one's own culture determines how well the person understands himself or herself as an essential part of the sub-cultures, local cultures and the negotiation between traditional and emerging cultures one belongs to.

Culture-Bound Syndromes and Emergence of Personal Culture

Cultural mediation of personal identity uses the construction and use of signs to transcend any here-and-now situated activity context by way of subjectively constructed personal meanings or 'personal culture' (Valsiner 2007, p. 60). The distinction between 'culture-bound' and 'universal' mental disorders works at this level of cultural internalization of a person's affective processes. According to DSM-IV, 'Culture-bound syndromes are generally limited to specific societies or culture areas that are localized, folk, diagnostic categories that frame coherent meanings for certain repetitive, patterned and troubling sets of experiences and observations. There is seldom a one-to-one equivalence of any culture-bound syndrome with a DSM diagnostic entity' (cited in Marsella 2000, p. 407). Marsella (2000) also observes that culture-bound syndromes entered Western psychiatric literature in the late nineteenth century as Western physicians working in colonies of Asia, Africa and South America reported strange and 'exotic' disorders that appeared distinct from disorders reported in Europe and North America. Reports of European travellers and adventurers and other historical journals also report the presence of many disorders which does not fit into the DSM classification of mental disorders.

Gopal (2008) mentions about the crisis of 'unknown' causes of mental diseases reported in the archival data from 1890 to 1900 of Calicut mental asylum at Madras presidency while tracing the historical evolution of mental illness in Kerala. He observed that Western physicians are unable to understand most of the symptoms which are culturally embedded and alien to them that made its reported percentage to be 40.22 among moral (26.12%) and physical causes (33.65%) (pp. 267–70). The report of 1890–1900 also shows that 80% of the causes of mental illnesses were unknown. Against this background it can be implied that lack of understanding about what causes insanity to natives would have resulted in culturally inappropriate diagnosis and treatment methods purely from an organic approach of Western psychiatry. What causes mental illness in a developed country sometimes may be understood as divine and supported by one's culture in a developing country. For instance, the practice of certain ritual art forms in South Indian culture includes the elements of possession and being possessed by a deity is considered to be a blessing in one's community. This should not be considered as pathological and to be treated as per Western standards.

While personal culture is interdependent with the inter-personal communicative processes, self-construction of individuals take place at a deeper personal cultural sense. Labelling culture-bound disorders with respect to ethnic specifications entails the uniqueness of any culture irrespective of which agency classifies them. Basu (2005a, b) while stating about mental health as a cultural practice criticizes DSM-IV as most of the conditions described are culture-bound to Euro-America with an exception of five psychiatric syndromes. They are schizophrenia, bipolar disorder, brief reactive psychoses, major depression, bipolar disorders and a range of anxiety disorders from panic states through phobias to obsessive compulsive disorders. Questioning this data base from different knowledge systems that exist in our culture, cross-culturally existing mental disorders may lose its identity and not be valid. Therefore, the etiology and symptom manifestation of anorexia nervosa (which is regarded as specific to industrialized societies) and schizophrenia (which is continued to be considered universal) occur in the internalization and externalization of collective and personal cultural meaning systems of a person.

The exploration into the cultural roots of disorders identifies the unstable base of Western psychiatric classification which questions the premises such as same etiology leading to different disorders; different etiologies causing same disorders and similar treatments used for disorders with different etiologies and expressions. For instance, the authors themselves observed that multiple usages of the same psychopharmacological drug, meant for a particular disorder, being prescribed for many other disorders. A pharmacological categorization of mental illness followed in the medical reckoner, available in any medical shops, is also different from that of DSM-IV.

Different etiologies, symptom patterns and treatment responsiveness of disorders in different cultures expand the limitations of a universal classification further. The universality versus relativity of truth in the construction of selves of individuals in a given culture is of particular importance here. Western psychiatry holds the view of a universal reality and maintains a strict and dominating place in deciding what should be the 'right' way of mental health practice. The emergence of a personal culture encompasses the experiential milieu in which a normal and abnormal self originates, elicit meanings, expresses and responds to other selves in the culture. A universal position ascribed by the Western psychiatric classification decontextualizes the symptoms and disorders which clearly represents an imbalance in power and leads to erroneous diagnosis and treatment.

Incorporating Culture into Psychotherapy in Mental Health Practices

Progression of mental health services in India takes different phases in its historical journey. Today's medical pluralism existing in the country encompasses embracing of world culture as we have multiple medical systems such as biomedicine, ayurveda, unani, siddha, naturopathy, yoga, Chinese and Tibetan medicine and a variety of folk traditions. 'The emergence and arrival of different medical systems, their acculturation into various communities, as well as the way they synchronized and contested with the indigenous are quite unique to Indian medical and cultural history' (Sujatha and Abrahama 2012). The available literature takes into account the record only since the colonial period which is reasonably well documented under the British rule. Kumar (2005) reports that the mentally ill were not treated separately although traditional Indian systems of medical sciences such as ayurveda, unani and siddha were well practiced in this country until the arrival of Europeans in the 18th and 19th centuries. The dualistic classification of illness into mental and physical has come along with the biomedical model of Western medicine whereas the culturally rooted Indian medical systems followed rather a holistic conceptualization of health and illness (Thomas 2009). Ayurveda has recognized forms of mental illnesses and treatment methods which are indigenously accepted. The value of inner peace and mental harmony are emphasized through *panchakarma* and yoga and meditation techniques. An individual's overall development in the traditional healing practices stresses on the equal significance to be given to body, mind and soul. Western psychiatry has brought a new conceptualization of illness which even nullified the existence of indigenous forms of healing in our culture and set a standard to measure its process of conduction through strict scientific reasoning alien to the natives.

Colonization has then controlled the different phases of mental health services in terms of development of infrastructure for basic health services, establishment of mental hospitals and the enactment of Lunacy Act in 1858. The custodial approach in building up 'asylums' rather largely followed a pattern of treatment and concepts of mental illness that of Britain and Europe. A shift in the development of mental health policy from custodial to preventive, promotive and curative services which led to the formulation of National Mental Health Programme for India in 1982 was an attempt to bring in national attention to psychiatric care. National Rural Health Mission programmes record very little effort to improve mental health services at the national, state or regional levels (Kumar 2005, p. 8). Community-based mental health approach, thus initiated in some of the centres in this country, is again strongly influenced by the mental health movements in the West. Although these models incorporate culture into psychotherapy, its effective adaptation and transferability and the development of culturally appropriate strategies is still an unanswered question. While incorporating counselling and psychotherapy into the indigenous healing methods is acceptable to the natives, the community psychiatry approach adapted from the West is power-centred which only provides a very minimal scope for complete inclusion of indigenous understanding of mental health and illness.

Cultural factors with its epistemologies and ontologies influences an individual's personality, construction of self, social role expectations and consciousness patterns. Psychopathology is also shaped through preferred breeding patterns, nutritional practices, climate and biologically related factors (Marsella 2000 p. 409).

Literature in the social and cultural conceptualization of mental health and illness observed growth in widespread research on indigenous theories of psychiatry. Acknowledging works of Girindarsekhar Bose, ways of proper implementation of historical and cultural perspective in research on Indian psychiatry is stressed by Amit Ranjan Basu consistently throughout his writings. Any attempts to map Indian psychiatry largely remained 'linear, positivistic and evolutionary' according to Basu (2005a, b) and historical methods for enquiring indigenous psychiatric knowledge remains ignored. Only by questioning the acclaimed history of Western psychiatry in counselling and psychotherapy training and practices which is a borrowed paradigm, a new genre of psychiatric knowledge emerged. Mental health research should focus their studies on the construction of mental illness in our country as well as its history and culture.

The need for locally based research with qualitative research methodology also brings hope as an emerging trend in cultural awareness about various healing aspects. Halliburton's study in 2003 in searching for pleasantness in treatment focuses on the significance of the positive and negative aesthetic qualities of different therapies existing in Kerala in southern India. He adopted semi-structured and unstructured interviews for knowing the illness histories of 100 patients and 20 healers about their methods of treatment. Informants were undergoing any one of the three forms of healing for mental illness—ayurvedic, allopathic and religious healing. Patients reported adverse reactions to allopathic treatments and in some cases asserted that they enjoyed ayurvedic procedures. Some informants with long-term illnesses had chosen to live in the process of therapy and reside indefinitely in the aesthetically engaging environment of a mosque, temple or church after pursuing medical therapies for years. Halliburton calls for reconsideration of the quality of the process of therapy from the subjective experiences of the patients and concerns about the aesthetic process of therapy. While examining the limitations of the concept of 'cure', he questions the goals of healing in some therapeutic settings. Exploring possible connections between ideologies of therapy, methods of therapy and patients' reported experiences, he asserts that it is essential to relook at the goal of allopathic practice in 'curing' mental illness. Towards the end of his research, Halliburton calls for broadening our understanding of the variety of the ways of coping with an illness to include care, living with a problem, curing and attaining a higher state.

In her research about the logical foundations of medical sciences such as allopathy, ayurveda, homeopathy and naturopathy, Thomas (2009) proposed the need for a theory/model to be developed incorporating the similarities and differences in these systems in relation to the practice of Western psychotherapy. Conceptual understanding of mental illness theorized in terms of the classification, etiology, diagnosis and treatment in various healing methods used for mental illness offer a multidimensional perspective to approach the health-illness deliberations.

Needless to say, Kakar's (1982) study by travelling all over India also gathered public's attention in observing and understanding the rich curative culture merged locally around us. Many of his books unravels the cultural construction on Indian psyche by analysing various facets of Indian identity and sexuality through sources as diverse as first person accounts, participant observations, case studies, Indian myths and legends, and popular cinema. Kakar's attempt to explore the cultural character of the Indians through their childhood, family dynamics and social realities renew studies on cultural psychology and classical psychoanalysis in India.

A UGC-funded project on psychocultural elements in the indigenous healing practices of mental illness in Karnataka summarizes the relevance of knowing the history and practice of ritualized art performances, possession cults, religious centre based practices, magico-religious practices and various local medicinal healing forms in effective treatment of mental illness (Varghese et al. 2011a, b, c). Analysis of Bengali texts/periodicals acknowledges the presence of the existence of a vernacular psychiatry and the classification of insanity through sexual discourses (Basu 2004). Various ritual art forms, community practices, religious healing centres and mental hospitals existing for the treatment of mental illness in Kerala is subjected to be explored by Gopal (2008) in order to understand the historical evolution of 'madness' in Kerala.

It has been observed that even though counselling and psychotherapy practiced in this country still hold a universal bio medical model of health and illness, the emergence, development and observation of the studies on indigenous healing practices carry a context-sensitive outlook to mental illness. Cultural determinants of psychopathology as a fundamental reality challenge mental health practitioners to broaden their conceptual models to include cultural, environmental and spiritual forces, and to explore the utility and value of indigenous models of psychopathology (Marsella 2000 p. 409). Western knowledge of mental health practice has to be revised with the emphasis on indigenous practices and knowledge systems. Even after the emergence and establishment of modern Western science of psychiatry in our training and practice of mental health post independence, there are hundreds of non-modern therapeutic systems still prevalent which will never become extinct with the kind of popularity it has among natives.

Good cultural understanding would help to develop an effective mental health policy. Table 17.1 indicates a comparative study conducted by WHO of the treatment outcomes of schizophrenic patients in developed versus developing countries.

It has been quite evident that the outcome of treatment of schizophrenia is better in our country compared to the developed ones. Acknowledging the existence and power of indigenous healing systems and negotiating with the mainstream medicine should be brought to the mainstream training and research on psychotherapy. Cultural integration, cultural dislocation, migration, moral standards, racism, sexism are certain stressors that shape psychopathology in some cultures. Mental health services need to be pluralistic due to the cultural differences brought by

Table 17.1 Five-year outcome of WHO study of schizophrenic patients in developed versus developing countries

Location	Percentage with best outcome	Percentage with worst outcome
Developed countries		
1. Aarhus, Denmark	6	40
2. London, UK	5	14
3. Moscow, Russia	6	21
4. Prague, Czechoslovakia	9	23
5. Washington, DC, USA	17	23
Developing countries		
1. Agra, India	42	10
2. Cali, Columbia	11	21
3. Ibadan, Nigeria	33	10

Adopted from Desjarlais et al. (1995). Table 2.2, p. 42 cited in Basu (2005)

religion, caste, age, gender and class on the construction of illness. While gender mainstreaming is a strategy put forward by WHO in opening up the issue of gender to everyone in all the endeavors, adopting a culture and community-based approach to mental health programmes in our country is not difficult to achieve.

Developing a Culturally Informed Approach for Counseling and Psychotherapy

A culturally informed approach in mental health practice transforms Western classification in diagnosis and treatment. The vocabulary we use in all the languages for representing the universal mental health categories and the interpretation of non-verbal signs are inevitable requirements for a mental health professional to design appropriate therapeutic tools. Basu (2005a, b) ardently criticizes the modern Western knowledge of medicine which is mostly controlled by the big multinational corporations and stresses the sensitivity a culture- and- community-based approach would bring into the mental health needs of Indian population. Marsella (2000) compels the mental health professionals to consider cultural factors in our case conceptualizations and deliberations and calls for conducting culturological interviews as it is to conduct conventional psychiatric and psychological examinations (p. 410).

In their qualitative study on cultural dimensions of clinical depression in Bangalore, Raguram et al. (2001) observed that patients were dissatisfied and disappointed with allopathic physicians whom they had previously consulted for their problems, who seemed to them not to appreciate their needs and expectations in treatment. Subjectivity of the symptoms and disorders and its personal significance need to be attended by the clinicians as they are shaped by cultural notions concerning the human body/mind in health and in sickness. They call for a cultural epidemiological framework in mental health practise which integrate *emic* and *etic* perspectives.

Therapeutic relationship followed in the Western-based psychotherapy widens the distance between the 'doctor' and the 'patient' who speak different languages whereas the healer in a cultural context is not unlike of the patient (Varghese et al. 2011a, b, c). Transcending this power-centralized Western approach in relationship to a closer perspective make the mental health professionals broaden their clinical gaze and base their clinical formulation on the experience and meanings of the patients. Multicultural counselling approach addresses the diverse nature of clients and cultural implication of their symptoms and experience but do not criticize the basic premise of the psychotherapeutic practices. Culturally informed counselling and psychotherapy intended to design culturally relevant psychotherapies which will be a new breed among the diverse healing systems and practices.

Suffering is viewed in traditional healing practices primarily as a state of mind, a subjective experience, not taking into account the causes of the problem (Anand et al. 2001). Healers develop their own psychological theories which are implicit in their healing practice. It has also been proposed for a paradigm shift in the training of counsellors, psychologists and psychotherapists which should be intended to reduce the gap between the discipline of psychology and alternative therapies as they are close in its goals, philosophy and moral vision. As the Rogerian person-centered therapy places client as the agent for initiating behavioural change, traditional healing systems in India perceive healing powers reside primarily within the patient's mind (Kakar 1982) rather than in the validity of a particular scheme or technique.

Current Initiatives

Mental health practitioners, these days are more aware about the significance of cultural implications on mental health. Community-based programmes implemented in our country are showing good results and, in UK, the question of having separate psychiatric services for ethnic minority has also been argued (Basu 2005a, b, p. 8). Innovative initiatives followed by the private sector by the NGOs adapt cultural learning in understanding mental illness. BELM and SCARF, Chennai are centres that promote cultural workshops and discussions to sensitize the mental health professionals and non-professionals regularly. The leadership from the medical/non-medical mental health professionals in terms of developing non-medical models for issues of rehabilitation, drug dependence and child mental health care is something noteworthy in this regard. Connecting, a nongovernmental organization located in Pune and Bapu Trust for Research on Mind and Discourse, Pune under the leadership of Bhargavi Dawar who herself is a survivor are two such centres which facilitates alternate ways of psychotherapy and rehabilitation services. White Swan Foundation for Mental Health in Bangalore is a not-for-profit organization that offers knowledge services in the area of mental health. They provide patients, caregivers and others with well-researched content that will help them make informed decisions on how to deal with mental health issues. The online content they have been providing through videos, talks, workshops, interdisciplinary discussions, cartoons, case studies and chat forums is well received and highly useful even for academicians, students and mental health practitioners.

Future developments need to focus on non-medical models and interventions largely which accelerates cultural inclusion of counselling and psychotherapy. Absorption of mental healthcare into the traditional healing systems, Ayurveda, unani, homeopathy, yoga, siddha, naturopathy etc. is another relevant leap. Health-related initiatives by professionals such as yoga centres, naturopathy centres spread across the country embraces holistic healing. Agencies that integrate psychological concepts and healing concepts is a 'new-age' trend found in metropolis these days and more number of people turn into such alternative therapies not covered by their medical insurance policies.

The mainstream academic training is more open towards cultural studies in psychology which is reflected in the curricula and research projects in cultural psychology, indigenous psychology, Indian psychology, Asian healing, health psychology, positive psychology, community psychology in various teaching programmes offered by universities across the country. A quick glance at the studies published from India on any topic showed a movement oriented more towards reporting Asian/Indian studies in research reviews of literature. Researches on non-traditional topics such as deprived populations, subaltern cultures, socially and culturally based phenomena are reporting in a more culturally sensitive manner. Funding for culturally relevant research projects is also a welcome symbol at the national level. It is also noteworthy to state that we have institutions and resource centres for continuing education.

Concluding Comments

Conceptual development of the silenced knowledge of Indian psychiatry explores the prospect of interdisciplinary research studies to understand various levels of discourses. Evolution of a model for apprehending cultural and social diversity would address *ahistorical* and *acultural* understanding and investigate the conceptual issues that are specific to indigenous knowledge of mental health and illness. Basing counselling and psychotherapy services on the question of subjectivity facilitates the clinicians to lean towards a patient's theory of health and illness which will help them to make effective diagnosis and treatment plans. Issue of survivors is another concern, acknowledging the alternative therapies they have experienced. Patients' turning towards alternative mental health care should not be viewed as unscientific rather a learning brought from the field of practice to the theory of practice. Integration of traditional knowledge into mainstream counselling and psychotherapy practices offer a new conceptual framework which will reconstruct the world of health and illness.

References

Anand, J., Srivastava, A., & Dalal, A. K. (2001). Where suffering ends and healing begins. *Psychological Studies, 46,* 114–126.

Basu, A. R. (2004). Emergence of a marginal science in a colonial city: Reading psychiatry in Bengali periodicals. *The Indian Economic and Social History Review, 41*(2), 103–141.

Basu, A. R. (2005a, November). Culture and mental health. *Health Action, 18*(11), 7–8.

Basu, A. R. (2005b). Historicizing Indian psychiatry. *Indian Journal of Psychiatry, 47*(9), 126–129.

Desjarlais, R., Eisenberg, L., Good, B., & Kleinman, A. (Eds.). (1995). *Mental health: Problems and priorities in low-income countries*. New York and Oxford: Oxford University Press.

Fraser, C., & Burchell, B. (2001). *Introducing social psychology*. UK: Polity.

Gopal, B. (2008). *The concept of 'madness' and its management: The Kerala scenario* (Unpublished doctoral dissertation). Department of Psychology, University of Calicut.

Halliburton, M. (2003). The importance of a pleasant process of treatment: Lessons on healing from South India. *Culture, Medicine and Psychiatry, 27,* 161–186.

Hofstede, G. (2011). Dimensionalizing cultures: The Hofstede model in context. *Online Readings in Psychology and Culture, 2*(1). https://doi.org/10.9707/2307-0919.1014.

Kakar, S. (1982). *Shamans, mystics and doctors: A psychological inquiry into India and its healing traditions*. Delhi: Oxford University Press.

Kim, U. (1997). Asian collectivism: An indigenous perspective. In H. S. R. Kao & D. Sinha (Eds.), *Asian perspectives on psychology*. Delhi: Sage.

Kumar, A. (2005, November). National rural health mission. *Health Action, 18*(11), 9–13.

Malinowski, B. (1944). A scientific theory of culture. Chapel Hill: The University of North Carolina Press.

Marsella, A. J. (2000). Culture-bound disorders. In A. E. Kazdin (Ed.), *Encyclopedia of psychology*. Oxford: APA/Oxford University Press.

Misra, G. (2003). Implications of culture for knowledge. In W. Berry, R. C. Mishra & R. C. Tripathi (Eds.), *Psychology in human and social development: Lessons from diverse cultures*. New Delhi, India: Sage Publications.

Misra, G. (2005). From disease to well-being: Perspectives from an indigenous tradition. In R. Singh, A. Yadav & N. Sharma (Eds.), *Health psychology* (pp. 281–302). New Delhi: Global Visions Publishing House

Raguram, R., Weiss, M. G., Keval, H., & Channabasavanna, S. M. (2001). Cultural dimensions of clinical depression in Bangalore, India. *Anthropology and Medicine, 8*(1), 31–46.

Sujatha, V., & Abrahama, L. (2012). *Medical pluralism in contemporary India*. New Delhi: Orient Blackswan.

Thomas, T. M. (2009). *Conceptual schemes of abnormal behavior: A study on the logical foundation of medical sciences* (Unpublished doctoral dissertation). Department of Psychology, University of Calicut.

Valsiner, J. (2007). *Culture in minds and societies: Foundations of cultural psychology*. New Delhi: Sage Publications.

Varghese, K. J., Gopal, B., & Thomas, T. M. (2011a). *Psychocultural elements in the indigenous healing practices of mental illness in Karnataka*. Report of a major research project submitted to UGC, New Delhi. Department of Psychology, Christ University.

Varghese, K. J., Gopal, B., & Thomas, T. M. (2011b). Revisiting psychotherapeutic practices in Karnataka, India: Lessons from indigenous healing methods. *International Journal of Health Promotion, 49*(30), 129–136.

Varghese, K. J., Gopal, B., & Thomas, T. M. (Script & Directors). (2011c). Spells, Possession and Madness (English, 45 minutes). Producer: Department of Psychology, Christ University (Funded by UGC).

Chapter 18
Cognitive Foundations of Community Mental Healthcare: The Role of Local Institutions and Practices

Raghubir Singh Pirta

Alternative Approach to Mental Health

Keeping in view the challenging scenario of mental health in India, Srinivasa Murthy (2007) underlined the development of know-how for community mental healthcare. Yet it is not clear how to accomplish this task, especially in the rural area. One way to achieve this goal is to use folk psychology approach (Allport 1954/1975) revitalized in cognitive (Olson and Bruner 1996) and evolutionary (Bering 2006; Shariff and Norenzayan 2007) sciences for analysing mental processes. This integration is promising since the revitalization of folk psychology in cognitive and evolutionary sciences underlines the functional aspects of beliefs in supernatural agents. These supernatural agents and associated concepts and rituals are central to folk healing practices in the villages. The institutions of deities are spaces for dialogues between the folk healers and the cognitive scientists. Rather, the more assuring aspect of this cognitive science of religious beliefs is the recognition of the salience of intuition in cognitive processing (Gervais and Norenzayan 2012; Pennycook et al. 2012). The narratives of people are largely intuitive, or people engage in storytelling which involves imaginary or personified figures including gods and goddesses.

In the last few years, we have been pursuing these ideas for developing an alternative model of mental health in India (Pirta 2005, 2006, 2012). It includes the resiliency-vulnerability dimension of clinical psychology, and the wear and tear of body and mind conceptualized as allostatic load (McEwen 1998; Ray 2004) in the holistic model of native cognition (Pirta 2003, 2007, 2009). Such an enterprise at this preliminary level involves exploration of some important aspects of the beliefs in supernatural agents more or less universally associated with health; these are as follows.

R. S. Pirta (✉)
Department of Psychology, Himachal Pradesh University, Shimla 171005, India
e-mail: rspirta@gmail.com

G. Misra (ed.), *Psychosocial Interventions for Health and Well-Being*,
https://doi.org/10.1007/978-81-322-3782-2_18

First, diversity of the supernatural agents involves locating the deities in a territory where people live in a community and relate with these deities in various ways. There is a lexicon of concepts about these supernatural cognitive agents associated with almost every institution of deity which regulate many essential aspects of the life of the community, in fact it is an order that governs the interactions and relationships among members.

Second, it is important to explore relationships among different supernatural agents, environmental objects and the social agents which form the structure of the institution of a deity. A detailed understanding of the organization of the institution and its practices has significance to facilitate processes for the well-being of the local community.

Third, the next task is to explore the developmental aspects of the beliefs in supernatural agents which involve ingredients of community mental healthcare. Moreover, there are positive (e.g. well-being) and negative (e.g. dissociation) aspects of mental health that emerge from various aspects of beliefs in supernatural agents linked to an institution of deity.

Fourth, at the mental level we have to figure out the dynamics of relationships among the cognitive processes having supernatural bias. The memory processes underlying the storage, organization and retrieval of these supernatural agents need exploration by designing appropriate studies.

The first part (Section "Collective, Supernatural, and Its Narrative") of this chapter presents three aspects of an alternative approach to mental health. After briefly looking into the community mental health viewpoint, we suggest a paradigm for initiating studies into the realm of supernatural agents in human mind, and then point out some approaches which help us in this endeavour. The second part (Section "Socio-psychological Context for Health and Well-Being") of the chapter describes the socio-cognitive context for health and well-being of people based on our work in Himachal Pradesh, India. The findings are summarized according to the four aspects of the supernatural agents as mentioned above: *diversity, institution, development and representation*.

Collective, Supernatural, and Its Narrative

A rather challenging feature of the community mental health tradition in India is its embedding in sacred institutions. Even more engaging feature is the integration of a variety of supernatural agents in the mundane life contributing through some extremely intricate ways to maintain cohesion in a community. Therefore, it is imperative to explore this tradition for the development of innovative ways of alleviating human mental suffering. But this effort needs a humble spirit of care for fellow beings (Hoch 1977), which is even more enduring to rural masses having their own meaningful worlds. In mainstream mental health there are faint signs of this empathic attitude. There are two opinions about it. For a majority, the role of traditional healers in mental health in India is substantial, but it has to be integrated in and/or replaced by modern psychiatry. It was articulated nearly three decades ago by Kapur (1975) and is implied in recent perspectives on mental health (Agarwal et al. 2004). But a minority is of the opinion that the mental health in India has a basis in popular belief systems (Chakraborty 2001), therefore, the endeavor should be to build our policies in consonance with it. On these lines, Wig (2004) envisions small mental hospitals near the community where care is taken to avoid alien concepts and there is more emphasis on methods of healing based on the Indian philosophy amply rich on understanding functions of the mind. From a different perspective, based on Sri Aurobindo's philosophy, Sundararajan et al. (2013) suggest healing centres (e.g. Hindu-inspired *ashramas*) instead of hospitals and clinics.

Though the majority view that emphasizing empowerment of mental health through modernization is perceived as colonization, in the minority view advocating indigenous methods of healing entails fear of hollow claims. This dilemma is not imaginary but obvious from contemporary mental health practice (Pirta 2012), and one way to alleviate such fears is to explore the universe of supernatural agents deeply rooted in the Indian psyche.

Community Mental Health Viewpoint

A pioneering psychiatric study of a village in India concluded that while villagers were loyal to their traditional healers who invoke supernatural agents, they were not averse to new remedies of mental health (Carstairs and Kapur 1976). There is evidence for community mental healthcare in ancient societies all over the world, much before its advent in the mainstream. This is particularly true for Indian society where alleviation of mental health problems and restoration of happiness in a community find mention in ancient texts (Balodhi 1989; Neki 1984). Balodhi (1989) noted that ayurveda has an elaborate theoretical and applied system in the area of mental health and illness. According to Balodhi, the mental therapy in ayurveda has three subgroups—divine therapy, rational therapy and psychotherapy. The divine therapy seems common among the masses in India and consists of (a) *mantra*, chanting of words; (b) *mani*, the touch of precious stone; (c) *mangala*, benediction; (d) *bali*, self-denial/sacrifice; (e) *upahara*, greetings; (f) *homa*, fire sacrifice; (g) *niyama*, observance; (h) *prayashchita*, atonement; (i) *upavasa*, fasting; (j) *pranipata*, submission; (k) *aushadha*, drug; and, (l) *yatragaman*, pilgrimage. The communities in India have some kind of indigenous healing systems to meet the basic needs of people with psychological problems (Srinivasa Murthy 1998).

The present community mental health movement has its roots in the United States and has two objectives: (a) access to high-quality care for all citizens and (b) the allocation of more resources to community level mental health programmes (Sharfstein 2000). This approach began in the 1960s, with Barton's (1966) conceptual framework. In this view: (a) community is more than a geographical area, it offers its residents many kinds of services and fills a variety of needs; cultural traditions and customs of ethnic groups in population are important; (b) sociocultural factors influence behaviour and interpretations of psychopathology; (c) mental health professionals need sensitivity to the community they serve; and (d) power structure of individual community can be understood in relation to various social programmes.

Nonetheless, the village as a community in India has an edge over the concept of simply a community in America, the country of the origin of community mental health. From the theoretical viewpoint the village in India has a long tradition of social support reinforced by religious institution on one hand and attachment among families through kinship on the other. The institution of deity characterizes almost each village or complex of villages in India and each has potential of a center for community mental health (Pirta 2005, 2006).

Our aim should be to open dialogues between various levels of explanations on mental health. In this endeavor, I shall first outline the essentials of the paradigm which are acceptable to community of scientists when we engage in the study of supernatural elements in human cognition, and then describe the approaches that are helpful in these studies.

A New Paradigm in Mental Health

The WHO in its Report on Mental Health in 2001 concluded that there was need to integrate the biological, social and mental factors for a new approach to public health. Broadly, there are two aspects of individual the mental and the physical or the mind and the body. The report (WHO 2001) has summarized research that supports the mutuality of body and mind. For example, women with advanced breast cancer live longer after supportive group therapy, the depression predicts the incidence of heart disease, and AIDS patients accepting their realistic death die sooner.

There are two aspects of mind and body interaction. That the body affects mind is obvious, but the second pathway, the mind affects body is difficult to demonstrate. Psychologists still follow the paradigm of classical physics where the agent is passive. For a quantum physicist the agent is active, having free will or intentionality, and psychologists must follow this dictum. In view of quantum physicist Sudarshan (1982), 'mind is an interface between the public world described by the physical sciences and the private world of personal experience and individuality.' In this case, the task of psychologist is to understand the latter part, experiences of the being, whereas the quantum physicist would help him to describe mind in terms of 'physic-chemical laws' (Sudarshan 2002, 2003).

The mental phenomena were subjected to rigorous enquiry in the 1950s under the leadership of D. O. Hebb, which provided sound basis for a neuropsychological theory. For him, *a stream of thought* was the product of phase sequence, activity in groups of various cell assemblies, whereas the stimulation of a group of neurons forming a cell assembly could be the equivalent of an *idea* or *image* (Brown and

Milner 2003). Later, Luria defined neuropsychology as the study of the effects of brain processes on mental processes, and his work provides the theoretical basis for cognitive planning (Das et al. 1996), and development of neuropsychological battery (Gupta et al. 2000). The essential feature of the neuropsychological approach is to explore how brain processes lead to mental processes in some particular cultural context.

The challenge awaiting psychology is how mind changes brain, a cornerstone of psychotherapy. It is time to replace the stimulus-response paradigm by a new holistic paradigm—mind-brain-mind. Schwartz et al. (2005) in an exhaustive analysis conclude that quantum physics has importance for a study of mind-brain link, and underline quantum Zeno effect as the key concept. The Zeno effect came into prominence in a paper of Misra and Sudarshan (1977), and is conventionally defined as the 'effortfully controlled intentional action.' In other words, a person consciously or actively controls certain intended mental activities, which in turn influence brain. Experimental psychologists have shown the importance of mental effort in cognitive functions (Kahneman 1973, 2003).

There are a number of therapeutic studies, which attempts to understand the mind-brain interaction borrowing principles from quantum physics, and underline the phrase 'change the mind and you change the brain' (Paquette et al. 2003; Schwartz et al. 2005). The joint work of these scientists from different fields has brought convincing evidence that *mind does really matter* (Beauregard 2007). This new work has great promise for treatment and practice in clinical psychology.

It occurred to a brain scientist R. W. Sperry that there may be a downward control where our higher mental processes become an intrinsic force and thus assume causal properties. In this macromental paradigm, the higher level mental phenomena such as beliefs and values cause material changes crucial for human affairs. The subjective belief 'is no longer a mere impotent epiphenomenon of brain activity' but also 'a shaper of both individual and social behavior' (Sperry 1991). And the most important beliefs are about life's purpose and meaning, and about God and the cosmic scheme. An important objective of macromental outlook where mind-brain forms an integrated whole is to take ultimate beliefs out of supernatural uncertainties into a realm consistent with science (Sperry 1992).

The scope of mind-brain interaction expands tremendously as focus changes from mental illness to mental health. After an exhaustive review of the various models of mental health developed over the last thirty years, Vaillant (2003) concludes 'mental health must always be broadly defined in terms that are culturally sensitive and inclusive'. Ray (2004) has outlined the role of four important systems, the mind, the endocrine system, the nervous system, and the immune system for a holistic paradigm of health and illness. This paradigm claims to explain how belief becomes biology.

Scientists from various disciplines are looking into the functional aspects of supernatural agents to understand the dynamics of various supernatural cognitive elements and their association with thinking, feeling and behaviour (Bering 2006; Boyer 2003). In addition, an important aspect of the institution of deity is to keep cohesion in a group. This is an interesting hypothesis and needs examination according to contemporary models of group selection in evolutionary biology (Nowak 2006). The evolutionary concept of group selection is analogous to Mahayana Buddhism with regard to the phenomenon of altruism. In the former case of group selection, an individual has predispositions to behave in a way that curtails his fitness but increases the fitness of the group as a whole. In the latter case, Mahayana Buddhism, the individual learns to follow certain social norms and practices by which he develops self-sacrificing behaviour to reduce the sufferings of others.

Cognitive Approaches to Study Supernatural Agents

Purzycki and Sosis (2011) write 'Supernatural agent concepts are found in every human society. From gods and ghosts to ancestor and animal spirits, supernatural agent beliefs exhibit not only many essential similarities but also remarkable differences across cultures' (p. 78).

In this section, I shall briefly refer to three approaches fashioned during the development of cognitive science: folk psychology, narrative analysis and dialogical interchange. Although folk psychology was introduced in 1916 by Wundt, known as father of experimental psychology, with cognitive revolution in the 1950s there was a revival of folk psychology. The main thesis, according to Olson and Bruner (1996) being that 'our interactions with others are deeply affected by our everyday intuitive theories about how our own minds and the minds of others work' (p. 10). Such lay theories or folk psychologies, Olson and Bruner underlined, involved *'certain wired in human tendencies' and 'they also reflect certain deeply ingrained cultural beliefs about the mind'* (p. 10). They further noted that folk psychology is the study of mind or how mind works.

Over the last several years, investigators are referring to two ways of cognitive processing, broadly the two systems of knowledge acquisition. A cognitive psychologist is not focusing exclusively on 'rational' mind, but the notion of knowledge involves two metaphors (Olson and Bruner 1996): Apollonian and Dionysian. It is stated that an Apollo is incomplete without Dionysus. Obeyesekere (2004) brought this metaphor into limelight by suggesting involvement of these two processes in Buddha's enlightenment during the meditative askesis. This hypothesis of Obeyesekere, following William James, underlines that there are other forms of consciousness, outside the normal cognitive faculties, which are alien modes of thought. These other forms of consciousness range from contemplative trance during meditative askesis (the Apollonian type) to uncontrolled states such as spirit possession or shamanic trances (the Dionysian type). The latter are rather more common in the Indian landscape. While some of these Dionysian states are pathological, they are indeed sources of knowledge for the common folk in crucial times. According to Obeyesekere (2004), this thinking occurs when the thought wishes ('It-thinking'), not when the individual wishes ('I-thinking'). These states of consciousness involve complex rituals designated to deities varying with culture.

The knowledge gained by a family or a group during these trance states has functional significance (Pirta 2005, 2006, 2012).

The inquiry into the knowledge function of various trance states has yet to begin (Pirta 2014), however, the other ways of knowledge acquisition, besides the rational, that has been pursued include folk psychology, narrative analysis and dialogical interchange. While in folk psychology (Bering 2006; Boyer 2003) investigators are exploring the supernatural beliefs, narrative analysis deals with mundane cognitive aspects of desires, thinking, feeling, beliefs, myths and social interactions in time and space. Second, the narrative accounts focus on how these intentional states lead to various activities performed by a person (Bruner 1991). It is essentially organizing one's experiences like storytelling. They become comprehensible to others in the light of folk psychology that is intrinsic to a culture and follows largely canonical ways of communication.

In a narrative there is violation of folk psychological canon (Bruner 1991). The canon version of self-narrative has a single author (or I, the knower) who tells a story about himself or herself (or Me, the known) as an actor, and there is an action directed toward a goal using some means (instrument) in particular context (scene). Hermans (2006), however, argues 'that people had not simply one story to tell, but rather different or even contradictory stories which seemed to emerge from different positions in their selves'. These ideas emerged, recalls Hermans (2006), when some of his clients spoke of imaginal figures in their lives, which involved: supernatural beings, strongly idealized persons, animal-like figures, monsters, a supreme being, or other anthropomorphic figures. These case studies were instrumental in conceptualizing that the self can take multiplicity of I-positions which can engage in mutually influencing dialogues in the landscape of mind. However, in some unique cases, referred in psychiatry as multiple personalities, these multiple voices become pathological. In these cases, the normal self is taken over by one or more imaginal figures. And thus at any time it is the voice of the normal self or the voice of an imaginal self (a deity or spirit). There is no dialogue between the two voices. On the other hand, dialogical interchange assumes a mutually influencing dialogue among different voices of self. For example, a woman while taking a decision about her son's marriage may have a dialogue in her mind from the position of a caring mother, a woman seeking blessing from her deity, as a citizen conscious of cultural norms and a parent managing resources of a family.

It is now overwhelmingly clear that processing of information (as emphasized above during knowledge acquisition) involves two distinct processes: System 1 which is fast and effortless; and, System 2 which is effortful and slow, in information processing (Kahneman 2003). The former involves intuitive decision making, whereas the latter results in rational decisions. According to Hermans (1996), following Bruner and other investigators, the human experiences are organized according to two modes of thought. The arguments (propositional thinking or System 2) are means to convince someone of their truth; on the other hand, storytelling (narrative thinking or System 1) mode of thought has an imaginative quality. The memory processes assumed to lie beneath these two systems are: episodic memory in storytelling or narrative thinking, and semantic memory in propositional thinking. These two cognitive systems have significance for understanding the role of imaginal figures including the supernatural agents. For, especially the System 1 or intuition is believed to be an alternative source of knowledge (Obeyesekere 2004), it gains further credence presumably due to its association with the trance states, the latter being a significant part of rituals associated with supernatural agents (Pirta 2014).

We have been exploring the institution of deity in some parts of the state of Himachal Pradesh in India to study the role of supernatural agents in different aspects of the life of people in the villages. The ethnographic and folk psychology approaches were followed to collect culturally relevant information, followed by experimental investigation of memory processes underlying supernatural beliefs of people in the context of mental health. The information so collected has been reported in various studies, and is briefly described here in four sections according to the objectives mentioned in Section "Alternative Approach to Mental Health".

Socio-psychological Context for Health and Well-Being

Although psychiatrists have shown concern about the role of cultural context in mental health (Carstairs and Kapur 1976; Hoch 1977), mainstream psychology has been evasive. The current scenario of psychology in India appears one that is characteristic of an agnostic, who is not able to decide which way to move, East or West. A relatively long chapter on clinical psychology by Chattopadhyay (2010) in the fifth ICSSR (Indian Council of Social Science Research) survey of psychology, surprisingly, fails to acknowledge the scope of spiritual embedded approach in clinical practice. Whereas, in the fourth ICSSR survey Kapur (2001) has underlined the need for dialogue with 'religious healers/mystics', she even made a distinction between the approaches of the great tradition (e.g., Ayurveda) and the little tradition (folk healing) to mental health in India. Continuing with this line of approach, Rao (2010) in her review of current researches on the use of yoga, meditation and spirituality in psychotherapy observed that there were indications towards an Indian model of psychotherapy. The two eminent psychologists of India, Sharma and Misra (2010), however, concluded that as far as health psychology is concerned, the current research on 'religion/spirituality' was scarce.

Himachal Pradesh, the tiny Indian state in the Himalaya has unique integration of traditional and modern life patterns that appears complementary to each other. Sometime back in the 1980s when social conflicts engulfed many states of the Indian Himalaya, Himachal Pradesh was peaceful. A theory prevailed that the calmness in the state was due to people's apathy to modern developmental processes; moreover, the unquestioning belief of people of Himachal in their deities was considered escapism. But it was not true. The spectacular progress of Himachal Pradesh (Dreze and Sen 2002) unfolded a new story. Although Dreze and Sen (2002) attributed the progress of Himachal Pradesh to a strong tradition of local cooperative action, they did not identify the institutions that promote it. But there

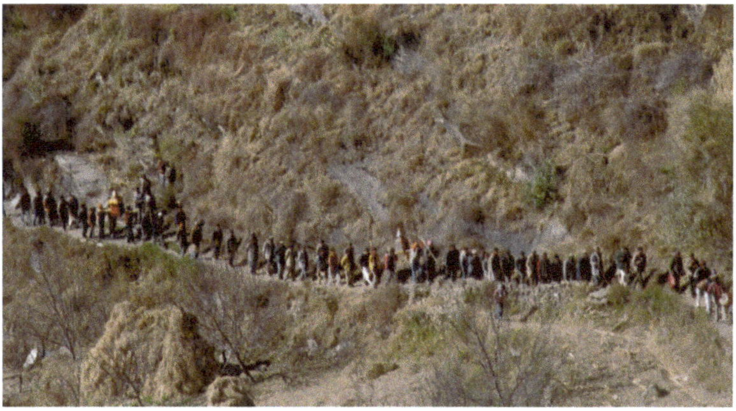

Fig. 18.1 The deities carried in palanquins from one village to the other. *Source* Author

was a suggestion that the institution of deity provides a context for cooperative action (Pirta 2007). We further support this thesis that besides providing a context for cooperative action (Fig. 18.1), the institution of deity is closely associated with the physical, social and psychological well-being of people.

To provide mental health in rural areas is challenging but it has opportunities as well (Srinivasa Murthy 2004). The financial constraints and lack of skilled human resources are the biggest challenges in mental health in India. But on the other hand, opportunities lie in harnessing the well-knit social support system in the villages and alternative mental healthcare systems, especially those located in the temple premises (Raguram et al. 2002). These institutions of deities have historical, environmental and evolutionary aspects. In addition, they have social, psychological and spiritual dimensions. Some of these aspects involving the supernatural agents and crucial for health and well-being of people are described in the following four sections: diversity, institution, development, and representation.

Diversity of Supernatural Agents

Socio-cognitive context of a group of people or a community has relevance for a sense of belongingness and ownership in decision-making processes facilitating health and well-being of its members. In a highly acclaimed stance, the global forum of scientists in the Millennium Ecosystem Assessment (MA 2005) recognized the dependence of human well-being on material welfare, health, good social relations, security and freedom. Even though globalization brings new opportunities, the transition can be wrenching (Bardhan 2006; Bhugra and Mastrogianni 2004). Rural communities need to strengthen the local social institutions to enhance their inner resources to meet these challenges effectively.

We illustrate the uniqueness of cognitive diversity with regard to supernatural agents by taking an example of two pastoral communities of Himachal Pradesh, the Gaddis and the Kanaoras (Pirta 2009). These pastoral groups occupy different niches in the upper region of Himalaya where they have their permanent homes. However, they move farther up in the Himalaya in summer and descend to plains of western India during the winter. This pastoral system is known as transhumance.

In the Himalayan ranges, transhumance along with trade has played significant role in the life of Kanaoras. The transhumant Kanaoras (known as the *arungzetsa*) used to take their sheep and goats deep into the Tibetan plateau, and over the centuries inculcated Tibetan Buddhism in the Hinduism. On the other hand, the access of Gaddis to higher altitudes of the Himalaya was limited; they only follow Hinduism (Fig. 18.2). As a result, the diversity of the supernatural agents among the Kanaoras is much more complex than the Gaddis.

The Great Lotsawa (translator), also known as Ratnabhadra (AD 958–1055) was behind the expansion of Buddhism from Kashmir to Arunachal. In Kinnaur (or Kanaor) it is not unusual to find coexistence of local deities, the deities of the great tradition (e.g. Kali and Shiva), and the Buddhist monasteries with innumerable deities. Of particular significance is the doctrine of the dependent origination (*pratityasamutpada*). This concept is analogous to the basic ecological relationships among the living and non-living objects.

For the Gaddis the abode of Shiva is Manimahesh, whereas Kanaoras visualize Shiva in Raldang Kailash. While one may find a feast of supernatural entities in the monastery of Nako, on the other hand, Chaurasi, the temple complex at Bharmour, is a little cosmos of supernatural entities drawn from the great tradition of Hinduism. Chaurasi, besides a place of pilgrimage, has association with folk healing practices. Traditionally, the migratory herds of sheep and goats of Gaddis would stop at Chaurasi to pay obeisance to Lord Shiva (Pakhretia and Pirta 2011).

The Chaurasi myth of the great tradition of Hindus involves Brahma's primordial incest (Ramanujan 1983), but at the folk level the temple complex depicts the cycle of 84 lakh births and deaths (*Chaurasi lakh juni*). It is a problem of human existence, the fear of death and afterlife (Bering 2006; Norenzayan and Hansen 2006).

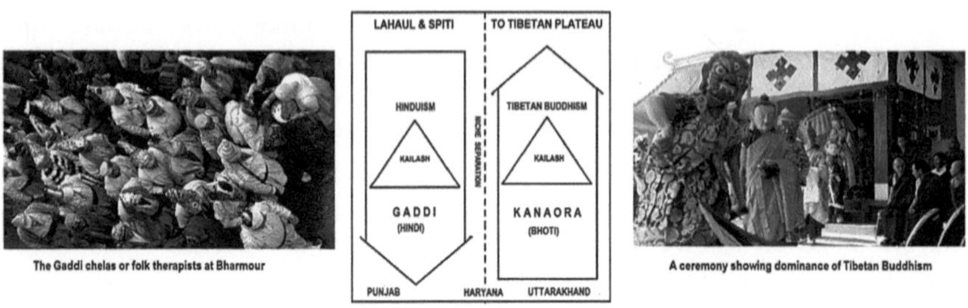

Fig. 18.2 Folk healing systems of two pastoral groups, the Gaddis and the Kanaoras. *Source* Author

The Institution of Deity

In the villages of India, social organization and well-being of people involve communal decision-making processes in which local deities participate through their spokespersons. A spokesperson of the deity is known by various names such as *gur*, *chela*, or *mali*. He or she goes into trance state when possessed by the deity. Some important aspects of the institution of a deity known as *Shadi ra Deo* from the Jubbal valley of Shimla district in Himachal Pradesh (Pirta 2005) are described in this section to illustrate the case. The institution is ancient, but we have important documentary evidence on its economic, social and other aspects since 1955.

The important social unit in a *gaon* or village is *ghar*, the household or family. A *gaon* consists of a number of ghar. Each ghar has one or more members who represent one or more generations, who are largely dependent upon the land owned by each ghar. In each gaon one or more castes live together performing various roles complementary to each other and essential for various functions in the gaon or the adjacent gaon. For example, members of a ghar specialized as musicians or *toories* would cater to the needs of several gaon in the area.

Decision-making process in various aspects of life is complex and takes place at the level of the individual, the ghar and the gaon and the institution of deity (Fig. 18.3). The ghar is more than a physical structure. It has physical, social and psychological properties for the survival of the inmates who are close kin. These activities occurring inside the ghar have close linkages with higher institutions. The gaon, next level institution is of immediate importance where the ghar also plays a significant role. However, the centre and the state also affect the functioning of the gaon through political, social and developmental processes, particularly the *gramsabha*, a unit of the *panchayat*, the village council.

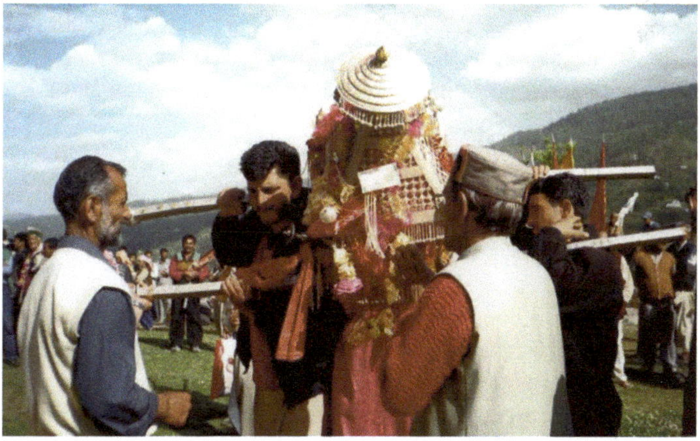

Fig. 18.3 The deity Shadi ra Deo participates in decision making. *Source* Author

In our focal village Dakaod, the total number of ghar increased from 16 in 1955–56 to 39 in 2002–03. They can be traced to two kin groups, respectively belonging to *khashia* (rajput) and *bhat* (brahmin) castes. Each ghar of Dakaod obeys the *kara* of Shadi ra Deo, the rules and regulations of the deity. The kara is an unwritten order, which is assimilated by the individual as he grows up in the gaon. Each ghar equally contributes in the form of manual service, agricultural produce (*jhakhadi*) and monetarily (*phant*). The contributions also come as offerings in the form of gold, silver, articles and cash (*bhaint*).

The territory of Shadi ra Deo includes almost half of the Jubbal valley starting from Khada Pathar and extending towards east up to Shadi village, the place of its origin (Pirta 2005). The river Bishkalti divides the valley into *shilli* and *parali* sides dotted by about 30 villages. The area was earlier a part of the princely state of Jubbal but now comes under Jubbal *tehsil* in the Shimla district. The temples (*deothi*) for Shadi ra Deo are in five villages and they worship the deity according to their turn, which comes every fifth year, starting from Shadi, and clockwise Chamaroo, Dakaod, Purana Jubbal and Kiari. The year of worship in each village is known as *bharanshi*. The *bharanshi poojan*, the worship of Shadi ra Deo is a collective decision of the gaon involving each ghar. They invite the deity from the preceding village on the occasion of the *Jagara* festival. All the five *bharanshi* worshipping villages and people from other villages participate in Jagara poojan (also known as *panjvi ki raat* or fifth day after the *Amavasya* or new moon that generally falls in the month of September). This is the last day of *bharanshi poojan* in a village, and next day the deity remains as a guest of the village.

During the *Jagara* function, the deity possesses the mali, and takes the ceremonial bath or *nahan* (Fig. 18.4). The deity thanks the villagers who worshipped the bharanshi, blesses them and also resolves any personal or social conflict brought to his notice. Early next morning, the members of the prospective village visit the deity and extend invitation of the *bharanshi*. They give assurance that they are happy to invite the deity and will abide by the kara. The deity gives his consent, and the next day the whole village, one member from each family, comes to take Shadi ra Deo to their village. The procession starts in the afternoon and reaches the next village by the evening. While the deity is decorated for movement to the other village, all the items that accompany the deity are documented, and a copy of the list is handed over to the next village.

Developmental Aspects of Supernatural Beliefs

I will describe here some concepts prevalent in the institution of Shadi ra Deo (Pirta 2006). One learns specific ways of behaving, thinking and feeling while growing up as a member of the institution of deity.

These learning experiences occur in an atmosphere charged with emotion, at a time when a child's cognitive abilities are not well developed. Parents seek blessings of the deity for their child in socially sanctioned ways. These events may

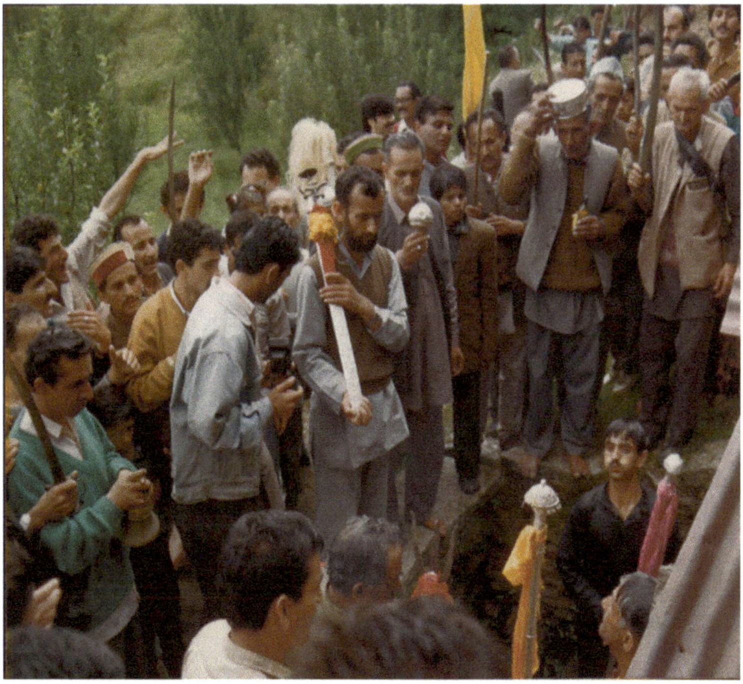

Fig. 18.4 A mali in trance during the ceremonial bath of Shadi ra Deo. *Source* Author

form part of emotional memories which come under non-declarative memories (the implicit associations). As the child grows there is priming by mother, other members of the family and by age mates about the rules and regulations of the institution, which constitute the *kara* or order. The child also internalizes the functional implications of the concepts about the sacred space, social structure around the deity and the divineness (*saot*) of the deity.

Through imitation and observational learning, receiving positive reinforcement on certain occasions and being a witness to the negative consequences of polluting the sacred, a child implicitly and explicitly develops the schemata of the institution of the deity in mind. At times these supernatural figures emerge through personification. Various ecological, social and mental aspects of the schemata get enriched as the individual grows up and the deity's figure perhaps manifests in his imagery as protector, savior, helper and companion (see Section "Exploration of the supernatural in Mind" for these enduring schemata). Furthermore, it is possible that internalization of the roles of the institution not only enhances attachment to the deity, a person may take the role of deity's functionary (*kardar* or *thane*) and one may become the spokesperson (mali) of the deity.

After some experience, a mali of the deity performs the task of healing, besides participating in other decision making to maintain the kara or order of the institution. In the beginning the possession (*tyari*) takes place during the deity's festivals. The person under these initial possession episodes has very high affective arousal accompanied by seemingly irrelevant motor activities and verbalizations. The content of the memories during these verbalizations is emotionally charged and the whole episode appears to be governed by non-declarative memory processes. Alternatively, in literature such episodes are classified as the Dionysian type involving intuitive processes. Later, the person gets possessed only during social and therapeutic rituals and the aim is to sort out the problems of members of community. However, after the person gets possessed frequently and becomes the socially accepted spokesperson of the deity or *deoramali*, his behaviour is controlled and the statements are coherent.

The healing by the mali is apparently similar in some ways to a behaviour therapist. A common belief is that not to follow the kara, the order of the deity, is to annoy him, which means inviting trouble for the family. The central concept is *dosh* or annoyance of the deity. These cognitions are also reinforced by the universal system of oral and written prescriptions in scriptures such as through the *Bhagvat Katha*. Numerous stories, life histories of saints, personal experiences narrated by people, all provide rich material that leads to the development of cognitive schemas where variety of positive and negative expectations become attached to the deity. On the basis of person's expectations from his deity and person's perception of his actions, we may observe four types of behaviour patterns (Table 18.1).

Although both, the mali and the behaviour therapist suggest some cause of the problem, they do not insist on it, the whole emphasis is on learning new relationships with the terrestrial (physical and social) and the non-terrestrial environment. A correctional measure is suggested, which involves manipulation of environmental events in such a way that they act as positive and negative incentives. The verbal reinforcement of the mali and the therapist has significance. But the mali has more control on the environmental contingencies than the therapist. The mali may manipulate the social (institutional) aspects as well as the beliefs in supernatural agents. In both kinds of therapies the cause and cure are external to the subject. Moreover there is an attempt to start reconciliation process between the two parties but the clients or parties have choices open to them. Thus the probability of a response in both kinds of therapies can be predicted in almost the same way. The response may increase or decrease according to the nature and the delivery or withdrawal of the reinforcement (Table 18.2).

A mali of the deity and a behaviour therapist are successful to the extent that they are able to manipulate the contingencies of the environmental stimuli. If some person or party accepts the deity's decision, he would be free from the assumed annoyance or dosh of the deity. But he may have to do something for the

Table 18.1 Four types of behavior patterns

Prospect from deity	View of own action	
	Positive	Negative
Positive	Secure	Insecure
Negative	Ritualistic	Fearful

Table 18.2 Increase or decrease in the behaviour of the client

Reinforcement by the mali or the therapist	Nature of the reinforcement	
	Positive	Negative
Delivery	Increase	Decrease
Withdrawal	Decrease	Increase

appeasement of the deity and on some occasions to satisfy the demands of other good or bad spirits. In case the other party is not ready to abide by the deity's decision, a unilateral sanction is enforced, and the other party or individual may then be liable for further annoyance of the deity. Occasionally, the deity suggests *chhuan* or severing of all physical and social relations with the disobeying party, which may be a close kin.

Exploration of the Supernatural in Mind

Some recent developments to understand the caregiving function of supernatural agents have immense significance in mental health. It is a common observation that people seek proximity to their deities. They show distress when there is an attempt to severe the relationship of a person or a group with their deity. When people engage in new activities or have to move away from their native area they seek the blessings of the deity. And, people approach the deity or recall him on perceiving a threat. The preceding four aspects, proximity seeking, separation distress, secure base and safe haven, respectively, are the salient features of the attachment relationship between the infant and the caregiver (Bowlby 1969/1997).

In fact, researchers have applied attachment theory of Bowlby to study a person's attachment to God or some deity. Central to Bowlby's attachment theory is the idea of internal working models (IWMs), the cognitive linkages that develop between the caregiver and the infant during the formation of social bond (Ainsworth et al. 1978). These IWMs of self and others are integral part of memory processes. They are perhaps the representations of caregivers and related environmental features in the mind of the child, which subsequently guide child's behaviour. Therefore, one way to understand the IWMs of an individual is exploration of memories. Table 18.3 shows a familiar design for the retrieval of memories related to attachment relationship with the deities (Kumari and Pirta 2009).

In a study scrambled sentence test (Shariff and Norenzayan 2007) was used for priming the subjects about god, and the secure base concept was introduced in the mind of subjects through script method (Kumari and Pirta 2009). The priming group differed from the no-priming group on the measure of latency (in sec) and number of memories recalled; though the former took longer time to recall the first association (Fig. 18.5), the number of memories recalled was greater. In other words, priming with god and subsequently a script of secure base (moving out as

Table 18.3 A design to study mental representations of supernatural agents

PARTICIPANTS	
PRIMING	NO-PRIMING
DISTRACTOR TASK	
SCRIPT OF GOD AS A SECURE BASE	
DEPENDENT VARIABLES [latency; memories; categories; items]	

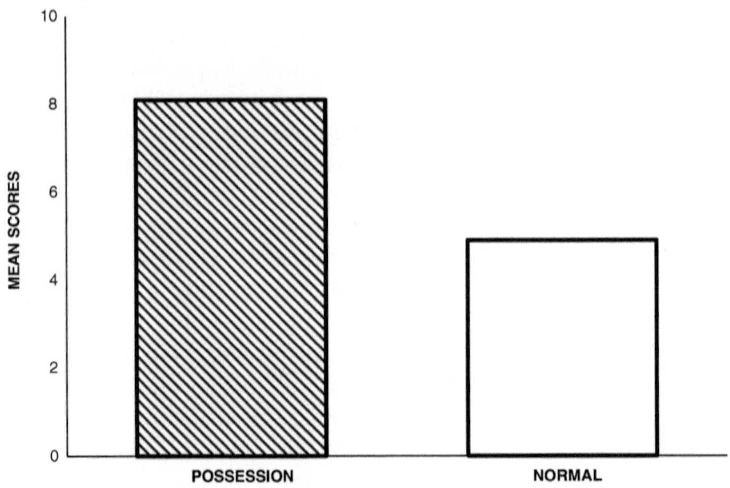

Fig. 18.5 Latency of the recall of first association after priming with secure base script. *Source* Author

deity is there to take care) elicited more associations but some form of inhibition prolonged the time to recall the first association.

A psychological phenomenon closely associated with the institution of deity is people undergoing trance when presumably possessed by these supernatural agents. In trance or possession, a person exhibits elements in psyche (through recall or

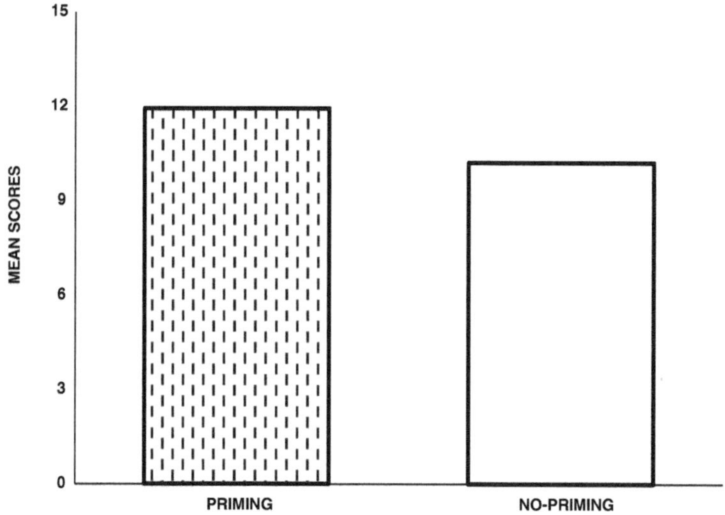

Fig. 18.6 Latency of the recall of first association in two groups after safe haven script. *Source* Author

interaction) that are embedded in specific local institutions, varying from village to village, affected by the social milieu. Therefore it is important to explore the cognitive representations or rather memories or verbalizations of people undergoing trance after possession by deity. These trance states are different from the trance states of a *mali* (*gur* or *chela*), the spokesperson of the deity. While the latter has therapeutic quality, the former type of trance is an indication of social or individual problems experienced by the person, and is referred to as pathological trance.

People undergoing pathological trance have poor general well-being and show neurotic tendency (Thakur and Pirta 2009). We also explored the question whether there was any difference on the recall of cognitive representations (associations or memories) of god as a safe haven (seeking deity when there is external threat) between the possession (pathological trance) group and the comparison group? The latency of recall of the first memory (Fig. 18.6) and the total number of memories recalled by the possession group were significantly higher from the comparison group. In other words, a person is likely to approach or recall the deity under a threat. This is evident from the greater recall of memories or associations by the people experiencing pathological trance and supports our assumption that these people needed help from their local deity. The longer time to recall the first association (latency in sec.) by this group, however, indicates some inhibitory processes during retrieval of information.

The findings of these studies are at best exploratory in nature, however, the design and methods suggest that they have significance for understanding the cognitive basis of supernatural realms in particular contexts. Having studied the socio-ecology of Ladakhis, Crook (1997, 1998) made a detailed analysis of the phenomenon of possession in the region, and observed that the dissociative possession has remained poorly understood either by the therapists or by the psychologists.

Conclusion

In India, psychological enquiry requires an adequate orientation to understand belief in the supernatural, on one hand, and its role in mental health on the other. Perhaps a key to this new look on supernatural beliefs lies in the functional approach. This approach is most appropriate for creating an environment for initiating reconciliatory dialogue between believers and non-believers in the supernatural. In addition, this dialogue, for which sufficient groundwork is now available, would certainly make way for a new paradigm for research since supernatural elements in every culture have allied in enabling human psyche, a quest significant for psychology.

References

Agarwal, S. P., Goel, D. S., Ichhpujani, R. L., Salhan, R. N., & Shrivastava, S. (Eds.). (2004). *Mental health: An Indian perspective 1946-2003*. New Delhi: Elsevier.

Ainsworth, M. D. S., Blehar, M. C., Waters, E., & Wall, S. (1978). *Patterns of attachment: A psychological study of the strange situation*. Hillsdale, NJ: Erlbaum.

Allport, G. W. (1954/1975). The historical background of modern social psychology. In G. Lindzey & E. Aronson (Eds.), *The handbook of social psychology* (2nd ed., Vol. 1, pp. 1–80). New Delhi: Amerind.

Balodhi, J. P. (1989). In pursuit of Indian *Shastric* sources for community mental health. *NIMHANS Journal, 7*(1), 49–54.

Bardhan, P. (2006). Does globalization help or hurt the World's poor. *Scientific American India, 1* (11), 68–75.

Barton, W. E. (1966). Trends in community mental health programs. *Hospital and Community Psychiatry, 17*, 253–258.

Beauregard, M. (2007). Mind does really matter: Evidence from neuroimaging studies of emotional self-regulation, psychotherapy, and placebo effect. *Progress in Neurobiology, 81*, 218–236.

Bering, J. M. (2006). The folk psychology of souls. *Behavioural and Brain Sciences, 29*, 453–498.

Bhugra, D., & Mastrogianni, A. (2004). Globalisation and mental: overview with relation to depression. *British Journal of Psychiatry, 184*, 10–20.

Bowlby, J. (1969/1997). *Attachment and loss. Volume 1: Attachment*. London, UK: Pimlico.

Boyer, P. (2003). Religious thought and behaviour as by-products of brain function. *Trends in Cognitive Sciences, 7*(3), 119–124.

Brown, R. E., & Milner, P. M. (2003). The legacy of Donald O. Hebb: More than the Hebb Synapse. *Nature Reviews, 4*, 1013–1019.

Bruner, J. (1991). Self-making and world-making. *Journal of Aesthetic Education, 25*(1), 67–78.

Carstairs, G. M., & Kapur, R. L. (1976). *The great universe of Kota: Stress, change and mental disorder in an Indian village*. London: Hogarth.

Chakraborty, A. (2001). Mental health of Indian women: A field experience. In B. V. Davar (Ed.), *Mental health from a gender perspective* (pp. 34–60). New Delhi: Sage.
Chattopadhyay, P. K. (2010). Clinical psychology. In G. Misra (Ed.), *Psychology in India. Volume 3: Clinical and health psychology* (pp. 1–106). New Delhi: Pearson.
Crook, J. H. (1997). The indigenous psychiatry of Ladakh, part I: Practice theory approaches to trance possession in the Himalayas. *Anthropology & Medicine, 4,* 289–307.
Crook, J. H. (1998). The indigenous psychiatry of Ladakh, part II: narrative and metanarrative in the cultural control of dissociative states in the Himalayas. *Anthropology & Medicine, 5,* 23–42.
Das, J. P., Kar, B. C., & Parrila, R. K. (1996). *Cognitive planning. The psychological basis of intelligent behavior.* New Delhi: Sage.
Dreze, J., & Sen, A. (2002). *India: Development and participation.* Oxford: New Delhi.
Gervais, W. M., & Norenzayan, A. (2012). Analytic thinking promotes religious disbelief. *Science, 336,* 493–496.
Gupta, S., Khandelwal, S. K., Tandon, P. N., Maheshwari, M. C., Mehta, V. S., Sundaram, K. R., et al. (2000). The development and standardisation of a comprehensive neuropsychological battery in Hindi (adult form). *Journal of Personality and Clinical Studies, 16,* 75–109.
Hermans, H. J. M. (1996). Voicing the self: From information processing to dialogical interchange. *Psychological Bulletin, 119*(1), 31–50.
Hermans, H. J. M. (2006). Moving through three paradigms, yet remaining the same thinker. *Counselling Psychology Quarterly, 19*(1), 5–25.
Hoch, E. M. (1977). Psychotherapy for the illiterate. In S. Arieti & G. Chrzanowski (Eds.), *New dimensions in psychiatry: A world view* (Vol. 2, pp. 75–92). New York: Wiley.
Kahneman, D. (1973). *Attention and effort.* New Jersey: Prentice-Hall.
Kahneman, D. (2003). A perspective on judgment and choice: Mapping bounded rationality. *American Psychologist, 58*(9), 697–720.
Kapur, M. (2001). Mental health, illness and therapy. In J. Pandey (Ed.), *Psychology in India revisited. Developments in the discipline. Volume 2: Personality and health psychology* (pp. 412–472). New Delhi: Sage.
Kapur, R. L. (1975). Mental health care in rural India: A study of existing patterns and their implications for future policy. *British Journal of Psychiatry, 127,* 286–293.
Kumari, A., & Pirta, R. S. (2009). Exploring human relationship with God as a secure base. *Journal of the Indian Academy of Applied Psychology, 35*(special issue), 119–124.
MA. (2005). Millennium Assessment Website: http://www.ma-secretariat.org [update: http://www.Millenniumassessment.org/en/index.aspx].
McEwen, B. S. (1998). Protective and damaging effects of stress mediators. *The New England Journal of Medicine, 338*(3), 171–179.
Misra, B., & Sudarshan, E. C. G. (1977). The Zeno's paradox in quantum theory. *Journal of Mathematical Physics, 18*(4), 756–763.
Neki, J. S. (1984). Psychotherapy in India. Traditions and trends. In A. De Sousa & D. A. De Sousa (Eds.), *Psychiatry in India* (pp. 333–352). Bombay: Bhalani Book Depot.
Norenzayan, A., & Hansen, I. G. (2006). Belief in supernatural agents in the face of death. *Personality and Social Psychology Bulletin, 32*(2), 174–187.
Nowak, M. A. (2006). Five rules for the evolution of cooperation. *Science, 314,* 1560–1563.
Obeyesekere, G. (2004). The Buddhist meditative askesis: A variety of the visionary experience. *Harvard Divinity Bulletin, 32*(3), 7–10.
Olson, D. R., & Bruner, J. S. (1996). Folk psychology and folk pedagogy. In D. R. Olson & N. Torrance (Eds.), *The handbook of education and human development: New models of learning, teaching and schooling* (pp. 9–27). Oxford: Blackwell.
Pakhretia, S., & Pirta, R. S. (2011). Cognitive foundations of mental health in Gaddi community: Role of sensual, affectional and supernatural elements. *Journal of Psychosocial Research, 6*(1), 53–61.
Paquette, V., Levesque, J., Mensour, B., Leroux, J.-M., Beaudoin, G., Bourgouin, P., et al. (2003). "Change the mind and you change the brain": Effects of cognitive behavioral therapy on the neural correlates of spider phobia. *Neuroimage, 18,* 401–409.

Pennycook, G., Cheyne, J. A., Seli, P., Koehler, D. J., & Fugelsang, J. A. (2012). Analytic cognitive style predicts religious and paranormal belief. *Cognition, 123,* 335–346.
Pirta, R. S. (2003). Native cognition of sustainable development in the western Himalaya. *Psychological Studies, 48,* 30–42.
Pirta, R. S. (2005). Community mental health approach in rural areas: Developing the traditional institution. *Journal of Personality and Clinical Studies, 21,* 91–108.
Pirta, R. S. (2006). Community-based approach to mental health: The traditional healing. *Journal of CommunityGuidance & Research, 23*(2), 161–177.
Pirta, R. S. (2007). *Ecology and human well-being: Nature and society in Himachal Pradesh.* Delhi: Shipra Publications.
Pirta, R. S. (2009). *Pastoralism and the tribesman of mountain: The arungzetsa of Kanaor.* Delhi: Shipra Publications.
Pirta, R. S. (2012). Some aspects of empathy in the process of psychotherapy: Learning from Indian tradition. *Psychological Studies, 57,* 336–347.
Pirta, R. S. (2014). Yoking gnosis and logos: On the knowledge function of some exceptional mental states for well-being. *Psychological Studies, 59,* 166–179.
Purzycki, B. G., & Sosis, R. (2011). Our Gods: Variation in supernatural minds. In U. J. Frey, C. Stormer, & K. P. Willfuhr (Eds.), *Essential building blocks of human nature* (pp. 77–93). Berlin, Heidelberg: Springer.
Raguram, R., Venkateswaran, A., Ramakrishna, J., & Weiss, M. G. (2002). Traditional community resources for mental health: A report of temple healing from India. *British Medical Journal, 325,* 38–40.
Ramanujan, A. K. (1983). The Indian Oedipus. In L. Edmunds & A. Dundes (Eds.), *Oedipus: A folklore casebook* (pp. 234–261). New York: Garland Publishing.
Rao, K. (2010). Psychological interventions: From theory to practice. In G. Misra (Ed.), *Psychology in India. Volume 3: Clinical and health psychology* (pp. 317–359). New Delhi: Pearson.
Ray, O. (2004). How the mind hurts and heals the body. *American Psychologist, 59*(1), 29–40.
Schwartz, J. M., Stapp, H., & Beauregard, M. (2005). Quantum theory in neuroscience and psychology: a neurophysical model of mind/brain interaction. *Philosophical Transactions of the Royal Society B: Biological Sciences, 360,* 1309–1327.
Sharfstein, S. S. (2000). Whatever happened to community mental health. *Psychiatric Services, 51,* 616–620.
Sharma, S., & Misra, G. (2010). Health psychology: Progress and challenges. In G. Misra (Ed.), *Psychology in India. Volume 3: Clinical and health psychology* (pp. 265–316). New Delhi: Pearson.
Shariff, A. F., & Norenzayan, A. (2007). God is watching you: Supernatural agent concepts increase prosocial behavior in an anonymous economic game. *Psychological Science, 18,* 803–809.
Sperry, R. W. (1991). Search for beliefs to live by consistent with science. *Zygon, 26*(2), 237–258.
Sperry, R. W. (1992). Paradigms of belief, theory and metatheory. *Zygon, 27*(3), 245–259.
Sundararajan, L., Misra, G., & Marsella, A. J. (2013). Indigenous approaches to assessment, diagnosis, and treatment of mental disorders. In F. A. Paniagua & A. M, Yamada (Eds.), *Handbook of multicultural mental health: Assement and treatment of diverse populations* (pp. 69–87). Oxford: Academic Press.
Sudarshan, E. C. G. (1982). Evolution of mind. *Journal of Time Space and Knowledge, 1,* 5–30.
Sudarshan, E. C. G. (2002). One quest, one knowledge. In W. M. Richardson, R. J. Russell, P. Clayton, & K. Wegter-McNelly (Eds.), *Science and the spiritual quest* (pp. 247–252). New York: Routledge.
Sudarshan, E. C. G. (2003). The promise of quantum computing. *Current Science, 84*(4), 504–512.
Srinivasa Murthy, R. (1998). Rural psychiatry in developing countries. *Psychiatric Services, 49,* 967–969.
Srinivasa Murthy, R. (2004). Mental health in the new millennium: Reseach strategies for India. *Indian Journal of Medical Research, 120,* 63–66.

Srinivasa Murthy, R. (2007). Mental health programme in the 11th Five Year Plan. *Indian Journal of Medical Research, 125,* 707–711.

Thakur, S., & Pirta, R. S. (2009). Mental health and cognitive representations of people experiencing spirit possession. *Journal of the Indian Academy of Applied Psychology, 35*(2), 203–209.

Vaillant, G. E. (2003). Mental health. *American Journal of Psychiatry, 160,* 1373–1384.

WHO. (World Health Organization). (2001). *The world health report: 2001: Mental health: New understanding, new hope*. Geneva: World Health Organization.

Wig, N. N. (2004). Mainstreaming mental health. In S. P. Agarwal, D. S. Goel, R. L. Ichhpujani, R. N. Salhan, & S. Shrivastava (Eds.), *Mental health: An Indian perspective 1946–2003* (pp. 341–343). New Delhi: Elsevier.

Part IV
Social Perspectives

Chapter 19
Social-Psychological Interventions to Change Disability Attitudes

Ajit K. Dalal

Physical disability is a major challenge for India, where more than 40% of the world's disabled population lives. Since independence of India from the British rule, government agencies, NGOs and community organizations have been actively engaged in the rehabilitation of disabled people. Many policy and administrative measures were taken to promote education, employment and medico-social rehabilitation by central and state governments. When 1986 was declared as the Year of the Disabled by the UNO, many international agencies also joined in the campaign to improve the quality of life of these people. The charity-based rehabilitation model was replaced in favour of social integration model, and numerous government policies and programmes were initiated to mainstream disabled people. In 1995, a comprehensive 'Persons with Disabilities Act' was passed by the Parliament, which was followed by 'National Trust Act (1999)' and a policy document 'The National Policies for Persons with Disabilities (2005). As a signatory of the United Nations Convention on the Rights of Persons with Disabilities (2008), the Indian Government has shown its commitment to frame policies to protect and promote human rights of disabled people. These measures and changing social environment have impacted the status of these people, as today there are more opportunities for education and employment for them than ever before.

To meet the goals of their mainstreaming and well-being, it has been increasingly realized that a change in societal perception and thinking about disability is imperative. Negative disability related attitudes of community, funding agencies, implementing bodies, teachers, employers, etc., have been one major impediment in improving the quality of life of people with disabilities. Negative attitudes towards people with disability include derogatory stereotypes, beliefs that people with disability have a lesser position in society, and that they have a diminished capacity

A. K. Dalal (✉)
Department of Psychology, Allahabad University, Allahabad, India
e-mail: ajitkdalal@gmail.com

G. Misra (ed.), *Psychosocial Interventions for Health and Well-Being*,
https://doi.org/10.1007/978-81-322-3782-2_19

to equal participation due to their physical impairment. Such attitudes lead people to maintain social distance from disabled people and spare them from social responsibilities.

To understand the implications of such negative attitudes, it is important to refer to the WHO's (2001) three-dimensional model of disability in terms of human functioning impairment, activity limitations and participation restriction. *Impairments* are problems in the functioning of the body—it could be some loss of functioning or malfunctioning at physical, neural or cognitive level. *Activity limitations* are problems in the capacity to perform activities, sensory or mental, simple or complex nature. And finally, *participation restrictions* are environmentally imposed limitations of a person across a range of personal, professional and social activities. These three dimensions of disability arise from an interaction between health condition of an individual and his or her physical, social, and attitudinal environment. The WHO model of disability thus lays greater emphasis on attitude change to ensure equal opportunities to participate in all domains of social life for disabled people.

This chapter discusses these disability attitudes, examine their implications for social integration and explore the possibilities of attitude change. The chapter will focus on Indian scenario as a case in point.

Meaning of Disability Attitudes

Attitudes are defined in terms of its three components—beliefs (evaluation), affects (feelings) and behavioural tendencies (Myers 2005; Stephen 2003).

Belief component forms the basis of our understanding of the world around us; they help in integrating previous experiences, make future interactions more predictable and meaningful. Beliefs simplify, amplify and organize our experiences. A generalized belief system is called a stereotype.

Feeling component refers to a whole range of emotions we express towards any person, group or object. People show a wide range of emotions—from fear, anger, indifference, sympathy to admiration and adoration in everyday life.

Behavioral component refers to how people tend to act in a particular context. Such actions could be actual, implicit or intention to act in a particular way. The behaviour could vary in terms of intensity, frequency and duration.

In the context of disability attitudes, these three components have specific meanings. A positive attitude towards persons with disability would refer to a belief that these people could be productive members of the society, that these people can and should decide what is good for them, and that it is possible for them to lead a normal life. At the affective level, positive attitude would imply an increased sensitivity towards their positive attributes and accepting them as members of one's own group. At the behavioural level, positive attitude implies creating conditions which can facilitate their efforts towards the goal of self-reliance and towards equal participation in the socio-economic development of the community (Dalal and

Pande 1995). It seems that negative attitude is one of the major reasons why people are generally apathetic and show low motivation to get involved in disability rehabilitation programmes.

Social and psychological theories have convincingly argued that the way people behave is often dictated by the attitudes and beliefs they hold. The social participation is dependent on the attitudes and beliefs which people have about health, disease and disability, and, about the factors contributing towards the success of a rehabilitation initiative. The situation becomes even worse when negative attitudes are internalized by persons with disability. This could result in low self-esteem, depletion of their psychic resources needed to cope with the challenges of disability (Pande and Tewari 2011). For successful rehabilitation, it is imperative that persons with disability arrive at a positive construction of their own self and are able to sustain hope and optimism.

Attitudes are learned responses and, therefore, amenable to change. Our past learning and experiences are the basis of attitude formation. An unpleasant encounter or information will contribute to the formation of negative attitudes. Attitudes have a self-serving bias, i.e., attitudes which are functional are less likely to change. Conversely, attitudes that become dysfunctional are more amenable to change (Kraus 1995). Consciously and unconsciously we form attitudes which are adaptive and useful. Again, the attitudes which are rooted in socio-religious belief system are less likely to change. Myths, legends, scriptures and folklore are all part of the cultural belief system that shape our understanding of physical disability.

Another important feature of disability attitudes is the 'spread effect'. Wright (1964) found that a negative evaluation of the condition of disability spreads to influence the evaluation of other non-impaired characteristics. Such spread effect—the power of single characteristic to evoke other inferences about a person—was demonstrated in many studies (Hewstone 1994). These studies evidenced that the term 'disability' can evoke many responses about other presumed dispositions of a person with disability. These responses are not transitory; they indicate the respondent's generalized views about disability. People generalize from the physical characteristic to affective and behavioural characteristics. Such stereotypes could be coherent and fit in people's own naive theories of disability. These are based on culture-specific popular misconceptions amplified by literature, poetry, paintings, music, movies, etc. Wright (1983) has stated that because of this spread, the degree of disability is often perceived as more severe and disabling than it actually is.

A related issue is the meaning of positive attitude. The research suggests that people with disability and those who do not have any disability differ significantly in their perception regarding what constitutes a positive attitude. For a disabled person positive attitude may mean either dispensing away with the special category of disability entirely, or promoting attitudes that defend their civil and special rights. For a non-disabled, positive attitude may demonstrate a desire to be nice, helpful and place the disabled person in a situation where they get special attention (Makas et al. 1988). Therefore, it is possible that in being nice, caring and helpful, the non-disabled may be perceived by disabled persons, as exhibiting a negative rather than a positive attitude towards them.

Negative attitudes are expressed sometimes subtly, sometimes bluntly, and sometimes viciously. People, who find it socially undesirable to express such attitudes publicly, develop their own indirect ways of expressing them. Sometimes it takes time to identify such negative attitudes, as they may be camouflaged in social niceties. For example, an employer offering a physically challenged employee an easy, risk-free and less difficult job may be manifesting a negative attitude, a belief that such an employee has poor abilities. In the similar vein, a person having patronizing attitude would give money to 'help those poor little crippled children'. Research on community attitudes has evidences of paternalistic and patronizing attitudes towards people with disability and its consequences for their inclusion in various life domains, such as employment. Other studies, however, have also found evidences of positive attitudes such as respect, trust and participation in social and professional domain.

Last but equally important, such attitudes and beliefs are often internalized by persons with disability to conform to social expectations. Their beliefs in their own ability may be low, show more dependence, low self-esteem and confidence. Often people with disability face the conflict of performing according to the expectations of the society on one hand, and expressing their real aspirations, on the other. They are expected to behave normally, while constantly reminded of their non-normality through interpersonal interaction, architectural barriers and restricted vocational choices (Holmes and Karst 1990). Whether the conflicting situations are seen as primarily imposed from the outside, or as stemming from internal conflicts will determine where the resentment will be targeted.

There are a number of disability surveys in India which have churned out statistics about prevalence, causes, education, employment and rehabilitation in different regions. There are a few national surveys conducted by Census, National Sample Survey (NSS).

Prevalence of Negative Attitudes

There are a number of disability surveys in India which have churned out statistics about prevalence, causes, education, employment and medical rehabilitation of the physically disabled in different regions. There are a few national surveys, conducted by Census, National Sample Survey (NSS) Organization, collecting the basic data about the prevalence of physical disability in India. Attitude surveys are few and that too have focused on specific population or region. Most of these attitude surveys are post-dated to the UN Year of the Disabled Persons (1986). Many national and international agencies conducted attitude surveys to examine the status of disabled people in the Indian society. These surveys have found overwhelming evidence of negative attitude and marginalization of people with disability in India.

Much of the early literature on disability in India has pointed to the importance of the concept of karma in attitudes to disability, with disability perceived either as punishment for misdeeds in the past lives of the PWD (Dalal 2002; Miles 1995).

That this finding is stable is shown in a later survey in Uttar Pradesh and Tamil Nadu (2005), in which about 50% of households with disability and without disability attributed disability to divine retribution. This could be one of the reasons that the overall attitude people hold towards children with disability is that of patronizing nature, as found in an earlier study (Berman et al. 1984). However, attribution to karma does not lead to passive acceptance of disability. It induces hope, positive construal and desire for right action (Dalal 2000a; Ghai 2001) in the face of hardships faced due to physical condition.

In a comprehensive attitude survey (Dalal et al. 2000) an attitude measure 'Disability-Attitude-Belief-Behaviour' (DABB) was developed to study attitudes of people in two rural communities in North India. Attitudes of community, family and people with disability were examined and their consequences for rehabilitation were studied. The overall attitude was negative for all the three groups. Family and community members considered disability as 'central' to the disabled person's negative feelings, self-concept, social comparisons and relationship. Also, having a disability was considered synonymous with needing help and social support for their daily living and livelihood. This was also found that people with disability internalized these negative attitudes about themselves and believed that they cannot do much to improve their lot. Also, those with disabilities often go through conflicting mental states; where on one hand they align with the perpetrators who exploit and harm them, and on the other hand, they resent the same group for frustrating their aspiration to access existing resources.

It may be mentioned in this context that dominant traditions and cultural values, at times, create attitudinal conflicts for people with disability. Studies have also shown that people with disability go through attitudinal conflict. This is particularly the situation in case of people with disability who do not conform social norms and prescriptions. Chib (2002), for example, was both lauded and criticized for her decision to live independently. Such people are denied their right to self-assertion, identity and development (Karna 2000). As noted by Ghai (2010), '… society's attitudes and perspectives toward disabled people have always been complex and are often catalysed by the prevailing culture, religion, government and economic conditions' (p. 150).

This scenario points to the necessity of moving individual attitudes to community and target group attitudes which are more relevant in this context. Dixon and Mark (2012) calls for this shift in attitude research objective, from changing negative attitudes to social change, i.e., from individual's prejudice reduction to collective attitude change. In this reconceptualization, prejudice is viewed as perceived social norm, rather than as an individual's personal attitude and emotion. Dixon and Mark suggest that to change disability related attitudes, the critical target is not what an individual personally thinks or feels about another people with disability, but rather what they perceive other members of their group think or feel.

Concomitants of Negative Attitudes

Here in this section we will focus on three concomitants of prevalent negative attitudes which society has towards people with disability. These are prejudice, stereotypes and discrimination. These three consequences, in turn, provide the broader framework within which disability and people with disability are treated by society. Such outcomes are contingent on the way biology of impairment interact with cultural norms and expectations to develop its own social construction of disability. Groce (1990) argued that societies develop their own characteristic patterns of managing disability, depending on how they view disability and their own role in dealing with it. Historical events, sacred texts and social institutions form the basis of social construction of disablement and the way people share the responsibility of rehabilitation. Once formed these constructions and practices have propensity to endure the vicissitudes of time and technological changes (Dalal 2011).

The greater the prejudice toward disabled people, the fewer the opportunities they have to earn a living, and the poorer and more destitute they become, thus reinforcing the prejudice and stigmatization. Disability is often considered to be an abnormality, a deviance, where the focus is on physical and mental state of the individual. There are negative stereotypes and prejudices about the disabled persons, as found in various studies conducted in India and elsewhere (Dalal et al. 2000).

Negative attitudes and discrimination exist in a vicious circle. Stigmatizing disability allows or encourages discriminatory attitudes. These attitudes are often reflected in stigmatizing disabled persons, subjecting them to discrimination in different domains of social life. Discrimination can occur in terms of access to public utilities, physical access to government or by private institutions, in education, housing, and health facilities, including water, grazing land, irrigation facility and the like in rural areas. Even when attempts are made to break the pattern of negative attitudes and discrimination by enacting laws, disabled people suffer stigma and experience social isolation. It should not be forgotten that disabled people have hardly any say in enforcement of various laws and in implementation of various schemes. It should not be forgotten that more than 80% disabled people belong to lower strata of the society.

Attitude Measurement

A number of scales exist to measure attitudes towards disability. These measures differ on varied aspects, intended for different types of disability, sample and objectives. Literature search revealed that most of them were prepared in the same manner as other attitude scales in the academic setting. Most of the scales have been designed as a part of research activities in academic institutions. An urban bias in these scales is also evident. Two most popular scales in early decades were: the Attitude towards Disabled Person Scale (ATDP, Yuker et al. 1960) and Interaction with Disabled Persons Scale (IDPS, Gething and Wheeler 1992), to measure the attitudes of both disabled and non-disabled persons. (Yuker 1994) listed 325 studies which had used their scale in past 25 years. A large number of such scales were developed in later years. One such comprehensive scale developed in India was Disability-Attitude-Belief-Behaviour (DABB) measure developed by Dalal et al. (2000). This battery of measures has combined measures related to beliefs, affect and behaviour, taking both qualitative and qualitative measures to be administered on different categories of people.

Most of these survey measures of disability attitude are self-reporting measures. Such measures are likely to be affected by social desirability bias. There is always a possibility of furnishing fake and misleading information, hiding one's rear attitude. Such attitude measures are developed on college students whose attitudes are likely to be different from those of the general population. These attitude measures are often based on restricted definition of disability attitude. Often, they simply reveal whether the attitude is positive or negative. Such measures are not very diagnostic and have field application.

Realizing that the existing verbal tests do not really convey the attitudes which people actually have, search for alternative measures of disability attitude continued. Several indirect and projective tests to map attitudes were developed in which vignettes and pictures were used. In other instances, qualitative methods are used to map disability attitudes. Most of these measures have methodological problems and are often ambiguous in their interpretation.

In more recent time, a breakthrough is made in the measurement of disability attitudes. (Greenwald et al. 1998) and many other researchers have demonstrated on the basis of experimental evidences that human behaviour is more under the control of unconscious mind than previously thought. They made a distinction between explicit and implicit attitude. Whereas explicit attitude is inferred on the basis of conscious and direct responses to verbal stimuli, implicit attitudes are indirect and initiated by subliminal stimuli. Implicit attitudes and stereotypes are those that are triggered automatically at the unconscious level, not mediated by conscious activity. The test relies on response time because faster responses equate to pairings that are more strongly associated in memory. In other words, if a testee associates men with positive words more quickly than with women, then that testee has a closer implicit association between men and positive attributes than women and positive attributes. That implies a more positive implicit attitude towards men than women. This measure has been successfully used to measure implicit disability attitude of different cross-sections of respondents.

In many studies implicit attitudes toward disability were tested using the Implicit Association Test. Archambault et al. (2008) found that 76% of the sample showed an implicit preference for those who have no disability. The negativity was consistent across genders, ethnicities, age groups and political orientations, making it a widespread and permeating bias. Again, they found a very week correlation between implicit and explicit disability attitudes. That this negativity bias in subliminal attitudes toward disabled persons is pervasive is many recent surveys (Pruett and Chan 2006; Vaughn 2009).

To conclude, some recurring findings from the studies of implicit bias are: (1) implicit bias is pervasive; (2) implicit bias diverges from the consciously reported preferences and beliefs of the same individual; (3) implicit bias predicts consequential behaviour; and (4) implicit bias is malleable and its effect on behaviour might be mitigated through conscious efforts.

Consequences of Negative Attitudes

Such negative attitudes which people have towards people with disability have far reaching consequences. It may not be possible here to cover all aspects of their lives which get affected by society's perception and attitudes. To bring about a change in society's perception of 'disabled', different nomenclature has been used by NGOs, government, professionals, such as 'people with disability', 'differently-able', disabled, physically challenged, persons with special needs, etc. However, merely changing labels have not helped in changing perceptions and attitudes of people in general. People may not be using derogatory expressions for disabled people in public, changing negative attitude is still a major challenge before the society.

Some significant consequences of these negative attitudes are discussed here.

Education and Employment

Elwan (1999) noted that the disabled children in developing countries who often are discriminated in schools, have low expectations from themselves, experience low expectations from teachers and others, and fail to get the support they need for equal participation. As adults, discrimination also tends to exclude them from employment and income-earning opportunities, leaving them in perpetual poverty (Hoogeveen 2005; Lwanga-Ntale 2003; World Bank 2005). This initial exclusion and lack of growth opportunities create a downward cycle of economic well being that can follow disabled people throughout their lives. As Sen (2000) has noted that not only do people with disability have difficulty earning an income but the disability also 'makes it harder to convert income into the freedom to live well' (p. 4). Sen further added that these people also find it difficult to convert available 'social facilities into actually usable opportunities' (p. 5).

The National Sample Survey (2002) found that 55% of the disabled in India are illiterate; only 9% have completed higher secondary education. Only 11% of disabled people in the age group 5–18 years have enrolled in special schools in urban areas; in rural areas it is less than 1%. In August 2004, the NCPED put out a report titled 'Research Study on Present Education Scenario'. The report had found that only 0.51% of disabled students were in mainstream educational institutions at the school level and 0.1% at the university level. These data are consistent with the overall scenario in the developing countries where about 90% children with disability do not go to school (UNESCO Report 2003). This is, in spite of the fact that 3% seats in all educational institutions are reserved for disabled people in India.

This dismal scenario has to be seen in the light of the fact that the Government of India had started the scheme of integrated education for the disabled way back in 1974. It was a major shift in the government policy from special schools to integrated schools for providing education to the disabled children. Except for the severely handicapped, other handicapped children were to be integrated in the ordinary schools with the help of special teachers, aids and resources. Funds were made available to suitably modify the buildings to make them more accessible. In later years, instead of effectively implementing this scheme and engaging in the exercise of removing its lacuna, this scheme was disbanded to be replaced by new international campaign for 'inclusion education' promoted by UN Convention on the Rights of the Child (1989), World Conference on Education for All (1990) and other follow-up activities. Based on tempting ideals of 'right to education as a basic human right', improving the 'quality of education for all' inclusive education became the guiding principle for formulating educational policies in many developing countries. Inclusive education marks shift in services from 'care of the disabled child' to his/her education and personal development. How this policy change has affected the quality of education of the poorest strata of the society is yet to be ascertained. Many surveys have revealed that less than 3–4% children with special needs had access to education (Mukhopadhyay and Mani 2002; Singh 2003). Current propositions and arguments about inclusive education have remained at the level of theory and no concrete steps or processes have been systematically developed so far to work out any implementation plan (Singal 2006). In 2009, the Indian Parliament passed 'Right to Education' Act to provide free and compulsory education to all children, including disabled children. It is yet to be seen how this Act will change the scenario.

The World Bank Report (2008) observed that while Indian economy was booming, employment of disabled people was falling way behind. The report noted a 5% drop in the employment rate of disabled people in the decade leading up to 2002. The fall in the employment rate of working age disabled people was from 42.7% in 1991 to 37.6% in 2002, uniform across all education and job levels. In the public sector, despite 3% job reservation since 2003, only 10% of the posts have been identified as 'suitable' for the disabled people. The data are more dismal in the case of private sector. In late1990 s, employment of disabled people among large private firms was only 0.3% of their workforce. In case of the MNCs, the situation is far worse, with only 0.05% of the workforce constituting disabled people. One can guess that employment of rural people with disabilities would be almost negligible. The World Bank Report (2008) further shows that assessment of people with disabilities for their capability to succeed on the job is low. Surprisingly, these assessments are shared by people with disabilities also.

Despite the most optimistic outlook for change in employment opportunities for women with disabilities, the present reality is that the best hope for productive work may lie in the domain of self-employment, probably in cooperative activities. Apart from economic independence, work is an essential means of enabling a person to develop a sense of identity and self-esteem. Thus, gainful employment is an important means of promoting social integration of women with disability.

Access to Health and Rehabilitation Services

Negative attitudes are an additional health hazard for people with disability who are already in need of health and rehabilitation services. They are more vulnerable and disadvantaged as compared to others also due to their reduced access to safe and potable drinking water, nutrition, proper housing, sanitation, and hygiene. Lack of education and employment add to their vulnerability.

How much of India's population has physical disability, is anybody's guess. The Indian Census of 2001 has revealed that 2.1% of the population has significant physical or neural disability. The National Sample Survey Organization (NSSO) conducted in 2002 reported that 1.8% of the population has a disability (NSSO 2003). Both these surveys seem to be gross underestimation. Leading Indian disability NGOs argue that 5–6% of the population has disability; WHO estimates a global prevalence rate of 10%. None of these surveys and estimates present reliable picture of the prevalence of disability in India. The lack of reliable estimates and underestimations has impact on the kind of policies and provisions framed for people with disabilities.

Furthermore, physical disability is taken as a category, a static state located within the individual, in his/her functional limitations. A standard criterion is to classify anyone who has 40% or above functional impairment as disabled, for all categories of disabilities. Consequently, rehabilitation services primarily focus on providing people with disability aids and appliances, immunization, etc. Rather than addressing the problems of physical and social barriers, most of the government budget is earmarked for aids and appliances and medical assistance. Data show that only 2–3% people with disability benefit from such largesse of governmental agencies and NGOs.

Around the mid-80s India's policy planners and disability NGOs abandoned the purely medical model of rehabilitation in favour of a CBR model, which emphasized social integration and rehabilitation of people with disabilities with the community support (Dalal 2000b; WHO 2011). Hopes were ripe that CBR will lead to public awareness and will involve community leaders for creating job opportunities for rural disabled. In later years, the government adopted CBR as its official programme and resources were channelized to promote CBR as a viable replacement of institution-based rehabilitation. It was an adoption of the social model of rehabilitation that draws a clear distinction between physical impairment and disability. Society disables people with impairments by its failure to recognize and accommodate difference, and through the attitudinal, environmental and institutional barriers it erects and fails to dismantle. This 'social model' of disability contends that it is not the individual that has to change, but society that should make radical changes through systems, services and attitudes.

CBR attempts to combine physical rehabilitation through medical care with empowerment, and social inclusion through participation of both, the individual with a disability and the community in the process of rehabilitation (Dalal et al. 2000). CBR emphasizes, above all, that disabled people have to be recognized as people—as human beings with equal rights. The advocates of CBR often claim it to be the best approach for inclusion and social integration of the people with disabilities. CBR depends heavily on the development of positive attitudes of the people involved. Positive attitude is essential for active community participation.

Social Exclusion

One major consequence of negative disability attitude is exclusion of people with disability from mainstream social life. ESCAP Report (1993) stated in the context of Asian and Pacific region, 'This is largely because negative social attitudes exclude persons with disabilities from an equal share in their entitlements as citizens. Such attitudes also curtail the opportunities of people with disabilities from social contact and close personal relationships with others' (p. 5). Miles (1996), on the basis of his survey in Pakistan and 30 other countries, noted that there is slow, progressive development from negative, stigmatizing and rejecting attitudes, through pity and compassion, towards willingness to accept the physically challenged persons on equal terms. Studies have shown that females than males tend to have more positive attitude towards the disabled and the younger generation has a more positive attitude than the older generation (Bakheit and Shanmugalingam 1997). However, any such general conclusion needs to be tested with more comprehensive empirical studies of attitudes and beliefs.

One of the reasons that exacerbate exclusion of the disabled people from the civic life is poor accessibility of public places. Though central and state governments in India have repeatedly pledged that public buildings would be made accessible for disabled people, the situation has only marginally improved in the last one decade. Ramps or lifts that accommodate wheelchairs, signs in Braille, audio commands at traffic signals, or toilets that wheelchair-bound people can use are still rare sights; in rural areas they are almost non-existent. Buses and trains are virtually out of bounds for people in wheelchairs. Various physical access audit reports have come to the same conclusion. This lack of accessibility has also serious implications for the education of children with disability. Most of the regular schools are out of their reach. There is hardly any transport facility, proper approach roads, toilets in schools which children with disability can use. The situation of women with disability is much worse. There is a critical need to build an enabling psychological and physical environment that is supportive of the ability of the woman with a disability to function, within the limits caused by the disability itself, and by social practices.

What we need are time-bound programmes with clear line of authority and accountability. Disability programmes and policies are caught in the complex bureaucratic web where there is no effective coordination between various agencies. It is an unending hurdle race for the disabled-rural-poor to cross legal and procedural barriers to avail the benefits of various schemes. We still need to figure out how did it change the lives of poor with disability? These and other developments of the last two decades did give the disability sector some new rhetoric, like empowerment, rights of the disabled people, inclusive development, etc. Such rhetoric, at times, substitute for actual rehabilitation activities. For many big disability NGOs, it marked a shift in focus from field projects to training, advocacy and awareness campaign. This made it easier for them to operate from their urban centres.

Social Interventions for Attitude Change

Attitude change is one of the most popular, yet challenging area of research in social psychology. A large number of studies are conducted to find methods and techniques of attitude change in the area of disability. Government, NGOs, disability groups, schools, media are all involved in the endeavour of attitude change. Many innovative ways of changing negative attitudes have been identified. Here, our purpose is not to catalogue them but to present the methods which we tried in our community projects (Dalal 2006; Dalal and Pandey 1995) and found quite effective, particularly in rural settings.

Empowering Activities

The Government of India has launched a number of schemes for the welfare of people with disability in the last five decades. Many government schemes, such as travel concessions, scholarships, disability pension, bank loans for self-employment, etc., were not accessible to the targeted groups, partly because of bureaucratic hassles, corruption and callousness. A disability certificate, which only the Chief Medical Officer of the district, or the Heads of Departments of the Medical College in Allahabad city were authorized to issue, is needed to avail these government schemes. For poor villagers, it was nearly impossible to procure these certificates on their own.

The venture of the CBR Village Committee was to organize three certificate camps. To organize these camps the Committee conducted a survey and identified about 350 physically challenged children and adults in the region. These persons assembled at a community centre on the day when medical officials, who were authorized to issue disability certificates, visited the project area. The team conducted the medical checkup and issued medical certificates to the deserving ones then and there. It helped 122 persons to get the certificate in the first phase. This certificate could be used by the physically challenged persons and their families to avail travel concession. For example, persons with disability gets 75% concession in rail and bus travel, and one of the accompanying persons was also entitled to the same concession. On the basis of this disability certificate few physically challenged persons got small loans from banks to start their own businesses. Availing these government benefits indeed made the physically challenged providers of certain benefits to their family and friends.

From Beneficiaries to Providers

Another activity which facilitated attitude change was an initiative taken by the children with disability to collect public donations for the relief of the flood victims. These children went from door to door in their neighbourhood appealing people to help victims of the flood that ravaged the nearby region. The physically challenged children prepared their own band and they took out processions to collect public donations. Though the money collected was not a big amount, children with disability were seen for the first time during these campaigns as contributing to a social cause, rather than being at the receiving end. This initiative by the physically challenged children was widely covered by local newspapers.

Breaking Mental Barriers

Our survey had shown that physically challenged and their families believed that disability severely restricts one's ability to be a productive member of the family (Dalal and Pande 1995). It was also found that people often describe disablement in terms of the activities which physically challenged cannot do. They attributed their condition to their karma (deeds) of the past lives. Often times, such prejudices and negative attitudes were functional, as it not only explained the suffering but also justified inaction on part of the family and community.

In our endeavour to shift attention from disabilities to abilities, the CBR Committee tried to create a condition in which people were required to discuss the abilities that these physically challenged had. The team organized focus-group discussions taking physically challenged unemployed youths, their families and other community members. The focus of the discussion used to be 'What work these youths can do?' for which there names could be recommended for the bank loan under the self-employment scheme of the Government. Since financial incentive was implicated in such discussions, participants often took more than usual interest in identifying the abilities in those whom they earlier thought 'cannot do anything'.

These focused discussions were helpful in identifying the strengths of the physically challenged applicants. These were listed in the recommendations of different focus-groups. As mentioned earlier, many of them got bank loan and became successful entrepreneurs. This initiative created many success models which not only inspired others, but also opened a public debate about what the physically challenged can do, and do well.

Community-Based Schooling

It had been realized for a long time that children with major disabilities had no access to education in the region. With some support from the Rajiv Gandhi Foundation, New Delhi, an integrated school was started in one of the villages with one teacher and 25 children, 15 of them with physical disabilities. The school was located on the premises of one of the office bearers of the CBR Village Committee. The children were imparted basic reading and writing skills and arithmetic. For most of the children with disabilities, this was their first experience of formal schooling. The school provided a forum for community members to come together, particularly the parents of physically challenged children. This community school became the centre of many community activities, and was consequently instrumental in breaking many misconceptions and prejudices about the children with disabilities. It also helped in bringing awareness in the community of the special needs of school-going children with disabilities. Many of these children later joined regular schools and did well.

Engaging Religious Centres and Healers

In India religious leaders and beliefs play important role in building attitude toward disabled people. Belief in theory of karma and divine retribution is widely prevalent and often endorsed by religious leaders. Disabled people and their families frequently visited shines, temples, mosques and consulted religious healers of their areas. These religious healers have a holistic way of dealing with human suffering; can inculcate hope that their situation may improve with right actions. We contacted some of these local religious healers and involved them in rehabilitation programme. The idea was not to change core beliefs of people but to dispel disability related misconceptions and superstitions. Their involvement did motivate disabled people and their families to be get more active in rehabilitation activities.

Attitude Change: An Ongoing Project

Disability attitudes and beliefs play an important role in the success of any rehabilitation programme. The fatalistic belief that disabled people cannot do much to change their lot, in fact, become a major impediment in involving disabled people and their families in rehabilitation activities. Fatalistic attitudes absolved family, community and officials of making concerted efforts to improve life conditions of the disabled people. With increasing number of disabled people coming for education and getting employment, these fatalistic attitudes are slowly changing.

It should be realized that many of these disability related attitudes are embedded in the cultural beliefs of a society and do not change in a short period and by piecemeal efforts. In a traditional society, like India, bringing a change in fatalistic attitudes needs long-term concerted efforts. Bringing about attitude change need to be part of the overall disability policies and action programmes. We need to think of innovative ways of dealing with negative attitudes and their deleterious consequences. Reinforcing positive attitudes, in this sense, is a long-term ongoing social project in India.

References

Archambault, M. E., Van Rhee, J. A., Marion, G. S., & Crandall, S. J. (2008). Utilizing implicit association testing to promote awareness of biases regarding age and disability. *The Journal of Physician Assistant Education, 19*(4), 20–26.

Bakheit, A., & Shanmugalingam, V. (1997). A study of the attitudes of rural Indian community peopletowards people with disability. *Clinical Rehabilitation, 11*(4), 329–334.

Berman, V. M., Dalal, A. K., & Anthony, L. (1984). Connotation of handicapped label in India. *Psychologia, 27,* 115–121.

Chib, M. (2002). Where is your helper? *South Pacific Disability Rehabilitation Journal, 14,* 139–145.

Dalal, A. K. (2000a). Social attitudes and rehabilitation of people with disability: The Indian experience. *Arab Journal of Rehabilitation, 5,* 15–21.

Dalal, A. K. (2000b). Poverty, development and disability: Some lessons from a community based intervention programme. In A.K. Mohanty and G. Misra (Eds.), *Psychology of Poverty and Disadavantage: A Fresh Look.* New Delhi: Concept.

Dalal, A. K. (2002). Disability rehabilitation in a traditional Indian society. In M. Thomas & M. J. Thomas (Eds.), *Selected readings in Community Based Rehabilitation: Series 2 -Disability and Rehabilitation in South Asia* (pp. 17–24). Bangalore: National Printing Press.

Dalal, A. K. (2006). Social interventions to moderate discriminatory attitudes: The case of the physically challenged in India. *Psychology, Health & Medicine, 11*(3), 374–382.

Dalal, A. K. (2011). Health care of the poor with disabilities: The challenges of social stigma and access to services. *Indian Journal of Physical Anthropology and Human Genetics, 29*(1 & 2), 109–115.

Dalal, A. K., & Pande, N. (1995). A community intervention programme for changing attitude toward disability. *The Social Engineer, 4,* 16–25.

Dalal, A. K., Pande, N., Dhawan, N., Dwijendra, D., & Berry, J. (2000). *The mind matters: Disability attitudes and community based rehabilitation.* Allahabad: University of Allahabad, India.

Dixon, J., & Mark, L. (2012). *Beyond prejudice*. Cambridge, UK: Cambridge University Press.

Elwan, A. (1999). *Poverty and disability: Survey of the literature*. New York: Social Protection Unit, World Bank.

ESCAP. (1993). *Asia and Pacific decade of disabled persons, 1993–2002: The starting point*. New York: United Nations.

Gething, L., & Wheeler, B. (1992). The Interaction with disabled persons scale: A new Australian instrument to measure attitudes towards people with disabilities. *Australian Journal of Psychology, 44*(2), 75–82.

Ghai, A. (2001). Marginalization and disability: Experience from the third world. In M. Priestly (Ed.), *Disability and the life course: Global perspectives* (pp. 26–57). Cambridge: Cambridge University Press.

Ghai, A. (2010). Psychology of disabled people. In G. Misra (Ed.), *Psychology in India, Vol. Clinical and Health Psychology* (pp. 107–184). New Delhi: Pearson.

Greenwald, A. G., McGhee, D. E., & Schwartz, J. K. L. (1998). Measuring individual differences in implicit cognition: The implicit association test. *Journal of Personality and Social Psychology, 74,* 1464–1480.

Groce, N. (1990). Comparative and cross-cultural issues. *Disability Studies Quarterly, 10,* 1–39.

Hewstone, M. (1994). Revision and change of stereotypic beliefs: In search of the subtyping model. In S. Stroebe & M. Hewstone (Eds.), *European review of social psychology* (Vol. 5). Chechester, England: Wiley.

Holmes, G. E., & Karst, R. H. (1990). The institutionalization of disability myths: Impact on vocational rehabilitation services. *Journal of Rehabilitation, 56,* 20–27.

Hoogeveen, J. G. (2005). Measuring welfare for small but vulnerable groups: Poverty and disability in Uganda. *Journal of African Economies, 14*(4), 603–631.

Karna, G. N. (2000). Disability rights movement: Conceptual framework and its implications for India. *Disabilities and Impairments, 14,* 15–22.

Kraus, S. J. (1995). Attitudes and predictions of behaviour: A meta-analysis of the empirical literature. *Personality and Social Psychology Bulletin, 21,* 58–75.

Lwanga-Ntale, C. (2003). *Chronic poverty and disability in Uganda.* Chronic Poverty Research Centre Working Paper. Manchester, UK: Institute of Development Policy and Management/CPRC.

Makas, E., Finnerty-Fied, P., Sugafoos, A., & Reiss, D. (1988). The issues in disability scale: A new affective and cognitive measure of attitude toward people with physical disabilities. *Journal of Applied Behavioural Counselling, 19,* 56–68.

Miles, M. (1995). Disability in an eastern religious context: Historical perspectives. *Disability and Society, 10*(1), 49–69.

Miles, M. (1996). Community, individual or information development: Dilemma of concept and culture in South Asia disability planning. *Disability and Society, 11*, 485–500.

Mukhopadhyay, S., & Mani, M. N. G. (2002). Education of children with special needs. In R. Govinda (Ed.), *India education report: A profile of basic education* (pp. 96–108). New Delhi, India: Oxford University Press.

Myers, D. G. (2005). *Social pschology* (8th ed.). New York: McGraw-Hill.

National Sample Survey. (2002). *Employment and unemployment 55th Round (1999–2000).* New Delhi: National Sample Survey Organisation.

National Sample Survey. (2003). *Prevalence of disability in India.* New Delhi: National Sample Survey Organisation.

Pande, N., & Tewari, S. (2011). Understanding coping with distress due to physical disability. *Psychology and Developing Societies, 23*(2), 46–57.

Pruett, S. R., & Chan, F. (2006). The development and psychometric validation of the disability attitude implicit association test. *Rehabilitation Psychology, 51,* 202–213.

Sen, A. (2000). *Social exclusion: Concept, application, and scrutiny* (Social Development Bank Paper, No. 1.). Manila: Asian Development Bank.

Singal, N. (2006). Inclusive education in India: International concept, national interpretation. *International Journal of Disability, Development and Education, 53*(3), 351–369.

Singh, J. P. (2003). *Disability status India* (p. XXIII). New Delhi: Rehabilitation Council of India.
Stephen, L. (2003). *Social psychology* (3rd ed.). New York: McGraw-Hill.
UNESCO Report (2003). *Global monitoring report: Gender and disability perspective*. Paris: UNESCO.
Vaughn, E. D. (2009). *The refinement of a multidimensional computer based implicit association test as a measurement of attitudes toward persons with disabilities* (Unpublished doctoral dissertation) Auburn University, USA.
WHO. (2001). *International classification of functioning, disability and health*. Geneva: WHO.
World Bank Disability Policy Center. (2005). *Disability and development and the world bank—A briefing summary on February 2, 2005*. Washington, DC: World Bank.
World Bank Report. (2008). *People with disability in India: From commitments to outcomes—Released in New Delhi on December 3, 2008*. Washington, DC: World Bank.
World Health Organization. (2011). *World Report on Disability*. Geneva: WHO.
Wright, B. A. (1964). Spread in adjustment to disability. *Bulletin of Menninger Clinic, 28*, 198–209.
Wright, B. A. (1983). *Physical disability: A psychosocial approach*. New York: Harper & Row.
Yuker, H. E. (1994). Variables that influence attitudes toward people with disabilities. *Journal of Social Behavior and Personality, 9*, 3–22.
Yuker, H. E., Block, J. R., & Campbell, W. L. (1960). *A scale to measure attitudes towards disabled persons*. Albertson, New York: Human Resources Foundation.

Chapter 20
The Rude, Rough, Friendless Rehab Road—Chasing Mental Health

Prateeksha Sharma

Introduction

The current conception of mental health is generally done in the context of psychiatric classifications. A common man is far removed from such technicalities of mental health, even though they may be impacted by it on a regular basis. By and large, the focus of all governmental efforts has been to increase the accessibility of people suffering to medication and increasing psychiatric infrastructure. From around the globe, there is a sea of evidence alarming the world about the rising incidence of mental illnesses, and making projections about the incidence of mental illness as the single largest reason for disability in the times to come. In such a one-sided propaganda how will anyone ever know that people can even recover, unless mechanisms are put in place to sensitize people about it? In a situation where mental health concerns presents a bleak scenario universally, modern medicine by itself cannot deal with the enormity of the problem. Expanding medical infrastructure and medicating patients have not diminished mental health problems anywhere. There is a need to infuse fresh thinking, to find alternative ways of treatment, and to lay greater emphasis on the preventive side.

Recovery from mental illnesses, though achievable and a legitimate goal, is a much neglected area, especially in the global South. While the richer countries of Europe, Australia and North America, are not only investing significant funds in recovery research, this effort is on in multiple locations, including university departments, non-profits, medical schools and community based efforts. They are willing to join hands and invite any participant for further research, if they find

P. Sharma (✉)
National Academy of Legal Studies and Research (NALSAR), Hyderabad, India
e-mail: hansadhwani.prateeksha@gmail.com

G. Misra (ed.), *Psychosocial Interventions for Health and Well-Being*,
https://doi.org/10.1007/978-81-322-3782-2_20

them capable of serious contribution. My own experience and dialogues with many academics in institutions of higher education/research have indicated to me their open-minded approach to inquiry, knowledge and a genuine commitment to solution finding. A parallel experience of academics in higher education in India has evoked minimal or no response whatsoever. It brings to fore a question which I invite the readers of this article to consider—what ought research to be, and what is its agenda? What knowledge contributes towards finding solutions for intractable problems in society and what pathways should be created to allow that knowledge to evolve and disseminate? In a seminal critique of current research trends, Gergen (2014a, b) questions the ethos of research which is merely a mirror of society, and contributes in no way to further solutions for problems that it sets out to examine. He proposes a radical shift in the orientation of research, which he describes as a move 'from mirroring to world making'. That research in which the agenda is simply to map an existing aspect of society is merely a mirror, looking glass. It does not go any further. But what if the purpose of research were to transform society in meaningful ways, as though contributing towards forming a new future?

Likely, a majority of readers would agree that mental illness is a question that fits the above description, whose solutions are not easy to find. If a way can be found out of mental illness by anyone, should it be considered a legitimate contribution to knowledge? Perhaps that solution finder need not be someone with an academic degree in medicine, psychology, or any allied discipline? What if the person is someone who has lived and recovered from a mental illness? Can their recovery be considered as an advancement in understanding human suffering, or would it fit in the category of 'luck', 'chance' or something equally dismissive? What happened in the field of HIV research and practice worldwide due to the contributors of people suffering or living with HIV as survivors, is a model for other stigmatizing conditions, to consider. They have struggled and brought to center-stage the focus that people who suffer have a humanity, a life and it needs to be valued and respected, not just treated as the recipients of services of healthcare, as passive actors. What they have accomplished in the past three decades is what has not been managed by those working in mental health in over three centuries. I was told this by a retired professor of psychiatry recently. My own experience is further testimony to the marginalization of those with lived and recovery experiences of mental illnesses.

In November 2010, I recovered from bipolar disorder that I was diagnosed with, due to a psychotic breakdown in November 1992. Recovery from any serious illness, though a personal accomplishment carries in it the seeds of social change, for that experience contributes to society's knowledge potentially. Society and individuals interact with one another alchemically, both transform one another. Just like the first man scaling Mount Everest was a significant event personally, it was also a great social achievement. Every triumph is as much a social as a personal victory. Whether we can cast recovery from debilitating illness as meriting social recognition is what society needs to consider. If there were a psychiatrist who could say that his patients recovered from schizophrenia or bipolar disorder, how would society construe him? The question is *whether one person's knowledge of recovery contributes to social good*. How should society utilize this knowledge? Does society owe any support to such a person, or does the person need to be satisfied about their victory as a personal triumph and start living life, post recovery, as though nothing ever happened?

In these past few years I interacted with a number of people who have recovered from serious mental illnesses and live just as 'normal' a life as anyone. In every story I found many a thing which furthers my knowledge. What a loss to society that though there are stories of recovery, their tellers are not more valued, acknowledged and made a reason for hope for others. We expend life, effort, time and resources in struggling to join the mainstream, to make ends meet, often despairing about the insignificance of our recoveries; knowing well what we can contribute to the social, in a respectable way. Is it stigma alone that makes someone prefer to remain quiet about a past of mental illness, or choose to deal with it as invisibly as possible? Or is it a deliberation by society as a whole to not consider voices of recovery as anything meaningful because they do not add to any further drama in the name of mental illness? They hold the potential to wean hordes of people away from medical interventions towards their social milieus for solutions, and ask the governments for better life, education and healthcare for everyone.

I currently work on two sides of mental health—preventive and recovery-oriented, via dialogues of a collaborative nature.[1] It is my conviction that a significant site of prevention of future mental breakdowns could be the schools. Since 2010, it has been my endeavour, as an emancipatory-researcher,[2] to promote mental health in my own neighbourhood[3] through a non-profit organization which I started. This organization has no regular funds, no infrastructure (except my home from where I operate). There is no other staff, just myself for the present. As a one-person organization I end up splitting myself between managing home, writing research, music (which has three sides to it—my own practice, teaching and learning) and managing the NGO.[4] In this chapter, I share my experience of trying to take my work forward and the challenges I encounter in the process. My experiences may provide some insights into how mental health is construed in urban India and the challenges it poses for a recent mental health worker who brings fresh (and possibly radical) perspectives into the field.

[1]It has its moorings in social construction, so the word collaborative and essentially it is a new method of counselling that I am working on.

[2]This is my preferred usage, over the phrase survivor researcher, for I consider myself emancipated from the linguistic dominance of psychiatric classification, which made me believe that I was a bipolar in disorder for two decades of my life.

[3]At the time of writing this paper, I was located in the north Indian state of Haryana, which is adjacent to the capital of New Delhi. I lived there from October 2007 to March 2014. The incidents I reported here were some of my interactions which happened both in New Delhi and Haryana.

[4]I am a performing artist as well.

The Narrative as Autoethnography

I narrate my experiences mostly through the form of autoethnography, due to its orientation towards self representation, in the task of representing a phenomenon. 'In autoethnographic inquiry, insights into the culture of interest are provided by the first-hand experiences of a cultural participant…In terms of underlying epistemology, this shift represent a major divergence from traditional empiricism, and indeed, all the above forms of qualitative inquiry. All these traditions make a clear separation between the observer and the observed, subject and object' (Gergen 2014a, b, p. 53). Autoethnography is about giving voice to one's own experience, to scrutinize it closely and to look at a culture through the lens of one person's experience. I have repeatedly tried to portray my experiences of mental illness related scenarios via first person narration. I am an 'insider', unlike a majority of researchers in mental health—having been on both sides of the fence, for years. This approach helps me as researcher to comprehend social reality through analysis of personal narratives. In this mode of analysis, the researcher's self is the subject matter of inquiry. McIlveen (2008) affirms that the defining feature of autoethnography is that it entails the scientist or practitioner performing narrative analysis pertaining to himself or herself as intimately related to a particular phenomenon. Autoethnography entails writing about oneself as a researcher practitioner, but it is not the same as autobiography in the literary sense. It is not simply the telling of a life, not that doing such would be simple. It is a specific term of critical enquiry that is embedded in theory and practice.

I repeatedly return to this narration in which I appear as actor, because via their retelling, I want to draw attention to the phenomenon, not necessarily my role in it. In the current representation, I cast a light on what scenarios anyone could be facing, if they were struggling to make a life of 'normalcy', post recovery from a stigmatizing mental illness. By sharing a common story of marginalization of ex-users or survivors of the psychiatric system, who need to be in the forefront of a mental health system as its heroes, I hope to not only shed light on our efforts, but also to invite a consideration of re-casting our roles, as a potential actors in the recovery of scores of others. It is the potential of contributing to a new future (Gergen calls it 'future forming orientation') that energizes my spirits every time I waver. Uotinen (2011) identifies autoethnography as a research method in which the researcher's personal experiences form both the starting point and the central material of study (p. 1308). It is through personal experiences I represent the cultural contexts of illness, recovery, and why the future of mental health would remain bleak, if newer forms of knowledge are not integrated into existing ones.

Dalal (personal communication, 28 May 2013) elaborates that 'autoethnography is a powerful research tool to understand culture, relationships and social structures. It helps us in peeling different layers of our personal life to understand the complex cultural web which defines what we are and explains our thinking and actions. In this sense it is different from autobiographical and diary research, where the main focus is to understand the person, as an embodiment of an ethnic group.' Social commentary and research are increasingly pointing to the narrative quality of lives, showing how the storying of the self is actively rendered and locally conditioned (Holstein and Gubrium 2000, p. 103). Commensurate with the ability of the researcher to comprehend the systemic nature of experience, autoethnography allows for its expression at a personal level, which mirrors a larger social reality. The purpose of this mirroring however, is to contribute towards a transformation of that social reality and not merely measure it.

This research is an autoethnographic inquiry of four personal narratives. These four encounters took place in the course of my engagement with mental illness, one way or another. Ellis says that 'with its emphasis on self-understanding, examining lives one at a time, and encouraging voice by person by person, autoethnography is a useful way-in addition to traditional social science analyses—to understand the world we live in; autoethnography is a constructive approach-in addition to changing laws or other macro-political structures—for changing and improving that world' (2009, p. 229).

My Feet in the World

By 'feet in the world' I refer to that identity in the public eye that we get defined by, and which consolidates my recovery via rehabilitation in occupational, social, financial and other areas of my life. In my 18 years of illness-recovery, the search for identity has been a difficult journey and I have variously searched for the defining moments which would be able to fix my identity, even for myself. Having successfully shed the skin of a bipolar identity behind, I have begun to feel a semblance of 'normalcy' and look forward to a productive-creative life.

In April 2010, with the support of family and friends, I founded a non-profit organization to work in the area of health and education, through the visual and performing arts.[5] I thought this is a neglected domain which has many long-term educational, spiritual and artistic implications for enhancing well-being of people. Though I had recovered from a difficult and debilitating condition, the likelihood of many recovering from the similar circumstances is limited. Not because the options available are limited; they are simply not visible. I was fortunate that I could access options, which I then utilized to my own advantage to re-train the mind in myriad ways. It is now a part of my endeavours to offer those insights and training to others who suffer from similar problems to improve their chances of recovery.

One attitudinal barrier that I frequently encounter is the perception of the former 'mentally ill'. It is difficult even for the most educated, to shed their prejudices about a label of mental illness. There are few who may be called 'survivors' of psychiatric treatment, fewer in India. Most of these 'user-survivors' are also activists in one or another form; largely as self-advocates. With many psychiatric

[5]I could not sustain myself and the non-profit for long, winding it off by 2017.

treatment is also an issue of human rights' violations; an issue of how society 'treats' its mentally ill, or who gets to be labelled as such. The dominant voices one gets to hear in the context of mental health, however, are those of psychiatrists and clinicians. There are practically no scholars/researchers in the field, who have also experienced serious, long-term mental illness and face the challenges of recovery and rehabilitation. Such a population nearly missing makes a person like me suspect in the eyes of a majority, who are not clear in what category to slot me.

What (New) Ideas Do I Bring to Mental Health

My idea is that if the visual and performing arts be made central to education, the process of education will stop being onerous for students and have an element of joy. Joy is what is conspicuous by its absence in the education system in India. If children are given an environment of fun and exploration they can learn a lot on their own, without getting stressed out. I also believe that maximum stress (therefore outcomes of mental illness, crime, violence, behavioural problems, substance abuse) comes from our school system. Schools are only an extension of a larger social reality, and a space where all social beliefs are further played out and reinforced, including notions of gender, patriarchy, social class, body image, caste equations, religious identities and more.

Instead of making learning so burdensome what can we modify in the school system to make it more fun, engaging and lively? With this in mind, I decided to meet someone in the government of India in the relevant ministry, hoping they would be able to see what I am referring to. I took an appointment, which came through with much calling and coordination and met the concerned person—someone of a senior rank, who is seen as a great supporter of the 'cause' of the mentally ill.

Before I met him I also shared with him, over the email my own story[6] of recovery from mental illness. Upon meeting me he was courteous, like any top bureaucrat but more than that he *also* saw in me another random person who had recovered from mental illness, instead of seeing me as someone who had some insights to offer about the subject. I cannot hold him responsible for his perception, for how is someone to ascertain anything about the former mentally ill? What would he have been thinking about me when I went to meet him? Could he ever have imagined that I was thinking of the Indian education system? I am quite certain, neither is anyone else. But the truth of my life is that that is where my whole heart lies—in preventive mental health—for I see a whole society spiralling into a tornado of emotional suffering due to something that could have been rectified at an early stage, within the schools.

---

[6]This was published in a Journal of Psychology. https://doi.org/10.1007/s12646-011-0126-6.

Sadly, instead of asking me why I had gone to meet him or inquire about the manner of my recovery, our dialogue turned out to be something entirely different. That gave me the idea about the value of lived experience to society as a whole. Over the years, that experience only got repeated from university-based academics to psychiatrists, students, parents of the current mentally ill to anyone. No doubt, bureaucrats would not have the time for individuals, but just a few months ago one of his junior officers had very pointedly warmed up to me after hearing me on a public platform and told me that now they had adequate funds and maybe I ought to come up with something worthwhile.

Mr. K: *I have read your paper and it is well written*
Me: *Thank you Mr. K*
Mr. K: *So what does your NGO focus on?*
Me: *We are looking at education and also how those with mental illnesses can be helped. I am just wondering if we can do a pilot project with some support which can show how mental health can be positively enhanced within the system of education.*
I do not think he even heard what I was saying. I felt like an idiot, with him attending to so many files that he was signing, the phone calls our brief interview was spattered with and the imminent appointments which his secretary had reminded him of.
Mr. K: *Oh I see. We do not work with NGOs by-the-bye. And in any case as far as the mental health issue is concerned we hope to reach its outcomes to the general public through the NRHM (National Rural Health Mission). And, whatever we have to do within the school system is to be done through the Sarva Shiksha Abhiyaan.*[7]
I looked at him and thought, 'This after all is the government. What would they know about the reality on the ground? Am I supposed to inform him of it? I am sure they have their own mechanisms to find out? Why would he believe me because I am someone who is only supposed to know about mental illness!'
I was disappointed. I know the government has no plan in place to prevent mental illness among school children, even though everyone knows that the age of onset of mental illness is 13–14, which is the schoolgoing age. So allocating funds for prevention and not knowing how to use the resources would not help anyone. I had hoped that by talking to me, not only as a recovered person but also as an artist I would be able to offer him insights in this direction, which stem from my own studies for the last several years. But I realized that government officers have no time for taking ideas that are coming unsolicited.

[7]A government scheme for universal primary education in India. Though it is undoubtedly the biggest mechanism to reach the benefits of education to the last child in the country, it has somewhat questionable outcomes that I am aware of, as I have had occasions to interact with their resource personnel on many a platform, including in advocating to them about art education.

Meta-autoethnography: The Devil's Advocate

I sent this paper to a friend for feedback and comments before submission for publication. He commented that the position taken by the government official as far as I was concerned was nothing wrong, if I were to see from his point of view. It made me also turn around and put myself in his shoes.

'For what,' said my friend, 'did he have as proof of you being capable of anything that he could look at you for?'

For a moment I could not but agree with this position, for what proof did I have that my recovery creates a pathway for others to follow or that I have any tangible insight to offer on the matter? In fact, most people who have recovered often ascribe a good bit of their recovery to their 'luck' and 'destiny'. I refuse to be so fatalistic so I got down to thinking of other ways to approach this dilemma.

However, my dilemma is two-fold. In addition to the fact that I have recovered personally and therefore know what pathway I took, I took nearly two decades to get here. In a way I sometimes count this time as 'lost time' because what I could have accomplished in these years I have nothing to show to them. One of the important things that I could not accomplish was how to create networks that would support my work either in music or in mental health. In the absence of both the challenge of daily living is still quite burdensome, fraught with a lot of work in a number of directions. Needless to say, remaining confined within domestic walls has reduced my stamina to work outside the home considerably.

I think it is not possible for any bureaucrat to look at any one person in any manner, except for a nuisance, if I relook the scene from his position. There are a number of people in India who have recovered from serious mental illnesses, who could become a resource for society is not something that they can easily think of. It also has the additional benefit of giving them employment and consolidate their recoveries further.

It was my hope that my story may be seen in a more universal manner, but now I feel that that cannot be accomplished by writing just one narrative of it. That brought me to the next level of research.

I paid five hundred for the taxi I had taken to make one side of this trip-an amount dear to me then. I was disappointed that people in positions of authority do not respond to new ideas, the manner I had hoped. In other words, they only understand that people have to become mentally ill and we need to provide medical care for them. Few are thinking of preventing mental illness in the first place-for the social origins of mental illness is not a reality for them, who attribute it to a biological basis.

As part of this struggle I have repeatedly tried to get a toe-hold in institutions of higher education, including in teacher training departments in several universities.[8] Till now no scope has emerged, nor willpower exercised to make that work tangible. The bigger problem is not that anyone thinks I lack in knowledge on the subject; everyone agrees it is valuable enough but how to 'pay' for my services. As someone who is an independent researcher, I cannot work for free, or for just my boarding and lodging paid for a few days of training. The unorganized nature of my work, on the margins of society, trying to find solutions for societal problems, is extremely taxing even for me.

How 'Open' Are Our Learning Environments

After this interview though I was extremely disappointed, I realized that in a more solution-focused country they would welcome people, even if they came from a completely different position. In our's the government is only looking at the implementation of programmes—there is no way anyone wants to understand the problem itself. For where is the time? Who has the resources? Who has the imagination to look at the problem in a systemic manner, when it is so much easier to reduce it to people's biological proclivities? What if they did, then also they would have to think of the mammoth scale of their implementation. So we end up cyclically creating huge structures, not to investigate their flaws in the initial stages to see how they effectively solve a problem and simply scale up the efforts, based on small successes, measured in questionable ways.

Chronologically the next thing to happen was my attempt at getting that 'label' for myself, so in future someday if I spoke with the authority of a Ph.D., perhaps people would pay more heed to my insights. The paper I had written had introduced me to the notion to social construction of mental health and I thought a more comprehensive inquiry was called for. I took about eight to ten months to study and prepare a research proposal for admission in a doctoral programme in an 'open' university in India.

In the course of writing this proposal I was unsure what department I could apply in. I explored a few possibilities which would permit an interdisciplinary inquiry in recovery from mental illness. But first I called the phone number given on their website of a department of disability studies (a label I had not accepted for myself till that day).

[8]In this effort several senior and retired academics have also assisted me to gain access in those departments imparting B.Ed. degrees. However, given their retired status they have not had the capacity to go beyond introducing me to the concerned people; who have frequently expressed great interest in the many sides of my work but never really got down to creating any access to their students.

Ring, Ring
Man's voice on the other end: *Who would you like to speak with?*
Me: *Can I talk to someone to discuss my Ph.D. study?*
Voice: *This is the disability department. Are you someone with a disability?*
Me: *Hmm…I think so. I have lived and recovered from mental illness.* (I feel ashamed to admit this to a stranger on the phone)
Voice: *Madam, are you visually challenged, hearing impaired or something like that or no?*
Me: *Well…no.*
Voice: *Look Madam, we have a certain mandate about who we recognize as disabled. And according to that classification you do not qualify for this category.*
Me: (horrified) *Look sir, I do not know what to say. Perhaps you do not understand. I am someone who has seen long-term disability…how can we decide that it is disability or not?*
Voice: *Perhaps you are not getting my point. May be you are quite right about what you are saying. All that I am saying is that our department does* ***not*** *recognize mental illness as a disability. Why do you not apply in the Medical Sciences department?*
Me: (crestfallen and reality beginning to dawn upon me) *No I cannot apply there because I want this to be a social science research and not medical view. Anyways I thank you.*

I put the phone down and called up another professor in the same university who I was hoping would agree to be a co-supervisor for my doctoral research. I had already decided about my main supervisor, a professor of Psychology from another university with whom I had developed my doctoral research proposal. Being an eminent scholar I knew I would not be lacking in guidance for research, as long as there was a department in which I was registered as a candidate. It was his suggestion to contact this university for my kind of interdisciplinary study.

Just a week before the submission of the proposal, I looked up their admission pre-requisites and figured out that I was falling short of one requirement. I had to have cleared my Master's exams with 55% marks, I had 52.4% The remaining criteria for getting a Ph.D. degree (at the time of degree being granted) included one publication in a peer—reviewed journal (I had at least three even at the stage of applying for Ph.D.) and I had to be a professional in another line of work to qualify on a certain track for admission (I was a musician, with CDs and newspaper cuttings from the press and records of qualifying radio auditions). I had done my Master's exams while in full blown 'mania' and that was 16 years before I applied for this course of study. I decided to meet the research head of the university as he may be able to resolve my dilemma. With great difficulty I got an appointment to meet him. I reached well before the appointed hour only to be told that he would be coming late that day. Since I had gone a far distance I had no option but to wait, as another visit of that sort would be difficult to plan. In the meanwhile I met the deputy research head, a genial lady who was very enthused by my research idea and proposal. She took it upon herself to introduce me to the Head. I waited for two and a half hours, before I was finally ushered into his presence.

He briefly heard me out and then casually said, '*I suggest you do this work in the social sciences department instead of inter-disciplinary studies.*'

My work was not one social science, it was an amalgam of music, mental health, sociology, psychology and therefore an interdisciplinary path was the most befitting for me.

This professor just looked at my thesis proposal, in his hand, the ten months of effort I had put into it and summarily told me, '*You should not worry about admission. We will get you in on a discretionary basis. The Vice Chancellor can give you a waiver on extraordinary grounds, because your case merits that.*'

My heart heaved a sigh of relief. It was not as if I was an unworthy candidate who was getting something she did not deserve, but a hard-fought battle seemed won.

I expressed my gratitude to him.

'*Look admission for you is a foregone conclusion. You should simply start your study and come back for admission six months later.*'

My heart sank. I had already spent close to a year preparing this research proposal. Starting the Ph.D. process another six months later meant he was postponing my entry by a whole year. I asked him why.

'*I think you should be in the psychology department and I do not think they are taking students this semester*,' he said.

Experience shows me how often people in positions of authority behave in seemingly autocratic ways in their approach towards those lower in the hierarchy. If a senior academic decides about the candidature of an applicant, it is unlikely the applicant stands any chance of entry into the institution.[9] A student or a potential student is someone who deserves the least amount of compassion in their minds. I was unsure how to interpret it. I looked at that man who was trying to assure me that I ought to begin my study in any case and come back for the formalities of admission six months later.

'*Meanwhile, you come back to meet me next week and let me introduce you to someone in the psychology department.*'

I felt confused with this whole turn of events but there was no scope for bargaining. I quietly came back, still hopeful that he had in any case told me to go ahead with my study, so it was only a matter of time before the doors of the university would open and let me in.

I decided to wait a while and see how things shape up. Just before starting my study actually, the week after meeting him, I tried to call him up and meet him to

[9]I have encountered this once long back at the time of my admission to college, when a clerk held back my admission just because I came a year late to apply, though I was within the qualifying cut-off of marks. Eventually after much deliberation, representation and cajoling though I got admission to the college, it made my entry experience a painful one, whose blemishes lasted for long and perhaps somewhere laid the foundation of my painful years in college that culminated in my 'breakdown'.

get a better grip on reality. He did not respond to my phone calls, nor replied to any email. I was perplexed. I had his mobile number, but I did not think it proper to call. He never responded and my dream of doing a Ph.D. got thwarted.[10] In any case, I resolved to go ahead with my research, even if it does not lead to a phd. I also tried to comfort myself in the words of another senior academic, who cautioned me against entering the university system, for it would demoralize me. Later I thought about the wisdom of his suggestion, for was I really up to dealing with this sort of rudeness after having come such a long way in my life? Did I really want to be re-visited by my anxieties and depressions that I had put behind me in my long years of struggle? If we are so closed in our approach to research why do we have 'open' universities? What are they really 'open' about?

So while waiting for those six months to pass, I started another research study about others with mental illness to examine its genesis and recovery, to examine the possibility of any patterns, if at all. All the groundwork had already been laid in the course of my study for the Ph.D. proposal.[11]

Watching a Social Construction

As part of my research I veered into social constructionism many years ago. Imbibing from it the post-modernist position of plurality of views, I habitually examine every phenomenon from multiple positions. In every 'abnormal' behaviour I am accustomed to examining the archaeology of the individual consciousness, trying to trace the roots of the visible behaviours. So when I met Janaki[12] I was open to all possibilities. A common connection had introduced her who referred to me as 'someone working in mental health'. Janaki was looking for ways to return back to some 'normalcy' from her sudden, catastrophic entry into the realms of the 'mentally ill'.

When she called me on the phone she sounded as though perfectly fine, with lively, alert voice. She also sounded very excited at the prospect of meeting me and hearing her enthusiasm I felt she could easily help me with some of the research, as I had no assistance.

She arrived with flowers in her hand! Big, white chrysanthemums—must be the first of the season. I was very touched to see that. I sensed she was keeping up appearances, for how 'unwell' she was I could only estimate upon meeting her. Having known the effects of psychiatric medication myself for close to two decades,

---

[10]Several months later another professor of English approached him to discuss my case, without knowing of this dialogue; and he was still adamant. She tried to think of many options but none seemed to work, because the whole issue came to what department I would fit into. I was doubly marginalized this way—marginalized once due to my illness and second time due to not being able to claim that I had been ill!

[11]I entered into Ph.D. research in July 2016, with a wholly different proposal and idea.

[12]Names have been changed to protect individuals concerned.

I could see her sedative stupor. She was pushing herself, but visibly unwell. In the course of my dialogue with her she frequently wept. I was unsure what to do. I knew she was ill, but I was helpless too, and could not do anything at the moment. She needed the work and had come to meet me in the hope that I could absorb her in my work, as an occupational mechanism for rehabilitation. Possibly she had many skills, but not related to research. I was not doing any work where she would be able to help. Having known the significance of work for reintegrating back into my own life, I understand its importance for others. McReynolds (2002) confirms that 'employment can serve as a normalizing factor since individuals who are unemployed and lack alternative societal roles are often stigmatized'. Janaki had come with a hope that as a survivor of a bi-polar disorder I will be able to steer her recovery as well, while she worked with me. While I was still struggling to get a firm foothold to make ends meet, how much could I offer in terms of help? I was unsure and not inclined to making false promises.

We kept in touch and I came up with an idea. In that month, I had journal access from a major publisher for a whole month, to download any number of articles from several of their published journals, for free. I had an idea of the quantum of time this would entail. So I thought it would be a good idea to engage Janaki for a few days and let her do the article downloading work. I could pay her for this work. I made her the offer and she readily agreed. Now the problem was that she did not have a computer with a high speed internet connectivity in her home. In that case, she would have to come to my home/office to do the work. I stayed in the suburbs to where travel was not easy. Would she be in a position to come and stay with me a few days and do this work? She said she would ask her mother. If she could then I would have to buy another computer because I could not stop my work, yet I had a little money in our non-profit kitty, which I could spend discretionarily.

When she agreed to come, I bought a second computer and got it going. On the day she was to come, her mother came with her, with another of her own colleagues. Meeting her mother was another view of her reality for me. She was a very simple, stocky, strong-built woman, who looked like a strong, working class person, and unlike her English-speaking urbane daughter was a plain vernacular-speaking lady, with no frills about her. Her difficult life was writ all over her and for a fraction I saw my mother in her, for her suffering due to her daughter's suffering was so much like my mother's, when I had been ill. I knew she had educated her girl with great effort, and made her come to a stage intellectually, socially and professionally which would be unacceptable to the segment they came from. Her milieu would not accept this girl of a single mother become a successful artist,[13] smoke, drink or wear clothes provocatively[14] and let her live in peace.

[13]She was in a master's course in art, from which she had to drop out just before completion of the course, due to a suicide attempt which had followed after an experiment with drugs and other substances.

[14]Which she came dressed in, a contrast to her mother and her office colleague. Perhaps if she had been with youngsters her own age it would not have been so visible even to me—but with the older people it stood out in bold contrast.

The mother and her colleague met me, made sure that they were leaving their child with someone trustworthy and assured themselves that it was well. I also assured them that I too had suffered, like Janaki and she may also recover, but it would take time. Her mother was frantic for recovery, willing to do anything for it. Naturally meeting me offered her a new hope which they had not had earlier—I suggested that they look for an alternative system of healing, as it seemed that Janaki was not doing well with the current medication.

Janaki came over to my house[15] for four days.[16] Looking at her and her functional communication, I thought she may be able to do the downloading work I had planned, while staying with me would give her a little change from her home environment. Due to her mother's job they had a one-room accommodation given to them, with food and other expenses paid for in a working women's hostel. In other words, they did not have to cook their food, maintain a kitchen or do anything to make a home operational. When I heard this I felt concerned, because such a scenario would never give any skills to a person to manage their own home.[17] What options did such a life leave her with to either lie in her room, or read, or watch TV, or go out and mingle with her own friends? Her social interactions, apart from her friends, were understandably an outcome of her mother's, because from the time she was one year old her mother stayed with her own brother's family.

Within an hour or two of her coming into my home, I realized I had made a mistake. The girl was in a stupor, what psychiatry would classify as 'hypomania'.[18] There was no question of her doing anything—she was like a little child constantly seeking attention. I appraised myself with the new reality, figured that no help was to be expected from her. If at all any it would be to let me work peacefully, which was not possible given how distracted she was and how she kept on drawing me into her conversations.[19] I told her she need not worry about any work but take it as

---

[15]I live alone with four dogs for the last several years. My sister lives a few houses away from mine and my parents live in Delhi. For all practical purposes I am a single person.

[16]At the time Janaki came another elderly friend of mine was staying at my house for the whole month and the guest room was occupied. So I requested my sister to allow her to stay in her house, while she would work in my house for the whole day, or whatever she would work.

[17]I consider these daily activities of running a home very significant for everyone—men and women, as they are activities which are required on a regular basis and one must be able to manage one's basic life issues before we become capable to accepting employments where we have to report to another person regularly. Management of day-to-day potentially stressful situations can be therapeutic and non-threatening especially within safe domestic spaces. Needless to say we also acquire many management skills along the way, as also a certain element of discipline.

[18]My own manic states have been very acute, so I can make out the difference between acute and less acute states.

[19]For the first time I felt as though the tables had been turned on me—for after two decades, I stood in the company of someone who was 'hypomanic', whereas I would have been the one experiencing it all these years. Strangely enough seeing her then, I just knew exactly how she would be feeling inside and I also suddenly knew how my family would have felt all those years when they saw me in similar or worse states. And though I knew what exactly could be done to engage her, did I have the time, the resources and the people around me who could assist me?

a little vacation and enjoy herself in my home and make herself comfortable and do what she could, but just let me study! There was no point in sending her back right now, as I would have to go and drop her and she had come mentally prepared to spend that much time. I let it be. But I told her clearly that since she would not be doing any work, she should not expect any payment for coming, which she tried to hit at me about by saying, 'Oh so you wanted to make me work for free'!

So she stayed and went back after three days, as a mishap with my sister[20] hastened her early exit. This was perhaps a mistake—for instead of heading back home, she went to meet some male friends of her's. I was troubled and faced a strange predicament. In my earlier dialogues with her she had shared with me about her sexual experiments with unknown strangers in Delhi, including going into a hotel with a hippie who vanished thereafter. I froze at the prospect of what could be happening. I called her mother up and she was equally worried then. With great difficulty she somehow reached back at after nine in the evening, having left my home at three in the afternoon, a distance she ought to have covered in three hours maximum.

It was clear that it was next to impossible for her mother to look after this girl. Knowing her current state Janaki would be putting herself through physical risk now and emotional damage later. I was concerned that when she 'wakes up' she would not be able to forget these traumae, because knowing her she just wanted to get married, 'settle down'. I felt that somehow the social milieu around her would not let her recover.

Somehow she made a switch over to homeopathy, but every form of medication requires other support mechanisms. I offered my counsel (for free). But her mother was concerned that I should give her employment. I told her that there was nothing she could do with me—I was not earning any money as part of my non-profit yet. The only money, whatever little I make is due to music teaching or concerts now and then. At this her mother snapped her communication with me.

From this I learnt that people sometimes think that others can help them at any cost, just because they understand the problem. What they do not realize is that they are themselves contributing to the pathological behaviour of their loved ones' 'illnesses'. Holding an outsider responsible for recovery, rehabilitation or anything else is not a mature way to deal with a mental illness. Ultimately, whoever recovers does so not because of an outsider, but due to developing an ability to determine and identify their support systems or newer pathways appropriately.

[20]My sister has also seen me for a long time in very acute psychotic states, so as an outsider she was good judge of telling me how well Janaki was faring. From her observations I knew that the girl was indeed very excitable, disturbed, scattered and dissipated. But my sister also pointed out to me that she had seen me in *worse states* than that.

Spreading the Net in the Community

Though I physically stayed in Haryana, my contacts there were limited to those within my vicinity, as I moved there only about five years back. At that time I had not recovered myself and spent a lot of time in study, music and so on. My decision to stay here eventually proved to be therapeutic and it was not really a part of any design. Therefore the best option for me was to approach another organization on the ground, and request them to assist me so that I could spread the scope of my work further. At the recommendation of a journalist I approached a big international organization that has global networks and scores of volunteers in every part of the world, including Haryana. I was told by the journalist that the people in this organization were very supportive and they would help me in taking my message of mental health further.

When I met the local head of the organization it looked like a favourable meeting to me.

Mr. S: *Madam I think you must see the work we are doing here and we will be only too happy if you take over the work.*
Me: *I will be happy to see the work, but let me tell you I have a certain area that I can work in and I think in our town there is a great scope for my work. May be if we could partner one another, we will be able to create something good in this town.*
Mr. S: *Yes, yes, I find you a very positive person too and I am sure there is much that can happen if two well-intentioned organizations work together.*

He took me around to show what they were doing. There was a big building complex coming up and they were already working in de-addiction. Plans were afoot to work in populations of the mentally handicapped; create employment and training opportunities for them. I tried to explain to him that mental retardation is not the same as mental illness. They even offered me the scope to work within their own complex, but first we had to have an agreement about our terms and conditions. He told me to write a letter which delineated the scope of our collaboration, with a proposal for how to execute it.

Among the skills I lacked one was proposal writing. It made me scared and uneasy, because I did not know how to deal with figures and numbers, or how to impute value to my work. Being an artist sometimes one can earn a big sum of money for a concert, sometimes you just sing for free—I do not know how to transpose this on any other situation. So I took nearly two months to write that proposal, by nailing every single detail of our work, including that we would train their volunteers for counselling in different populations and then also supervise their work and make sure that more and more people become skilled to handle counselling.

Though I overcame a big obstacle of proposal writing with this and sent the proposal to him on 24 December 2012, I never heard from him again. When we tried calling he always said, 'he is putting up the file in front of his seniors' and that is still to happen. In more than seven months, the file never moved beyond his table!

Such ignorance and apathy towards mental health made me think whether it is not such people who are also responsible for the sort of society we live in. Haryana is a particularly feudal place, with the lowest male/female ratio, the highest rate of female infanticide, almost the greatest number of crimes against women and rampant caste-related violence, especially in matters of marriage. The elderly are also severely disadvantaged here and sexual abuse is common. It is a particularly hostile place for women as I have known, living alone and therefore it was my plan to address this menace at a deeper level.

Conclusion

There is no failure if we learn from them. I am richer for these failures, though no doubt discouraged about the mental health scenario, or how rehabilitation can occur for those who have lost a 'critical' time in their lives, when they had to acquire skills of various sorts, or whether what they have acquired in terms of experiential knowledge is just a waste.

In an ocean of suffering, I find it incongruous to take up life as a musician, unless it helps in reducing human suffering in a tangible manner. The suffering of millions of people due to mental illness conditions is not something I can forget in a hurry, having spent years in the same mire. Recovery of one is a pointer to many, and that is the pathway that I am trying to lay down and consolidate via my work in different directions. I believe mental illness is a sign of someone trying to overcome the contradictions they face, to become a more authentic, healed and whole person. For that they need to start by questioning the manner they conceive of themselves and claim ownership on their lives and narratives. The seeds of change lie within.

It is ideas that provide the bedrock of change and new ideas always face resistance. Universities or academia is not the only place from where social change occurs. Ideas change when people change the ways they look at themselves or alter the belief systems about what they deserve, their entitlements and how they should deal with what surrounds them. My ideas about me changed when I moved beyond the linguistic identification of my suffering as a bipolar in disorder, to becoming an independent researcher and musician.

Yet to a world that measures a person by their academic degrees, people like me make little sense. Due to research and long term engagement with mental illness, the ideas with which I work with the so-called 'mentally ill' cannot be found in any degree-oriented enterprise. They partially come from experiential knowledge. Experiential knowledge emancipates us from the dominance of university-based knowledge, setting us free to heal, recover and help in the healing of others. University-based knowledge can only give us a label of an illness, not really take it back to give our whole, healed selves back. Universities can give us degrees to validate the knowledge further, but can they really create more healed individuals?

Reasons for hope, whatever I have, come from meeting those who currently suffer, for when they meet me they feel hopeful about their recovery. Nobody shies of telling me their deepest secrets, because we understand one another so differently. This is equally true of those who suffer from mental illnesses and those who are not there clinically. There is candor and faith and that gives me hope to go on, to hold another hand, to offer a little insight or listen patiently, because in listening with belief we just let others unburden. The belief that their truth is believable gives them confidence for newer outcomes, and constructions.

At the time of writing this I am over 43, with no regular income, a past that is largely shrouded in the haze of depressive glooms of wasted years, not academic or professional laurels, a future where nothing is tangible. Despite this for years, I bury my head in non-funded research, carried out amidst great distraction, household responsibility and with my family chipping into pay my bills, someone paying my rent, someone my food bill and someone else for my books. I keep alive a hope that my work will be useful and many will know that recovery is a certainty, not chance that could happen to a few lucky ones, and no more. My ideas and I have lived and worked alone for months and years, writing, reading, researching, thinking newer ideas, listening to illness narratives and analysing, discussing, joining new dots, examining a picture from various positions, to find a way for another to recover. So though the road is rude, rough and there is no certainty where my next step would land, nor someone to point a way forward, this is the road which I have to traverse —the road of belief. The recovery of one person is not a chance, there is a method in it, which needs to be found. The method cannot be disseminated by another, who has not walked the road. I may not do this work for a university degree or acknowledgement, but the road which is 'friendless' for most parts, has brought many a new friend to me; not the friends with whom I can celebrate life, but friends who trust me to speak the truth and can appreciate it—a reward in itself. This drives my current 'madness'—the search for a unifying voice among those touted 'mentally ill'.

References

Ellis, C. (2009). *ReVision—Autoethnographic reflections of life and work.* CA: Left Coast Press.

Gergen, K. J. (2014a). Pursuing excellence in qualitative inquiry. *Qualitative Psychology, 1*(1), 49–60.

Gergen, K. J. (2014b). From mirroring to world-making: Research as future forming. *Journal for the Theory of Social Behaviour.* https://doi.org/10.1111/jtsb.12075.

Holstein, J. A., & Gubrium, J. F. (2000). *The self we live by—Narrative identity in a postmodern world.* New York: Oxford University Press.

McIlveen, P. (2008). Autoethnography as a method for reflexive research and practice in vocational psychology. *Australian Journal of Career Development, 17*(2), 13–20. Accessed in USQ ePrints http://eprints.usq.edu.au.

McReynolds, C. (2002). Psychiatric rehabilitation: The need for a specialized approach. *International Journal of Psychosocial Rehabilitation, 7,* 61–69.

Uotinen, J. (2011). Senses, bodily knowledge, and autoethnography: Unbeknown knowledge from an ICU experience. *Qualitative Health Research, 21*(10), 1307–1315.

Chapter 21
Gender and Mental Health: Masculinity, Femininity, Modernity and Daily Hassles as Predictors of Subjective Well-Being

Jayanti Basu, Matangini Samanta, Sipra Basu and Mahua Bhattacharya

Gender as a Context of Mental Health

Gender is an enigmatic domain of study. Considering the brilliant brains and bodies devoted to its scientific exploration for the last 150 years, there should have been little more to add. Yet gender posits a perpetual riddle in personal, social and moral domains. The ambivalence is apparent in the present controversies within the Indian legal system about gender role transgression.

In one sense, the traditional gender prescription was simpler: the genital was the fixed and indisputable point of reference for determining both sex and gender role of a person. Femaleness and femininity, maleness and masculinity, sex and gender were the one and the same thing (Deaux 1985; Hofstede 1980/2001). Gender role identity was deemed as a natural corollary of the characteristics of the body; role enactment was controlled by normative sex roles. Whether people actually adhered to this norm in private life is, of course, an altogether different story.

Historically, the roles ascribed to women have always been more stringent, atrocious, designed to make them more responsible, more committed, less valued, less paid, barred from knowledge associated with exposure to the outer world, and hence more exploited (Unger and Crawford 1992). The modern world's first organized movement for women is attributed to 32-year-old Elizabeth Cady Stanton at Seneca Falls in 1948. Within two decades, the feminist agenda spread in Europe and other countries, and international alliances were formed. After the 1960s, the dissociation of gender from sex was formulated (Stoller 1968/2000). Over the last 40 years, we have generally accepted that sex refers to the biological structures of

J. Basu (✉) · M. Samanta · M. Bhattacharya
Department of Applied Psychology, University of Calcutta, Kolkata, India
e-mail: basumjt@gmail.com

S. Basu
Kolkata, India

G. Misra (ed.), *Psychosocial Interventions for Health and Well-Being*,
https://doi.org/10.1007/978-81-322-3782-2_21

femaleness and maleness, and gender to the psychological, social and cultural connotations associated with sex (Deaux 1985; Vindhya 2010). Thus, gender has come to be acknowledged as a social construction, contexted and embedded in culture, and amenable to learning and unlearning (Kimmel 2000). This conceptualization separates maleness from masculinity, and femaleness from femininity. From this perspective, masculinity refers to the stereotypical masculine traits related to power and instrumentality; femininity represents stereotypical female traits like expressiveness and emotionality. Either may reside in any individual, male or female. However, even this sex–gender distinction had its own critiques from within feminism. For example, Judith Butler (1990) eschewed the very concept of gender fixity implied in sex–gender distinction and considered sex as 'embodied gender'—the corporeal incarnation of discursively constituted (performative) gender.

India has taken up the feminist agenda in her own way. Women's independence was initiated during British rule and under the-then patriarchal frame, liberation of women initially came through men like Rammohan Ray and Iswar Chandra Vidyasagar. By the end of the nineteenth century, a few enlightened women came forward to build women's organizations. Women's work outside home and voting rights came gradually. Women's participation in the freedom movement further facilitated their involvement with women's causes (Basu and Ray 2003; Kaur 1968). Afterwards, strengthened by gender equality declared in the constitution of independent India, there have been no dearth of theoretical writing and activism for women (Chaudhuri 2005; Vindhya 2007).

Yet, prosperity in research and activism did not put an end to the conundrum called 'gender'. As a social construction, gender is also a multi-component concept. Archer (1980) has observed two basic components of gender-related roles and stereotypes, namely, (1) Gender Role Identity, referring to what an individual considers oneself to be in terms of perceived masculinity and femininity, and (2) Gender Role Attitude or the dimension of modernity–traditionality referring to the belief as to what the members of a given sex should do.

The feminists of the 70 s operationalized the segregation of sex and gender in behavioural domain; a genitally male person may possess measurable degree of femininity in identity, or vice versa. Sandra Bem's (1974, 1981, 1984) work on masculinity and femininity, and Spence's (1978) research on instrumental versus expressive traits liberated the early researchers from the notion that masculinity and femininity are opposite dimensions; they were recognized to be orthogonal and coexisting with equal vigour in one person. Thus, the concept of androgyny was introduced. This encouraged an upsurge in research relating masculinity and femininity as components of identity to different behavioural aspects.

Following Bem's or Spence and Helmreich's concepts, a number of Indian studies have worked with the variables of femininity and masculinity in relation to specific behaviour domains (Basu and Chakroborti 1996; Dasgupta and Basu 2011; Mittal et al. 2010). Unfortunately, a considerable part of such works seem to be rather isolated attempts without any comprehensive plan to delve deeper into the concepts, and the reader ends up with little insight gained from them. Thus, integrated probe into masculinity and femininity, especially in relation to mental health is lacking.

Gender Role Attitude is the declared view about gender typical acts. This is not about what one is, but about the belief regarding what women and men should do. Earlier research has indicated that Gender Role Identity and Gender Role Attitude are not necessarily correlated (Datta et al. 1995); a person may express modern view of gender equality, yet refuse to accept characteristics stereotypically associated with the other sex in oneself.

Negative and Positive Indices of Mental Health with Special Reference to Subjective Well-Being (SWB)

Since 1981, World Health Organization's conceptualization of health entails wellness. Previously, illness and wellness were considered as two poles of a single dimension. In the last four decades, their partial independence has been established (Diener et al. 1997) with increasing research thrust. SWB deals with issues like happiness, life satisfaction and morale (Ryan and Deci 2001; Reichhardt 2006). In 1997, Diener et al. enumerated the cardinal characteristics of SWB. It covers the entire range of affective existence from agony to ecstasy, defined in terms of the individual's internal experience, and is a long-term state.

In the last few years, research on positive psychology and well-being has flourished in India in the backdrop of cultural and religious heritage (e.g., Kumar and Kumar 2013, Maheswari and Singh 2009) and economic and cultural change (Biswas-Diener et al. 2013). The elusive concept of wellness has been studied and refined (Mehrotra et al. 2013). Variables like Subjective Well-being (SWB), happiness and hope have been scrutinized by different groups of participants including teachers (Sharma 2011), students (Pareek and Jain 2012), special educators (Sudha and Shahnawaz 2013), professional groups (Sahoo and Mahapatra 2009), under-trial prisoners (Khurana 1996). Factors of wellness have been studied in sociocultural and economic contexts in both urban and rural India (Agrawal et al. 2011; Kiran Kumar 2003; Linssen et al. 2011). However, while sex difference in wellness has been studied extensively, gender stereotype in connection with wellness in India has remained under-explored (Mukhopadhyay et al. 2007).

Sex Difference in Mental Health in Relation to Stress, Daily Hassles and Gender Role Stereotype

Gender balance in prevalence of mental disorders is long known to be asymmetric (Busfield 1996), women and men being vulnerable to different kinds of diseases. Certain disorders like depression, anxiety disorders, certain somatoform disorders and eating disorders are more notable, or at least diagnosed more frequently in women (Desjarlais et al. 1995; McIntyre and Hunt 1997; Russo 1990). Contrarily, addiction, alcoholism and antisocial personality disorders are prevalent among men all over the world (de Girolamo 2006; Russo 1990). Epidemiological studies conducted in various states of India including West Bengal (Duke 1970; Nandi et al. 2000; Venkataswamy Reddy and Chandrashekhar 1998) have consistently revealed that gender difference in prevalence of psychiatric disorders in India is similar to the West, although somatization is more common and eating disorder less prevalent in most communities (Isaac et al. 1996; Khandelwal et al. 1995).

Although salience of gender in mental health is applicable to men's health as well (Eisler et al. 1988), WHO, as early as in 2000 and 2004, had paid particular attention to the issue of women's mental health, as women worldwide are more deprived of health support. Literature further points out that while biological correlates of cognitive and emotional problems of women, like menstruation, child birth, lactation, menopause etc. are salient (Greendale et al. 2009), their negative impact on mental health is not so much due to the hormonal imbalance as much as to their personal, social and political implications (Lorber 1997; Sims 1994). Studies have consistently demonstrated that women's experiential universe is different from that of men; they are less exposed to external injury and trauma (Sabo and Gordon 1993) and more exposed to chronic and daily hassles and negative life events (Malik et al. 1992; Nolen-Hoeksema, et al. 1999). Thus, psychosocial stressors and gender role conjointly assume singular significance in mental distress and wellness of women.

Womanhood in India is not a unitary construct. Depending on the urban–rural, working–non-working, organized–unorganized sectors, not to say about marital and fertility status, caste, class and religious categories, there are innumerable socio-cultural and socio-political discriminations causing stressors and affecting mental health of Indian women. The pervasive concern with HIV-AIDs had added health and stigma-related dimensions to women's distress. Studies also imply distinctive characteristics of organized, unorganized and migrated sectors of women in workforce, initiating different dimensions of stress (Dave 2012; Mohanraj and Manivannan 2013). Researchers have demonstrated the impact of demographic status on mental health in low and middle-income countries of the world (Desjarlais et al. 1995; Patel 2007). Within India, specific issues relating socioeconomic and other demographic factors like tribalism to mental health have been discussed (Blue et al. 1995; Malhotra and Chhabra 1991; Trivedi et al. 2009). The size, depth and diversity of problems render any simple generalization problematic. However, one may safely conclude that women's health in response to societal discrimination is not necessarily a direct response to palpable torture; it is a symbolic interaction with the meaning of gendered experiences.

The exact operation of gender-related psychosocial characteristics in mental disorders have been investigated abroad by researchers for the last 30 years (Wichstrom 1999), and also in India (Suresh Kumar 1998; Vindhya 2001a), though consensus is still lacking. The generally identified factors held responsible for the greater burden of women are stress and hassles (Weissman et al. 1993), violence and abuse (Sugarman and Frankel 1996), sexist discrimination (Klonoff and Landrine 1997; Patel and Kleinman 2003), and finally, role conflict and multiple roles (Cleary and Mechanic 1983; Gove 1979). While detail discussion of such complexly interwoven sociocultural matrix of gender is beyond the scope of the present chapter, it remains important to acknowledge its contributory role for understanding and applying the research findings, especially in the context of traditional gender role stereotype vis-a-vis women empowerment. Advocacy, awareness building and intervention at the community level need to be the essential ingredients of women's wellness. Failing to appreciate such pragmatic aspects would result in lopsided planning and policy.

In psychological and psychiatric literature, stress contributing to negative mental health outcome have been conceptualized from two perspectives—major stressful life events over a time span, versus everyday minor hassles or negative occurrences (Mazure et al. 2000). Their modes of operation differ (Serido et al. 2004). Life event stressors signify irreversible stressful happenings like death of spouse, or failure in major examination. Daily hassles, on the contrary, are relatively minor events, like travelling by a crowded bus to office. It is recurrent in nature, often without provision for remission. Sometimes they may be perceived as more stressful than major events (Flett et al. 2006; McCullough et al. 2000). Studies have focused on the relation of hassles and positive indices of mental health. Kanner and Feldman (1991) studied the relationship of hassles and uplifts with adaptational outcomes. Robinson (2000) studied the role of daily life events in affective and cognitive components of well-being.

Gender role stereotype, as hegemonic expression of sociocultural polarization of the sexes, has been observed to strongly influence sex differences in mental health and illness. Women's and men's health-related behaviour and clustering of symptoms develop partially as a result of adherence to schematized stereotypes about self and other's gender-specific roles (Paykel 1994). Studies have focused on the processing of emotions in relation to gender role identity. It has been observed that femininity is associated with fear (Gallacher and Klieger 1995) and suppressed anger and assertion (Sawrie et al. 1991), particularly among women. Masculinity, in contrast, is associated with better processing of all emotions (Arrindell et al. 1993; Kopper and Epperson 1996). A section of the studies deal directly with disorders and deviations. Nathanson (1975) commented on the feminine role identity and illness behaviour. Neuroticism has been found to be associated with femininity among non-clinical samples (J. Basu et al. 1995; Krampen et al. 2006). Much of the available literature in this regard concentrates on explaining depression and eating disorders (Culbertson 1997). Systematic study of specific psychosocial determinants of these disorders pertaining to Indian culture is virtually non-existent.

In the above context, two studies were conducted to examine if Gender Role Identity and Gender Role Attitude, and Daily Hassles predict SWB in two different samples. The work was conducted in Kolkata, West Bengal.

Study I

Subjective Well-Being (SWB) of College Students

The specific objectives of Study 1 were to determine (1) whether SWB differs between the women and men college students and (2) which of the Gender Role Stereotype variables and Daily Hassle can successfully predict SWB of college students.

Method

Variables

The predicted variable of the study was **SWB** as a measure of one's quality of life. The predictor variables for the study were as follow:

(a) **Gender Role Variables including the following components**: (1) *Gender Role Identity* including Masculinity (M) and Femininity (F) and (2) *Gender Role Attitude* (GRA).
(b) **Daily Hassles** defined as the number of minor negative events as potential stressors occurring in the daily life of the subject during the last one month.

Among the other relevant variables, apart from the demographic parameters detailed later, major life events were controlled to isolate the role of Daily Hassle. A Life Events Scale was administered and those with more than five major life events in the past one year were excluded. Furthermore, the absence of psychiatric disorder was confirmed from information schedule and administering GHQ-28.

Participants

Participants were 200 women and 200 men Bengali Hindu unmarried college students, age between 19–22 years, residing in Kolkata for the last 10 years. They belonged to families with middle-income level, father being at least graduate, mother having passed at least school-leaving examination. Exclusion Criteria were: History of any acute or chronic physical or mental illness, history of any major break in family, for example, parental divorce or death before the age of 18, and more than five major life events in the last one year.

Students were selected through stratified sampling technique. Stratification was done in terms of sex of the students, locality of the colleges, broad academic streams (Science, Humanities and Commerce), and class (1st, 2nd or 3rd year). From a zone-wise list of colleges, 15 colleges from North, South, East, West and Central Kolkata were selected. The students were contacted through college authorities and Students' Unions. Those who volunteered were included as participants after screening. The men and women matched roughly on major demographic variables.

Measures

Apart from a detailed information schedule, the following measures were used for screening of the sample:

General Health Questionnaire (GHQ-28) by Goldberg and Hiller (1979) ***Adapted by Basu and Dasgupta*** (1996) HQ is a self-administered screening test aimed at detecting short-term changes in mental health in any individual above 12 years. The GHQ-28 containing 28 items was derived from factor analysis of GHQ-60. Each item has four response alternatives. Its sensitivity was found to be 0.8, and specificity 0.88. The GHQ-28 has been adapted in Bengali culture by Basu and Dasgupta (1996). Split-half reliability was 0.97 with sensitivity and specificity 1.00 and 0.88 respectively. Scoring for screening was done by GHQ method (0-0-1-1). Total score ranged from 0 to 28. Threshold for case identification was taken as 4/5, four signifying a non-psychiatric case and five indicating a psychiatric caseness.

Presumptive Stressful Life Events Scale (PSLES) by Singh et al. (1981) PSLES consists of 51 life events applicable to Indian adults. The participant indicates the life events occurring in last one year. The test–retest reliability of this scale at a gap of 1 month is 0.99. In the present study, those with more than five life events in the past year were excluded.

The predictor variables including the Masculinity, Femininity, Gender Role Attitude and Daily Hassles was assessed by the following measures:

Indian Gender Role Identity Scale B (IGRIS B) (Basu **et al.** 2012) ***to Assess Masculinity and Femininity*** The IGRIS has been developed roughly by following Sandra Bem's conceptualization of Masculinity and Femininity (Bem 1984), as well as by incorporating a number of modifications in response to numerous criticisms to Bem's work (Taylor and Hall 1982; McCreary 1990), especially related to evaluation of the desirability of gender typical traits (Basu 2010). A 30 item scale with 10 items each for assessing Masculinity, Femininity and Neutral traits and applicable for all age groups (IGRIS) was initially prepared as a short measure of Gender Role Identity. The scale had satisfactory construct and discriminant validity and high reliability. However, since GRI changes with age, three separate variants of IGRIS were also prepared for detailed evaluation of GRI among late adolescents, college students and general adults, known as IGRIS A, IGRIS B and IGRIS C respectively. All the variants had high construct and discriminant validity. The IGRIS A had 42 items, IGRIS B had 48 items, and IGRIS C had 54 items. In the present study, IGRIS B had been used for its salience with the college student sample. Reliability of the scale has been assessed by Split-half technique with Spearman-Brown correction, Cronbach's alpha and Test-retest after 1 month. For the M scale of IGRIS B, the respective reliability values were 0.88, 0.83 and 0.78, and for the F scale of IGRIS B, 0.77, 0.75 and 0.79.

Scanzoni's Sex Role Attitude Scale by Scanzoni (1975) ***Adapted by Rao and Rao*** (1983) This scale, developed by Scanzoni (1975) is a 20-item measure of attitude towards the gender role. The first 13 items assess the attitude towards wife role, the next five items assess the attitude towards mother role, and the last two items assess the attitude towards father/husband role. Respondents are asked to indicate their choice on a five-point scale. The total score ranges between 20 and 100. A lower score indicates traditional gender role emphasis, while a high score indicates modernity. Modernism is indicated by weaker concern with the traditional patriarchal ideology. Coefficients of internal consistency calculated by Cronbach's alpha were 0.74 for wife role, 0.68 for mother role and 0.62 for father role/husband role. The scale has been slightly revised by Rao and Rao (1983) for the Indian culture. Datta et al. (1995) adapted the scale in Bengali culture. The split-half reliability of the total scale in Datta et al.'s work was 0.79 and test-rest reliability was 0.75.

The Daily Hassles Scale of the Hassles and Uplifts Scale (Lazarus and Folkman 1989***) with Minor Cultural Modification*** The Hassles and Uplifts scale assesses everyday negative encounters called hassles, and positive encounters called uplifts within a time frame. It consists of three independent scales: The Daily Hassle Scale, the Uplifts Scale and the Combined Hassles and Uplifts scale. In the present study, only the Hassles scale was used with reference to the past one week. This scale consists of 117 items used to measure the frequency and severity of daily events that produce stress. The respondent responds on a four-point scale to indicate magnitude of hassle. Hassles frequency score was found to be stable over a period of nine months (0.79) and higher than the stability of the severity rating (0.48). Validity studies with outcome variables yielded correlations ranging between 0.30 and 0.65. Scoring can be done either by counting frequency or by severity rating. Here the frequency count technique was used.

An initial pilot study indicated that two items were not meaningful in the present group of participants for our culture: Auto maintenance (item 61) and Yardwork (item 112). After some preliminary trials, these two items were replaced with the following two: Maintenance of gadgets and household things (including gas booking, paying electricity bills etc.) and Problems with household helpers (maids, servants, drivers).

The criterion variable SWB was assessed with the following scale:

Subjective Well-Being Scale **(*Sell and Nagpal*** **1992)** The SWB Scale measures the feeling of well-being or ill being as experienced in various day-to-day life concerns. It consists of 40 items. Subjects respond on any of the three alternatives, namely, 'very much', 'to some extent' and 'not so much'. High score indicates greater wellness. The inventory measures 11 factorial dimensions, buta global score of wellness is also available from the scale and used in the present work. The reliability coefficient of the scale is 0.87.

Procedure for Data Collection and Scoring

A total of 452 data were collected in small group situations consisting of three–five students at a time at the college premises. The approximate time required for collection of each set of data was 1.5–2 h distributed over a period of two days. Incomplete and doubtful data were eliminated and finally 400 data were retained.

Analyses and Findings

- *Men enjoyed better SWB than women*. The means and standard deviations of the SWB scores for the women and men were 81.18 (8.00) and 83.80 (7.74) respectively. The mean difference was statistically significant as revealed from Independent samples t test, with $t(398) = 3.33$, $p = 0.000$.
- *Masculinity and Daily Hassles were the most significant contributors to SWB for both men and women students*. Step-wise Multiple Regression Analyses with Masculinity, Femininity, Gender Role Attitude and Daly Hassles as predictors of SWB revealed that Masculinity and Daily hassles were the most significant predictors for women ($R = 0.302$; Adj $R^2 = 0.082$; $F(1,\ 398) = 9.905$, $p < 0.01$), and for men ($R = 0.425$; Adj $R^2 = 0.173$; $F(1,\ 398) = 21.768$, $p < 0.01$). Gender Role Attitude and Femininity were not significantly associated with wellness.
- *The greater the Masculinity and less the Daily Hassles, better was the SWB of the individual*. The contribution of Masculinity was higher among men then in women (Beta coefficient being 0.236 for women and 0.405 for men). The impact of Daily Hassles was higher among women than among men (Beta coefficient being −0.183 for women and −0.133 for men).

Study II

Subjective Well-Being (SWB) of Young Adult Psychiatric Patients and Their Healthy Counterparts

The study examined whether the findings from the Study I, conducted with college students of healthy physical and mental disposition, could be generalized with young adult clinical sample and a comparable adult healthy sample. The specific objectives of the study were to determine (1) whether SWB differs between the women, (2) whether SWB differs between the clinical and healthy young adults, and (3) which of the Gender Role variables and Daily Hassle can successfully predict the SWB of college students.

Method

Variables

As in Study I the criterion variable was SWB and the predictor variables were Masculinity, Femininity, Gender Role Attitude and Daily Hassles. Apart from the demographic variables controlled in the selection of samples, those having more than 6 major life events in the last one year were excluded. For the clinical group, neuropsychological deficit, co-morbidity and medication were controlled.

Participants

Participants were 50 women and 50 men psychiatric patients and 50 women and 50 men comparable healthy Bengali adult individuals, from low and middle social class with age between 20 and 35 years. The female clinical group included 17 women suffering from depressive disorders (major depression and dysthymia), 18 suffering from anxiety disorders (generalised anxiety disorder and panic attack) and 15 suffering from somatoform disorder (somatisation disorder). The male patient group consisted of 16 men suffering from depressive disorders, 19 suffering from anxiety disorders and 15 suffering from somatoform disorder. The participants of the clinical group were contacted from various hospitals and clinics of Northern, Central and Southern districts of West Bengal. They were diagnosed through a double blind technique by one psychiatrist and one clinical psychologist as suffering from the specific Axis I disorders according to DSM IV-TR. After the patients were diagnosed by the hospital/clinic, they were also administered the Beck Depression Inventory and the State-Trait Anxiety Inventory for cross checking. Those with co-morbidity, underlying psychoticism or Axis II disorder as per DSM IV were excluded. They were assessed on the first day of their visit to the hospital and before they had started taking any psychiatric medicine.

The healthy group was selected from the visitors or accompanying persons to the hospital or clinic, or from general population. They were included only after being screened for freedom from any major physical or psychological disorder, and from any apparent neuropsychological deficit. They were free from pathological depression and anxiety as revealed from Beck Depression Inventory and the State-Trait Anxiety Inventory.

The women and men, and the clinical and healthy groups matched on the background variables.

Measures

For collecting significant demographical and medical history, a detailed information schedule was prepared to assess variables like demographic details, family pattern, social and financial positions. Besides, a brief Medical History Schedule was to be filled in by the participants. For the clinical group the same was filled by the family members accompanying the patient. Cases with uncertain and conflicting medical history were excluded.

For screening the participants for eligibility of inclusion the following measures were used:

Bender Gestalt Test II or BG II by Brannigan and Decker (2003) The Bender Gestalt test was originally developed by Bender (1938) as a short assessment of visual motor integration to provide information about neuropsychological functioning. The Bender Visual-Motor Gestalt Test, Second Edition (Bender-Gestalt II) has been developed by Brannigan and Decker (2003) offering a simpler global scoring procedure. The Bender-Gestalt II consists of 16 cards with a figure drawn on each of them. It has a copy and a recall phase. The validity of the test has been assessed against intelligence tests like Stanford Binet or WISC III.

General Health Questionnaire-28 or GHQ-28 by Goldberg and Hiller (1979) ***adapted in Bengali by Basu and Dasgupta*** (1996) It was ensured that the clinical groups had a GHQ score above 4 and the normal group had a score below 5.

Beck Depression Inventory or BDI by Beck **et al.** (1961)***, Adapted by S. Basu*** **et al.** (1995) BDI is a self-administering inventory to assess severity of depression. It consists of 21 items, each containing 4 or 5 statements ranked in order of severity. The respondents choose statements closest to their present mental state and assigned scores from 0 to 3. The total score ranges from 0 to 63. High score indicates greater depression. Applicability of BDI in Bengali population has been reported by J. Basu et al. (1995). For this version the split-half reliability is 0.81.

State Trait Anxiety Inventory by Spielberger and Vagg (1995) The State-Trait Anxiety Expression Inventory (STAI) was developed by Spielberger and Vagg (1995). Both the Trait Anxiety (A-Trait) and State-Anxiety (A-State) scales consist of 20 statements each. The A-trait scale measures anxious disposition by asking people to describe how they generally feel. The A-State requires subjects to indicate how they feel at a particular moment in time. In the present study, only A-Trait scale was used. Alpha co-efficient computed by Cronbach (1951) for the normative samples ranged from 0.83 to 0.92.

The predictor variables were assessed with the following tools:

Indian Gender Role Identity Scale C (IGRIS C) by Basu **et al.** (2012) This IGRISC is applicable to general adult population. This has 48 items with 16 items in each of the Masculinity, Femininity and Neutral scales. Reliability of the scale has been assessed by Split-half technique with Spearman-Brown correction, Cronbach's alpha and Test-retest after one month. For the M scale of IGRIS C, the respective reliability values were 0.86, 0.84 and 0.89, and for the F scale of IGRIS C, 0.79, 0.75 and 0.85.

Sex Role Attitude Scale by Scanzoni (1975) Same as in Study I.

Daily Hassles Scaleby Lazarus and Folkman (1989) Same as in Study I.

The criterion variable was SWB which was assessed through the **SWB Scale (Sell and Nagpal** 1992), as in Study 1.

Procedure

Data were collected either at the hospital or clinic, or at the office of the investigator. Each participant was administered the tests individually over three days distributed within a week.

Analyses and Findings

- *Analysis revealed no sex difference in well-being in this study, which differs from the findings of Study 1. However, the clinically ill group had less wellness than its matched healthy counterpart.* This was revealed from a 2 (gender) × 2 (groups) ANOVA examining whether the means of SWB differed significantly in terms of sex, clinical status and the interaction of sex and clinical status.

Levene's F tests for homogeneity of variances indicated satisfactory homogeneity. Effect of sex was not found to be significant: $M_{Male} = 66.56$, $SD_{Male} = 18.67$; $M_{Female} = 67.88$, $SD_{Female} = 19.37$; $F(1, 196) = 1.315$, $p = 0.253$. Effect of clinical status was found to be significant: $M_{Clinical} = 50.10$, $SD_{Clinical} = 7.32$; $M_{Healthy} = 84.34$, $SD_{Healthy} = 8.88$; $F(1, 196) = 885.019$, $p = 0.000$. The interaction effect also not significant, with $F(1, 196) = 0.639$, $p = 0.425$.

- *Masculinity was the only predictor of SWB in the clinical group, for both women and men.* Step-wise Multiple Regression Analyses with Masculinity, Femininity, Gender Role Attitude and Daily Hassles as predictor and SWB as predicted variable revealed Masculinity was the only significant predictor for women ($R = 0.311$; Adj $R^2 = 0.078$; $F(1, 98) = 5.148$, $p < 0.01$) and for men ($R = 0.450$; Adj $R^2 = 0.186$; $F(1, 98) = 12.178$, $p < 0.01$). Daily hassle, Gender role attitude, and Femininity were not significant predictors of wellness.
- *In the clinical group, greater the magnitude of Masculinity, greater was well-being.* The association of Masculinity with SWB was greater for men (Beta coefficient for women being 0.311, and for men 0.450).
- *As in Study I, in the healthy sample, Masculinity and Daily Hassle predicted SWB for both women and men.* Step-wise Multiple Regression Analyses with Masculinity, Femininity, Gender Role Attitude and Daly Hassles as predictor and SWB as predicted variable revealed that Masculinity and Daily Hassles were the most significant predictors for women ($R = 0.480$; Adj $R^2 = 0.197$; $F(1, 98) = 7.025$, $p < 0.01$) and for men ($R = 0.516$; Adj $R^2 = 0.235$; $F(1, 98) = 8.526$, $p < 0.01$). Gender role attitude, and Femininity were not significant predictors.
- *The greater the Masculinity and less the Daily Hassles, better was the Subjective Well-being of the individual.* The contribution of Masculinity was higher among men than in women (Beta coefficient being 0.328 for women and 0.370 for men) The impact of daily hassles was higher among women than among men (Beta coefficient being −0.305 for women and −0.293 for men).

General Discussion

Subjective Well-Being Across Clinical Status and Sex

As expected, in Study II, well-being was lower in the clinical group in comparison to the healthy counterpart. Sex difference in SWB was observed in Study 1, but not in Study 2. In Study I, men enjoyed better well-being than women. Greater wellness in men has been discerned in earlier studies abroad (Russo and Green 1993), and in India (Mukhopadhyay et al. 2007), although some have evinced no significant sex difference in well-being (Seghal 1999, 2000). In Study I, the age range was between 19 and 22 years; hence, groups were more homogenous. In Study II, the age range was between 20 and 35 years, the average age being higher. Therefore, one possibility is that the male advantage in well-being decreased with age. Furthermore, in Study II, about 52% of the participants were from lower class, unlike the middle class only of Study I. Such considerations suggest impact of sociodemographic factors in wellness.

Daily Hassle as Predictor of SWB

Daily Hassles have been observed earlier to be associated with reduced wellness (Tov 2012). In both studies, correlation of Daily Hassles with Well-being was higher among women than men. This suggests that women are more perturbed by everyday hassles, which in turn may be due to their gender role prescription. However, for the clinical sample of both sexes, Daily Hassle did not contribute significantly to the variance in Well-being. One possible reason might be that because of the illness, this group has already withdrawn from the daily work, and the burden of the illness overshadowed the burden of hassles.

Gender Role as Predictor of Subjective Well-Being: Primacy of Masculinity Model

Both studies demonstrated that Masculinity emerged as the singularly most effective predictor of well-being, thus generally supporting the Masculinity model of mental health. Despite gaps in research, the findings concerned with gender role stereotype and mental health may be grouped to support either the Androgyny model or the Masculinity model. The former was advocated by Bem, claiming that androgyny is a protection against mental illness and promotes positive outcome, like self-esteem, wellness and happiness (Bem 1974; Lefkowitz and Zeldow 2006; Spence and Helmreich 1978). In India also, Prakash et al. (2010) found androgyny to be psychoprotective. The Masculinity hypothesis, emerging mainly through meta analysis, attributes much of the positive outcome of androgyny to the presence of the masculinity component. The critical papers by Taylor and Hall (1982), Whitley (1983, 1984) and Whitley and Gridley (1993) demonstrated the predicaments of androgyny, and significance of masculinity as the key to mental health. Some studies indicated relationship of femininity to mental health, though the association with masculinity was always stronger than that with femininity (Whitley 1983). Masculinity promotes mental health, because it is associated with control over self and others, the power to execute, to decide. It is also possible that possession of masculine traits enables one to perceive wellness (Cloninger and Zohar 2011). The fact that modernity of attitude did not come up as significant for any group, suggests that attitude toward gender role enactment is less important than identity for promoting subjectively perceived well-being.

The present studies indicate that at least in the non-clinical samples, Masculine identity and Daily Hassles conjointly predict SWB. A few earlier studies have demonstrated the complex interrelationship between gender role stereotype, stress and mental health (Gianakos 2002; Hoffman and Su 1998). The present study endorses the above works, at least in the healthy samples.

Suggestions for Incorporating Gender Role Training in Mental Health Promotion

Our studies unequivocally supported the Masculinity hypothesis. Of course, masculinity does not mean maleness or manhood; but refers to the instrumental traits leading to assertion, power, leadership and decision making (Spence and Heimreich 1978). The finding may be interpreted to underscore that well-being lies in feeling empowered; in the ability to control one's inner and outer environment.

At this point, we may look into what message our culture imparts to us. Some scholars point out that the notion of a powerful femininity is observed in Indian Hindu tradition in contrast to western ones. Yet, if we look into Indian, especially Hindu heritage, we would find inconsistencies and ambivalence toward femalehood and femininity (Bose 2000). On the one hand, women have been glorified as derivatives of the 'Devi', the goddess, and rendered an ethereal position of being the 'Shakti'—the prime power. However, one must note that power of the 'Devi' is a masculine trait according to all present frames of Gender Role Stereotype. On the other hand, in mundane life, the same women have been denounced as the 'gateway to hell' for men, and their claim in all decision-making domains, including social, financial and educational spheres have been suppressed (Bhattacharji 1994). Thereby, the ideal superhuman femininity is powerful, a trait usually ascribed to masculinity; yet the humble femininity in women within households signify powerlessness. This inner contradiction between the ideal and the observed makes the psychological development of a girl child thorny, not only for the patriarchy induced selective deprivation and oppression, but also owing to the confused identity perpetuated by the culture. Simultaneously, women's sacrifice and tolerance of pain has been eulogized and designed to enhance her self-esteem, thereby tactfully suppressing her assertiveness and demand for material pleasures. Thus, femininity is clad with confusion, which might have cancelled out its positive and negative impacts on well-being, and ended up with statistically insignificant results.

It may be stated that in the Indian context, gender role training is still important for promoting wellness. This may be executed in two ways. The masculine traits may be encouraged in both women and men; these traits are actually instrumental ones and enhance affect self-esteem by increasing possibility of real life success. It would be advisable to dissociate assertion and power from masculine stereotype and project these as strategies for survival essential for both sexes and gender roles. Simultaneously, ambivalence around feminine traits like expressiveness and emotionality may also be scrutinized and destigmatized.

Often intervention for promoting women's mental health is formulated at micro level in medical terms. However, the broader socio-psychological aspects of intervention needs to be underscored, so that health or lack of health is not conceptualized at its clinical dimension only, and isolated from its interpersonal frame of reference. The present findings highlight the priority of social empowerment in promoting wellness. This needs to be designed at the macro level in terms of broader socioeconomic and work-family context so that women's access to material and health resources, including right over her own body, thoughts and emotions is enabled. It may be asserted that women's wellness improves in proportion to increase their empowerment, provided empowerment does not enforce linear patriarchal values, but is situated harmoniously with women's existential requirements. Needless to say, violence against women is also proportionally and negatively associated with empowerment, thus relating to women's quality of life. In the mental health sector, the service providers and social workers must be sensitized to the complexities of the gendered normativity in relation to wellness, and intervene at the community level through mobilizing not only individual, but also all available interpersonal and collective mechanisms. A disorder may sometimes be treated at the individual level; one person can be cured of some disease. But wellness cannot be delivered to one individual; staying happy requires collective happiness, which in turn requires sociocultural ambience promoting quality of life.

Vindhya (2001b) explained how women's mental health is compromised in transition from the personal to the collective normativity. Indeed, one implication of empowerment for well-being is to be watchful toward one's own bodily and psychological needs and to act towards healthy practices. This requires recognition of one's individualized identity. Undoubtedly self-sacrifice and altruism are virtues; but socially imposed norms of sacrifice on women as carers only for all family members, disproportionate eulogy of maternal role at the cost of neglecting own bodily needs, often result in self-denial, inadequate nutrition, lack of relaxation and reduced personal space among Indian women. That individual self-care is as important as family care is not yet instilled in Indian society adequately. It needs tobe reiterated that only a person possessing power to decide can choose to be altruistic; otherwise heraltruistic service becomes indistinguishable from servitude.

Davar (1999) viewed the problem of unequal epidemiology, discrepant aetiology and divergent symptom formation in line with cultural specificities. Her final destination was to construct a 'self' of Indian women through re-viewing their distress and coping under the rubrics of mental health and disease. Our present mental health policy may recognize gender difference in disorders, but ignores how such gender difference is construed through gender role and uneven distribution of hassles. Thus, the gendered self remains split and unorganized, lopsidedly bent toward desiring masculine power, without balancing it with tenderness. The burden of this misappropriation is borne mostly by women. To render femininity its due role in well-being, we must understand that since power and status go hand in hand, these two must be considered as a gender neutral corollary to health and well-being. It lies with the social scientists to come up with an interdisciplinary model of gender role training worked upon cultural heritage and modern requisites to reconceptualize wellness in Indian society.

Acknowledgements The study was partially funded by the Women Studies Department, University of Calcutta, and partially by the Department of Science and Technology, West Bengal.

References

Agrawal, J., Murthy, P., Philip, M., Mehrotra, S., Thenarasu, K., John, J. P., et al. (2011). Socio-demographic correlates of subjective well-being in Urban India. *Social Indicators Research, 101*(3), 419–434.

Archer, J. (1980). The distinction between gender stereotype and sex role concepts. *British Journal of Social and Clinical Psychology, 19,* 51–52.

Arrindell, W. A., Kolk, A. M., Pickersgill, M. J., & Hageman, W. J. J. M. (1993). Biological sex, sex role orientation, masculine sex role stress, dissimulation, and self-reported fears. *Advances in Behaviour Research and Therapy, 15,* 103–146.

Basu, J. (2010). Development of the Indian gender role identity scale (IGRIS): Psychometric properties and application. *Journal of Indian Academy of Applied Psychology, 36*(1), 25–34.

Basu, J., & Chakroborti, U. (1996). Effect of sex role identity on academic achievement of late adolescents in India. *Journal of Social Psychology, 136,* 257–259.

Basu, J., Chakroborti, M., Chowdhuri, S., & Ghosh, M. (1995). Gender stereotype, self-ideal disparity and neuroticism in Bengali families. *Indian Journal of Social Work, 56,* 297–311.

Basu, S., Chattopadhyay, D., Deb, A., Ash, S., Samajdar, J., Deb, Z., et al. (1995). Adaptation of the beck depression inventory into Bengali and its clinical validity. *Bulletin of the Indian Psychiatric Society, West Bengal, 5*(1), 5–9.

Basu, S., & Dasgupta, S. K. (1996). *Adapted Bengali version of General Health Questionnaire-28.* Calcutta: Department of Applied Psychology, Calcutta University.

Basu, A., & Ray, B. (2003). *Women's struggle: A history of the all India women conference, 1927–2002* (2nd ed.). Delhi: Manohar.

Basu, J., Dasgupta, S., Chakraborty, U., & Basu, S. (2012). Variants of the Indian Gender Role Identity Scale (IGRIS) for different age groups in Bengali population. *Journal of Indian Academy of Applied Psychology, 38*(2), 305–310.

Beck, A. T., Ward, C. H., Mendelson, M., Mock, J. E., & Erabugh, J. K. (1961). An inventory for measuring depression. *Archives of General Psychiatry, 4,* 561–571.

Bem, S. L. (1974). The measurement of psychological androgyny. *Journal of Consulting and Clinical Psychology, 42,* 155–162.

Bem, S. L. (1981). *Manual of Bem sex role inventory.* California: Mind Garden.

Bem, S. L. (1984). Androgyny and gender schema theory: A conceptual and empirical integration, *Paper Presented at Nebraska Symposium on Motivation.*

Bender, L. (1938). *Bender visual-motor gestalt test.* Alexandria: American Orthopsychiatric Association Inc.

Bhattacharji, S. (1994). *Women and society in ancient India.* Calcutta: Basumati Corporation.

Biswas-Diener, R., Tay, L. & Diener, E (2013). Happiness in India. In H. Selin & G. Davey (Eds.). *Happiness across cultures, Science across cultures: The history of non-western science* (Vol. 6, pp. 13–25). https://doi.org/10.1007/978-94-007-2700-7_2.

Blue, I., Ducci, M. E., Jaswal, A., Ludermir, B., & Harpham, T. (1995). The mental health of low income urban women: Case studies from Bombay, India; Olinda, Brazil; and Santiago, Chile.

In T. Harpham & I. Blue (Eds.), *Urbanization and mental health in developing countries*. Avebury: Aldershot.

Bose, M. (Ed.). (2000). *Facets of the feminism in ancient, medieval and modern India*. Delhi: Oxford University Press.

Brannigan, G. G., & Decker, S. L. (2003). *Bender visual-motor gestalt test* (2nd ed.). Itasca, IL: Riverside Publishing.

Busfield, J. (1996). *Men, women and madness*. Houndsmills, Hampshire: Macmillan Press.

Butler, J. (1990). *Gender trouble: Feminism and the subversion of identity*. New York: Routledge.

Chaudhuri, M. (2005). *Feminism in India (issues in contemporary Indian feminism)*. New York: Zed.

Cleary, P. D., & Mechanic, D. (1983). Sex differences in psychological distress among married people. *Journal of Health and Social Behavior, 24,* 111–121.

Cloninger, C. R., & Zohar, A. H. (2011). Personality and the perception of health and happiness. *Journal of Affective Disorders, 128*(1), 24–32.

Cronbach, L. J. (1951). Coefficient alpha and the internal structure of tests. *Psychometrika, 16,* 297–334.

Culbertson, F. (1997). Depression and gender: An international review. *American Psychologist, 52,* 25–31.

Dasgupta, S., & Basu, J. (2011). Marital quality and gender role stereotype. *Psychological Studies, 56*(4), 360–367.

Datta, S., Das, S., & Basu, J. (1995). Effect of gender role identity on gender role attitude of women. *Journal of Community Guidance and Research, 12,* 55–62.

Davar, B. V. (1999). *Mental health of Indian women: A feminist agenda*. New Delhi: Sage.

Dave, V. (2012). Women workers in unorganised sector. *Women's Link, 18*(3), 9–12.

de Girolamo, G., Polidori, G., Morosini, P., Scarpino, V., Reda, V., Serra, G., et al. (2006). Prevalence of common mental disorders in Italy: Results from the European study of the epidemiology of mental disorders (ESEMeD). *Social Psychiatry and Psychiatric Epidemiology, 41,* 853–861.

Deaux, K. (1985). Sex and gender. *Annual Review of Psychology, 36,* 49–81.

Desjarlais, R., Eisenberg, L., Good, B., & Kleinman, A. (1995). *World mental health, problems and priorities in low income countries*. New York: Oxford University Press.

Diener, E., Suh, E. M., Lucas, R. E., & Smith, H. (1997). *Subjective well-being: Three decades of progress-1967–1997*. Illinois: University of Illinois.

Duke, K. C. (1970). A study of prevalence and biosocial variables in mental illness in a rural and an urban community in Uttar Pradesh India. *Acta Psychiatrica Scandinavica, 46,* 327–359.

Eisler, R. M., Skidmore, J. R., & Ward, C. H. (1988). Masculine gender role stress: Predictor of anger, anxiety and health-risk behaviours. *Journal of Personality Assessment, 52,* 133–141.

Flett, G. L., Blankstein, K. R., Hicken, D. J., & Watson, M. S. (2006). Social support and help seeking in daily hassles versus major life events stress. *Journal of Applied Social Psychology, 25*(1), 49–58.

Gallacher, F., & Klieger, D. M. (1995). Sex role orientation and fear. *The Journal of Psychology, 129,* 41–49.

Gianakos, I. (2002). Predictors of coping with work stress: The influences of sex, gender role, social desirability, and locus of control. *SexRoles, 46,* 149–158.

Goldberg, D. P., & Hiller, V. E. (1979). A scaled version of the general health questionnaire. *Psychological Medicine, 9,* 139–146.

Gove, W. R. (1979). Sex differences in the epidemiology of mental disorders: Evidence and explanations. In E. S. Gomberg & V. Franks (Eds.), *Gender and disordered behavior: Sex differences in psychopathology* (pp. 23–68). New York: Brunner/Mazel.

Greendale, G. A., Huang, M.-H., Wight, R. G., Seeman, T., Luetters, C., Avis, J., et al. (2009). Effects of the menopause transition and hormone use on cognitive performance in midlife women. *Neurology, 72,* 1850–1857.

Hoffmann, J. P., & Su, S. S. (1998). Stressful life events and adolescent substance use and depression: Conditional and gender differentiated effects. *Substance Use and Misuse, 33,* 2219–2262.

Hofstede, G. (1980/2001). *Culture's consequences: International differences in work-related values*. Beverly Hills, CA: Sage.

Isaac, M., Janca, A., & Orley, J. (1996). Somatization—A culture-bound or universal syndrome? *Journal of Mental Helath, 5,* 219–222.

Kanner, A. D., & Feldman, S. S. (1991). Control over uplifts and hassles and its relationship to adaptational outcomes. *Journal of Behavioural Medicine, 14*(2), 187–201.

Kaur, M. (1968). *Role of women in the freedom movement, 1857–1947*. New Delhi: Sterling.

Khandelwal, S. K., Sharan, P., & Saxena, S. (1995). Eating disorders: An Indian perspective. *International Journal of Social Psychiatry, 41,* 132–146.

Khurana, A. (1996). Effect of Vipassana meditation on quality of life of undertrials. In Vimla Veeraraghavan (Ed.), *Certain perspectives of quality of life*. Delhi: Krishna publishers.

Kimmel, M. S. (2000). *The gendered society*. London: Oxford University Press.

Kiran Kumar, S. K. (2003). An Indian conception of wellbeing. In J. Henry (Ed.), *European Positive Psychology Proceedings 2002*. Leicester, UK: British Psychological Society.

Klonoff, E. A., & Landrine, H. (1997). *Preventing misdiagnosis of women*. New Delhi: Sage.

Kopper, B. A., & Epperson, D. L. (1996). The experience and expression of anger: Relationships with gender, gender role socialization, depression, and mental health functioning. *Journal of Counseling Psychology, 43*(2), 158–165.

Krampen, G., Effertz, B., Jostock, U., & Müller, B. (2006). Gender differences in personality: Biological and/or psychological? *European Journal of Personality, 4,* 303–317.

Kumar, A., & Kumar, S. (2013). Karma Yoga: A path towards work in positive psychology. *Indian Journal of Psychiatry, 55*(Suppl 2), 150–152. https://doi.org/10.4103/0019-5545.105511.

Lazarus, R. S., & Folkman, S. (1989). *Manual for the hassles and uplifts scale*. Palo Alto, CA: Mind Garden.

Lefkowitz, E. S., & Zeldow, P. B. (2006). Masculinity and femininity predict optimal mental health: A belated test of the androgyny hypothesis. *Journal of Personality Assessment, 87,* 95–101.

Linssen, R., van Kempen, L., & Kraaykamp, G. (2011). Subjective wellbeing in rural India: The curse of conspicuous consumption. *Social Indicators Research, 101*(1), 57–72.

Lorber, J. (1997). *Gender and the social construction of illness*. New Delhi: Sage.

Maheshwari, S., & Singh, P. (2009). Psychological well-being and pilgrimage: Religiosity, happiness and life satisfaction of Ardh–Kumbh Mela pilgrims (Kalpvasis) at Prayag India. *Asian Journal of Social Psychology, 12*(4), 285–292. https://doi.org/10.1111/j.1467-839X.2009.01291.x.

Malhotra, D., & Chhabra, R. (1991). Effect of psychological androgyny and stress on problem solving among tribals. *Psychologia, 37,* 104–119.

Malik, I., Bukhtiari, N., Good, M. J., Iqbal, M., Azim, S., Nawaz, M., et al. (1992). Mothers' fear of child death: A study in urban and rural communities in Northern Punjab, Pakistan. *Social Science and Medicine, 35,* 1043–1053.

Mazure, C. M., Bruce, M. L., Maciejewski, P. K., & Jacobs, S. C. (2000). Adverse life events and cognitive-personality characteristics in the prediction of major depression and antidepressant response. *American Journal of Psychiatry, 157,* 896–903.

McCreary, D. R. (1990). Multidimensionality and the measurement of gender role attributes: A comment on Archer. *British Journal of Social Psychology, 29,* 266–272.

McCullough, G., Huebner, E. S., & Laughlin, J. E. (2000). Life events, self-concept, and adolescent's positive subjective wellbeing. *Psychology in the Schools, 37,* 281–290.

McIntyre, S., & Hunt, K. (1997). Socioeconomic position, gender and health. *Journal of Health Psychology, 2,* 315–334.

Mehrotra, S., Tripathi, R., & Banu, H. (2013). Psychological well-being: Reflections on an Elusive construct and its assessment. *Journal of the Indian Academy of Applied Psychology, 39*(2), 189–195.
Mittal, U., Janjani, P., Hingar, A., & Pareek, S. (2010). Impact of gender identity on subjective wellbeing among educated non-working women. *Indian Journal of Social Science Researches, 7*(2), 47–55.
Mohanraj, P., & Manivannan, L. (2013). Occupational stress among migrated workers in unorganised sectors. *International Journal of Research in Management and Technology, 3*(1), 13–19.
Mukhopadhyay, S., Basu, J., & Rajan, I. (2007). Mental health, gender ideology and women's status in Kerala. In S. Mukhopadhyay (Ed.), *The enigma of the Kerala woman: A failed promise of literacy* (pp. 71–101). New Delhi: Social Science Press.
Nandi, D. N., Mukherjee, S. P., Nandi, P. S., & Nandi, S. (2000). Psychiatric morbidity of a rural Indian community Changes over a 20-year interval. *The British Journal of Psychiatry, 176,* 351–356.
Nathanson, C. (1975). Illness and the feminine role: A theoretical review. *Social Science Medicine, 9,* 57–63.
Nolen-Hoeksema, S., Grayson, C., & Larson, J. (1999). Explaining the gender difference in depressive symptoms. *Journal of Personality and Social Psychology, 77,* 1061–1072.
Pareek, S., & Jain, M. (2012). Subjective well-being in relation to altruism and forgiveness among school going adolescents. *International Journal of Psychology and Behavioral Sciences, 2*(5), 138–141. https://doi.org/10.5923/j.ijpbs.20120205.02.
Patel, V. (2007). Mental health in low- and middle-income countries. *British Medical Bulletin, 81–82*(1), 81–96. https://doi.org/10.1093/bmb/ldm010.
Patel, V., & Kleinman, A. (2003). Poverty and common mental disorders in developing countries. *Bulletin of the World Health Organization, 81,* 609–615.
Paykel, E. S. (1994). Life events, social support and depression, ActaPsychiatra Scandinavia. In J. Lonnqvist & T. Sahi (Eds.), *Depression: Preventative and Risk Factors* (Vol. 89 supplement 377, pp. 50–58). Copenhagen: Munksgaard.
Prakash, J., Kotwal, A. S. M., Ryali, V. S. S. R., Srivastava, K., Bhat, P. S., & Shashikumar, R. (2010). Does androgyny have psychoprotective attributes? A cross sectional community based study. *Industrial Psychiatry Journal, 19*(2), 119–124. https://doi.org/10.4103/0972-6748.90343.
Rao, V. V. P., & Rao, V. N. (1983). *Sex role attitudes: A comparison of sex-race groups*. San Antonio, Texas: Paper Presented at the meeting of South Western Social Science Association.
Reichhardt, T. (2006). Well-being research: A measure of happiness. *Nature, 444,* 418–419.
Robinson, M. D. (2000). The reactive and prospective functions of mood: Its role in linking daily experiences and cognitive wellbeing. *Cognition and Emotion, 14,* 145–176.
Russo, N. F. (1990). Overview: Forging research priorities for women's mental health. *American Psychologist, 45,* 368–373.
Russo, N. F., & Green, B. L. (1993). Women and mental health. In F. L. Denmark & M. A. Paludi (Eds.), *Psychology of women: A handbook of issues and theories*. Westport, CN: Greenwood Press.
Ryan, R. M., & Deci, E. (2001). On happiness and human potentials: A review of research on hedonic and eudaimonic well-being. *Annual Review of Psychology, 52*(1), 141–166.
Sabo, D., & Gordon, G. (1993). *Men's Health and Illness: Gender and the body*. London: Sage.
Sahoo, F. M., & Mohapatra, L. (2009). Psychological well-being in professional groups. *Journal of the Indian Academy of Applied Psychology, 35*(2), 211–217.
Sawrie, S. M., Watson, P. J., & Biderman, M. D. (1991). Aggression, sex role measures, and Kohut's psychology of the self. *Sex Roles, 25*(3/4), 141–161.
Scanzoni, J. (1975). *Sex roles, life style and child bearing*. New York: Free Press.
Seghal, M. (2000). Gender, personality and wellbeing. *Behavioural Medicine Journal, 3,* 43–49.
Sehgal, M. (1999). Self-efficacy, stress and health: Across-gender perspective. *Journal of the Indian Academy of Applied Psychology, 25,* 57–60.

Sell, H., & Nagpal, R. (1992). *Assessment of subjective wellbeing*. Regional Office for South East Asia, New Delhi: WHO.

Serido, J., Almeida, D. M., & Wethington, D. (2004). Conceptual and empirical distinctions between chronic stressors and daily hassles. *Journal of Health and Social Behavior, 45,* 17–33.

Sharma, A. (2011). Subjective well-being of retired teachers: The role of psycho-social factors. *International Journal of Psychological Studies, 3(1).* www.ccsenet.org/ijps.

Sims, J. (1994). *Women, health and environment: An anthology*. Geneva: World Health Organization.

Singh, G., Kaur, D., & Kaur, H. (1981). Presumptive stressful events scale (PSE-scale): A new life events scale for use in India. *Indian Journal of Clinical Psychology, 8,* 173–176.

Spence, J. T., & Helmreich, J. R. (1978). *Masculinity and femininity: Their psychological dimensions, correlates and antecedents*. Austin and London: University of Texas Press.

Spielberger, C. D., & Vagg, P. R. (1995). Test anxiety: A transactional process model. In C. D. Spielberger & P. R. Vagg (Eds.), *Test anxiety: Theory, assessment, and treatment* (pp. 1–14). Washington, D.C.: Taylor & Francis.

Stoller, R. J. (1968/2000). *Sex and gender: The development of masculinity and femininity*. London: Karnac Book Co.

Sudha, K. S., & Shahnawaz, M. G. (2013). Core self-evaluation as a correlate of subjective well-being among special educators. *Journal of the Indian Academy of Applied Psychology, 39* (1), 83–90.

Sugarman, D., & Frankel, S. L. (1996). Patriarchal ideology and wife-assault: A meta-analytic review. *Journal of Family Violence, 11,* 13–40.

Suresh Kumar, P. N. (1998). Age and gender related analysis of psychosocial factors in attempted suicide. *Indian Journal of Psychiatry, 40,* 338–345.

Taylor, M. C., & Hall, J. A. (1982). Psychological androgyny: Theories, methods and conclusions. *Psychological Bulletin, 92,* 347–366.

Tov, W. (2012). Daily experiences and well-being: Do memories of events matter? *Cognition and Emotion, 26,* 1371–1389.

Trivedi, J. K., Sareen, H., & Dhyani, M. (2009). Psychological Aspects of Widowhood and Divorce. *Mens Sana Monographs, 7*(1), 37–49.

Unger, R., & Crawford, M. (1992). *Women and gender: A feminist psychology*. New York: McGraw-Hill.

Venkataswamy Reddy, M., & Chandrashekhar, C. R. (1998). Prevalence of mental and behavioral disorders in India: A meta-analysis. *Indian Journal of Psychiatry, 40,* 149–157.

Vindhya, U. (2001a). Mental health care: A review of gender differences. *International Journal of Diabetes in Developing Countries, 21,* 86–96.

Vindhya, U. (2001b). From the personal to the collective: Psychological/feminist issues of women's mental health. In B. Davar (Ed.), *Mental Health from a Gender Perspective* (pp. 82–98). New Delhi: Sage Publications.

Vindhya, U. (2007). Quality of women's lives in India: Some findings from two decades of psychological research on gender. *Feminism and Psychology, 17,* 337–356.

Vindhya, U. (2010). Issues of gender in psychology: Traversing from sex differences to quality of women's life. In G. Misra (Ed.), *Psychology in India* (Vol. IV, pp. 173–226)., Theoretical and Methodological Developments New Delhi: ICSSR.

Weissman, M. M., Bland, R., Joyce, P. R., Newman, S., Wells, J. E., & Wittchen, H. (1993). Sex differences in rates of depression: cross-national perspectives. *Journal of Affective Disorders, 29,* 77–84.

Whitley, B. E., Jr. (1983). Sex role orientation and self-esteem: A critical meta-analytic review. *Journal of Personality and Social Psychology, 44,* 765–778.

Whitley, B. E. (1984). Sex role orientation and psychological well-being: Two meta-analyses. *Sex Roles, 12,* 207–225.

Whitley, B. E., & Gridley, B. E. (1993). Sex role orientation, self-esteem, and depression: A latent variables analysis. *Personality and Social Psychology Bulletin, 19,* 363–369.

Wichstrom, L. (1999). The emergence of gender differences in depressed mood during adolescence: The role of intensified gender socialization. *Developmental Psychology, 35,* 232–245.

World Health Organization (2004). *Gender and women's mental health.* Geneva.

World Health Organization report (2000). *Women's mental health: An evidence based review.* Mental Health Determinants and Populations. Department of Mental Health and Substance Dependence. Geneva.

Chapter 22
Delivering Quality Healthcare in India: Issues and Challenges

Manisha Agarwal

While the economic development in India has been gaining momentum over the last decade and a large proportion of the gross national product is spent on healthcare, the Indian health system is at crossroads today and its needs much more than the available resources. India's achievements in health outcomes are only moderate by international standards; India is ranked 118 among 191 WHO member countries on overall health performance (WHO 2000). In 2004, national healthcare spending was about 5.2% of nominal GDP. Together, this health infrastructure serves a population of over one billion, growing at about 2% annually (Bisht et al. 2012). The private sector accounts for more than 80% of total healthcare spending within India (Ram-Persaud 2007). In India, the government at various levels such as municipality, district and state offers primary, secondary and tertiary healthcare to its citizens at highly subsidized rates. These hospitals offer a wide range of outpatient and inpatient services, including a few superspecialty services. Each government hospital is organized into several clinical, investigation and administrative departments. From a pan-Indian perspective, presently, there are more than half a million doctors employed in 15,097 hospitals. Additionally, there are 0.75 million nurses, who look after more than 870,000 hospital beds. During the previous decade, the number of doctors increased by 37% and an estimated 30% medical practitioners held specialist qualifications (Mahal et al. 2002). Some of the major problems faced currently by the industry may be listed as:

- Many hospitals and healthcare providers are struggling with outdated information technology in India today.
- A major challenge for the nation and the healthcare industry would be not only to retain the healthcare workforce but also to develop an environment, which would attract those abroad to return (reverse brain drain).

M. Agarwal (✉)
Department of Psychology, Banaras Hindu University, Varanasi, India
e-mail: manisha12529@gmail.com

G. Misra (ed.), *Psychosocial Interventions for Health and Well-Being*,
https://doi.org/10.1007/978-81-322-3782-2_22

- The growing demand for quality healthcare and the absence of matching delivery mechanism pose a great challenge.
- There is an acute shortage of faculty of medical teachers all over the country. One of the pivotal factors to sustain the projected growth of the healthcare industry in India would be the availability of a trained workforce, besides cheaper technology, better infrastructure etc.
- Another challenge is to find good talent in India to provide ancillary healthcare services, especially the voice-based ones which require not only good English communication skills but also very good analytical skills.
- Amidst all the growth, the sector is also suffering from internal as well as external challenges; the major one being failure of human resource practices to decrease turnover of medical professionals in healthcare organizations. The high costs associated with excessive voluntary turnover rates of medical professionals are frequently cited as a key issue for the government and healthcare administrators.
- The assumption that urban health services are better equipped and organized due to greater availability of health professionals and healthcare facilities has led to the long neglect of urban health planning (Reddy 2013). The absence of a well-designed system of urban primary healthcare has resulted in fragmentation of health services, with the poor being denied basic care and the middle and upper classes overloading the secondary and tertiary care centres with problems that are best attended to in primary care facilities. Urban health now presents an unacceptable mix of marked inequities in health indicators, serious inefficiencies in service delivery and avoidable escalation of healthcare costs.

In this context, it is worth mentioning that the National Urban Health Mission (NUHM) targets the urban poor and other vulnerable groups and promotes their access to affordable and good quality preventive and primary services. It intends to develop a public investment plan for primary and secondary healthcare services in small, medium, large and mega-cities by clearly defining the roles of the Centre, State and Urban Local Bodies (ULBs). While integrating various vertical disease programmes, it will define 'essential healthcare packages' for each level of healthcare and design effective referral procedures.

Quality of Patient Care

Quality of patient care has become the major focus of healthcare organizations and in India it has generally been explored in terms of organizational and employee factors that enhance quality of patient care and devise programmes for its improvement. Organizational researchers have focused on the public sector, particularly hospitals, in an effort to link organizational characteristics to a number of important outcomes for patients and staff. Employees' satisfaction with their jobs and commitment to their organizations has been viewed as major determinants of organizational effectiveness. Concerns about employees' job satisfaction and organizational commitment are just as, or even more, critical in the knowledge-based sectors, such as the healthcare industry. This is particularly significant for India where a large number of people are dependent on the public health service system.

Few question why 'management matters' in delivering quality healthcare is inadequate. Migration of health professionals has also reduced the quality of health services. This has affected the workforce of healthcare and the quality of health service system is severely compromised by the shortage of staff and other resources. An overview of the research findings in healthcare organizations highlights the various issues that have arisen in this context for healthcare and organizational researchers globally with specific reference to the Indian scenario. There is no generic definition of quality and one can find quality defined as excellence (Garvin 1984), value (Cronin and Taylor 1992), confirmation to specifications (Garvin 1988) and meeting customers' expectations (Gronross 1984; Parasuraman et al. 1985). The *Oxford English Dictionary* defines quality as a noun meaning 'degree of excellence'. The Bureau of Indian Standards defines quality as the totality of features and characteristics of a product or service that bear on its ability to satisfy stated or implied needs.

There are different aspects and dimensions of quality. A number of studies have been conducted on this important subject. Among the several research studies undertaken in the variable of service quality, some of the important ones include studies on importance of customers' perception of quality (Teas 1993), the strategic benefits of service quality (Andrian 1995), tangible aspects of service quality (Carman 1990), assessing the effects of quality on customer satisfaction (Cronin and Brandy 2000) and measuring service quality (Cronin and Taylor 1992). The results of these studies reveal that service quality has a significant impact on satisfaction and behavioural intentions.

The transactional aspects along with human aspects of the personnel like expertise, friendliness, reliability, service value, etc., affect the service quality and relationship quality which in turn have significant influence on customer satisfaction and future interaction with the organisation. Healthcare providers in developing countries like India, are beginning to adopt some or all of the main three components of quality assurance, namely, quality design, quality control and quality improvement (Koeck 1997). Identification of the level and type of services required by the customers is a prerequisite for setting up quality measures, but assessing customers' need in an Indian health service context is uncertain.

Service selection is largely affected by customer income and their desire to select a particular quality level. India, a country with a population of about a billion, represents an immense variety of economic levels, social statuses and cultural groups. A mass of poor people, along with a large middle-class, constitutes nearly 80% of the population. The low income group hardly manages to access private nursing home services unless otherwise crucial to survival; they prefer government or charity-run hospitals. Upper-class people, on the other hand, can access nursing home services and other cosmetic health services. Øvretveit provided reasons for improving quality in the developing countries: patient dissatisfaction with higher costs (particularly concerning private care), patients are paying more for their care but are finding services do not treat them well or give them what they need, and so on. The public services are of very low quality in all care aspects. There is a need to find ways. It is important to start with an understanding of the real situation and the problems faced by healthcare professionals (West 2001).

Studies conducted on quality of patient care in India have been by and large directed at examining the effects of financial resources on the level of service quality provided by hospital organizations. For example, Bhat et al. (2001) found that the efficiency variations were more significant within district hospitals than within the grant-in-aid institutions. The overall efficiency levels of grant-in-aid institutions were higher than the district level hospitals. The grant-in-aid institutions were relatively more efficient than the public hospitals. Shah and Dhar (2007) identified HRD factors in healthcare and compared them across India and the USA. Twenty factors emerged which were analysed in terms of their varying importance, weightage and role in healthcare. The key factors commonly perceived by all doctors and all nurses were as follows: IT applications, relationship, efficiency, openness, and quality, elements of development, competence, effectiveness and ethics. Out of these only three were commonly perceived by all doctors, nurses and patients. These were IT applications, relationship and efficiency. Concern, commitment, consideration, spirituality and housekeeping were perceived significant only by the patients. Transparency was perceived by all doctors, while appraisal by all nurses. It is also interesting that four factors, namely, responsiveness, welfare, recognition and empathy, were not perceived either by all doctors, all nurses or by all patients. Only doctors in India perceived responsiveness and welfare as independent factors, while only nurses in India perceived recognition and only patients in the USA perceived empathy.

They suggested that IT applications and promoting much higher investment in the core healthcare sector should be strengthened and widened; quality circles should be set up in hospitals as part of a well-designed TQM plan in consultation with HRD experts. Quality circles may ensure promoting not only technical quality, but also functional and infrastructural quality in the hospitals in India. Special attention needs to be paid to improve teamwork and team spirit, as well as more interactive communication between doctors and nurses with a view to promoting a more collaborative environment and devise persuasive methods of creating awareness and collaborative sense of responsibility among doctors and nurses to voluntarily and steadily reduce the incidence of medical errors through extra care and concern at all stages.

Mehta (2011) has noted three factors of service quality, namely, promptness, medical aid and patient interest for service quality and amenities, clinical services and physical services. The study revealed that while service quality and patient satisfaction were more strongly associated with adherence and continuity of visit; service quality was positively associated with patient satisfaction which can be important for improving the outcomes in healthcare settings. In a recent study,

Agarwal et al. (2012) examined the impact of hospital organizational factors, namely, decentralization, coordination and work autonomy, on perceived levels of psychological contract fulfilment of medical employees and the reported quality of patient care in not-for-profit public hospitals which are (a) attached to a teaching institution and (b) those which are only involved in providing medical services (railways, non-teaching). The study was conducted on a sample of paramedical staff in both types of hospitals ($N = 200$) in northern India. Results highlighted the importance of 'co-ordination' as the salient factors that predicted perceived levels of psychological contract fulfilment and quality of patient care in both types of hospitals. Mediator effects of perceived psychological contract fulfilment on the relationship between the organizational factors and quality of patient care revealed that psychological contract fulfilment mediated the prediction of quality of patient care by decentralization and work autonomy only in the public (non-teaching) hospital but failed to mediate the prediction of quality of patient care by 'coordination' in both types of hospitals. Findings highlighted the significance of co-ordination among various specialities and departments in hospitals as the single important factor that can be promoted by hospital administrators for increasing perceived contract fulfilment among their paramedical staff and enhancing the quality of patient care.

Mental Health of Healthcare Professionals

A series of studies have been undertaken by economists, sociologists and psychologists to understand people's sense of well-being or distress (Cox et al. 2005; Kersley et al. 2006; Peccei 2004; Warr 2002). Therefore, the concept of employee well-being at work promotes advantages to organizations of having a healthy workforce. Hospital work often requires coping with some of the most stressful situations found in any workplace.

A hospital, unlike any other institute, is a complex and intricate organization. It needs the frequency matching and fine-tuning of all associated staff with the hierarchy. This level of adjustment and understanding often poses to be the most difficult in all situations to tackle, specifically in the Indian set-up. The Indian hospital industry, by and large, is managed by the medical professionals who excel in professional degrees and have a wide range of experience and practice. However, they do not possess an acclaimed managerial degree, and therefore lack the requisite skill and training to function as an efficient administrator. A hospital requires inter-disciplinary interactions, effective and efficient management of the available resources, coordination along the hierarchy, logistics and supply-chain related issues along with many other issues that are required to be instilled in a qualified professional in management and administration.

The public sector falls short to set up and operate world-class healthcare assets on its own as it is constrained by inadequate funds, limited micro-managerial expertise and an ever-standing shortfall of human resources (Sharma and Zodpey

2011). Healthcare professionals must deal with life-threatening injuries and illnesses complicated by overwork, under-staffing, tight schedules, paper work, intricate or malfunctioning equipment, complex hierarchies of authority and skills, dependent and demanding patients, and patient deaths, all of which are significant contributors to stress. High exposure to stressful events among medical personnel may manifest itself in several different outcomes including depression, anxiety, self-doubt, post traumatic stress disorder, loss of sleep and disturbed relationships with family. These factors may be important contributors to an unhealthy workplace in the hospital setting. Physicians under stress are more likely to treat patients poorly, both medically and psychologically. They are also more prone to make errors of judgment. The resulting stress-related mental impairment among these workers may result in sub-optimal performance and delivery of less than best care to their clients.

According to Caplan et al. (1975), the work of healthcare professionals is inherently stressful as it is acknowledged that being responsible for people rather than objects is a major source of occupational stress. Compared with other professional groups, healthcare workers are subjected to unique stressors associated with dealing with sick people, many of whom may have various degrees of deformity, or are suffering physical and mental ill health, and on some occasions they also experience the death of a patient. Stressors identified in the medical profession are to a great extent psychosocial in their origin (Agius et al. 1996). These factors highlight some of the vulnerabilities to stress to which employees of the healthcare professions are exposed over and above other professions.

Factors such as the well-known triple signs of 'ignorance, indifference, and carelessness' of physicians toward their own health have been pointed out. As a consequence, it would be expected that physicians should be at increased risk for emotional symptoms. Emotional withdrawal, social isolation, burnout, unhappiness, depression, denial of professional problems, irony and cynicism are some important consequences of physician stress (Ramirez et al. 1996; Wall et al. 1997). Studies using depression scales for evaluation of physicians' job-related affections or 'burnout' as an outcome measure revealed some significant relationships with psychological health status, particularly with depression (Simoens et al. 2002; Appleton et al. 1998; Sibbald and Bojke 2004).

All in all, psychosomatic health complaints have been found to be quite frequent among nurses (Escribá-Agüir et al. 1993; Piko 1999). All these negative aspects of the job of healthcare staff have major behavioural and health implications as a consequence (Piko 1999; Shamian et al. 2002; Trinkoff and Storr 1998; Wahlstedt and Edling 1994). There is accumulating evidence that hospital workers are at increased risk for ill-health and mental health problems (Alexopoulos et al. 2003; Eriksen et al. 2003; Rafnsdottir et al. 2004; Tómasson et al. 2004). According to Warr (2002), cognitive factors that affect the quality of life are likely to be linked to people's perception of their own level of well-being. Therefore, effective well-being (psychological) emphasizes the centrality of feelings about life. As a conclusion, primary healthcare physicians' job-related negative emotional perceptions were associated with reactions in terms of mental health problems (Uncu et al. 2007).

Therefore, the dynamics of employee well-being at work is pivotal in the understanding of the different domains that affect the quality of life at work. One study among physicians revealed that one-third of all doctors reported lowered standards of patient care that is associated with primarily stress-related origins, and tiredness were determined to be at fault for 48.8% of the incidents, where doctors provided a lowered standard of care to their patients (Firth-Conzens and Greenhalgh 1997). Grol et al. (1985) have shown that frustrations, tensions and annoyance with time pressures are linked to giving patients short shrift: physicians may write a plethora of prescriptions yet give a paucity of time to listening and explaining. Links have been made between healthcare professional distress and patient satisfaction and outcome (Hillhouse and Adler 1997; Leiter et al. 1998; Tarnow-Mordi et al. 2000). Shanafelt et al. (2002) in their study reported that 76% of 115 residents met the criteria for the burnout. Of those with burnout, more than half judged that they had rendered suboptimal care at least monthly compared with 21% residents who were not at a low ebb. Other researchers have been also studied with similar findings (Revicki et al. 1993). Because primary healthcare physicians' job related affective well-being matter, they were serving as gate-keepers for the health of the whole nation. Their negative moods and emotions related to their job will disturb the quality of the service and the *continuity* of patient–physician relationship (Uncu et al. 2007).

Indian researches in the area of healthcare and medical personnel have focused basically on stress and satisfaction of medical personnel, consumer satisfaction, quality management and cross cultural studies of these variables. Parikh, Taukari and Bhattacharya (2004) studied occupational stressors and coping mechanisms in nurses, and reported that occupational stress appears to vary according to individual and job characteristics, and work-family conflict. Common occupational stressors found among nurses were workload, role ambiguity, interpersonal relationships, death and dying concerns. Shift work was highly prevalent among nurses and a significant source of stress. Emotional distress, burnout and psychological morbidity could also be a product of occupational stress. Perceived control appeared to be an important mediator of occupational stress. Coping and job satisfaction were found to be reciprocally related. Nurses' common coping mechanisms included problem solving, social support and avoidance.

Sharma (2005) reported that doctors, especially government doctors, experience various types of role stress. She suggested that when an organization decides to diagnose and systematically analyse the status of mental-cum-physical health they should use exercise a stress audit. It involves an attempt on the part of the organization to study, explore and control various types of stresses that doctors experience by virtue of their organizational membership. Both private and government hospitals should consider conducting stress audits regularly so that affected doctors can be identified and their stress levels reduced, which will in turn improve the quality of work. Tankha (2006) conducted a study with the aim of investigating the effect of role stress in nursing professionals. The obtained results revealed that male nurses experienced significantly higher stress level as compared to females. Secondly, male nurses from private hospitals showed significantly higher level of stress levels than the government nurses on eight out of the ten dimensions of organizational role stress scale (Pareek 1983).

Saha et al. (2011), observed the prime sources of stress were underpayment, excessive workload, inadequate staff, and being involved in the emotional distress of that patients. They recommended that a proper workload management policy, adequate delegation of authority along with responsibility, recognition of efforts along with on-going training, stress and time management can go a long way in managing stress in these personnel. Dasgupta (2012) conducted a study on nurses in three large private hospitals of Kolkata to assess the relationship between role conflict, overload and ambiguity, disengagement and exhaustion and role efficacy. Results showed that an increase in role overload, role conflict, role ambiguity led to an enhancement in disengagement and exhaustion while enhancement in self efficacy led to a reduction in role overload, role conflict, role ambiguity, disengagement and exhaustion among nurses.

Job Attitudes of Healthcare Professionals

Researches in the area of healthcare and medical personnel have focused basically on stress and satisfaction of medical personnel, consumer satisfaction, quality management and cross cultural studies of these variables. Studies exploring the association between overall job satisfaction and job performance have found a minimal but consistently significant correlation between the two (Vroom 1964). Health professional's satisfaction has also been linked to patient satisfaction, physician performance (Kerr et al. 2000). Fisher et al. (2004) claimed that job satisfaction includes the positive feelings associated with the rewarding aspects of a job that can intuitively lead to improved work performance. Haas et al. (2000) reported that patients of physicians who rated themselves to be very or extremely satisfied with their work were more satisfied with their healthcare and most recent physician visit. Managed care controls may partly explain this relationship (Haas et al. 2000). Leggat et al. (2010) found that psychological empowerment fully mediated the relationship between high performance work system (HPWS) and perceptions of quality of patient care. Job satisfaction moderated the relationship between HPWS and perceptions of quality of patient care.

For primary care patients with pain or depressive symptoms, primary physician job satisfaction is associated with some measures of patient-rated quality of care but not health outcomes. Many primary physicians believe that managed care and market competition have eroded their satisfaction with medical practice (Stoddard et al. 2001; Murray et al. 2001; Grembowski 2005). Pain and depression patients of physicians with greater job satisfaction had greater trust and confidence in their primary physicians. Pain patients of more satisfied physicians also were less likely to change physicians in the follow-up period. Depression patients of more satisfied physicians had higher ratings of the care provided by their physicians. These associations remained after controlling statistically for managed care. Physician job satisfaction was not associated with health outcomes.

A number of studies have been conducted to study the relationship between role stress and job satisfaction in India (Chaudhary 1990). Chaudhury and Bannerjee (2004) reported that job satisfaction among the younger doctors was high, but fell abruptly after the age of 35 years, to again rise gradually in the fifth and sixth decades of life. Rameshan and Singh (2005) examined a case study of the customer orientation of primary health centers (PHCs) of a district in Uttar Pradesh they explored input level facilities and human resources available for providing services and attitude and behaviours of doctors and other staff towards customers (patients and attendants of patients) were studied from the perspective of the customers. Analysis suggested that customers wanted to improve services of PHCs through panchayat pressure, persuasion and leaders' intervention. Agitation was the relatively less preferred strategy, they also did not want to passively tolerate poor services at PHCs. Interviews also suggest that doctors and staff had their own grievances that affected their morale and performance.

Pestonjee and Mishra (1999) have examined the nature of role stress and job satisfaction among doctors and nurses, and to explore the relationship between these variables. They could not find any significant difference between the two groups, except in the management area of job satisfaction and the inter-role distance (IRD) dimension of role stress. Further, job satisfaction variables correlated negatively with all the dimensions of role stress in the case of both groups. Bhandari et al. (2010) undertook a study to assess the levels of job satisfaction among the healthcare providers in CGHS dispensaries. A standardised tool developed by Warr et al. (1979) was used to measure the healthcare providers' job satisfaction in the present study. For this study healthcare providers (n = 250) working in the CGHS dispensaries of Delhi were interviewed. This included 100 doctors, 50 nurses and 100 paramedics which included both pharmacists and lab technicians. The findings of this study indicated that the levels of job satisfaction were not very high among the healthcare providers who were interviewed.

Sudhaker and Gomes (2010) analysed nurses' job satisfaction through an examination of the relationship between job stress coping strategies and job quality indexes. The nurses had moderate-high levels of stress. The employers, therefore, must take occupational stress seriously, as at the end of the day the message is that occupational stress costs—in litigation, on out-of-court settlements, in sick pay and in having a de-motivated and underproductive workforce.

Agarwal and Sharma (2010) examined the effects of certain hospital workplace factors on job involvement among healthcare employees at the paramedical levels and quality of patient care in teaching and non-teaching public hospitals in North India. They found that employee perceptions of the workplace factors, namely, participation in decision making, innovative practices, perceived organizational support and role efficacy were significantly different in the teaching and non-teaching hospitals. The factor 'innovative practices' was a positive predictor of job involvement in the non-teaching hospitals but a negative predictor in job involvement in the teaching hospital. Job involvement significantly mediated the relationship between the perception of workplace factors and quality of patient care only in the non-teaching hospitals. Agarwal and Sharma (2011) further reported that despite significant differences in perceived workplace factors of the two types of hospitals, the levels of psychological well-being and job satisfaction of the participants were nearly similar in both types of public hospitals. The organizational factors, co-ordination and work autonomy were significantly predictive of job satisfaction and psychological well-being of healthcare employees, while process-related workplace factors, participative decision making and intra-professional relations emerged as significant predictors of psychological well-being and job satisfaction in both types of hospitals. Findings have significant implications for public hospitals which are currently facing competition from the state-of-the-art healthcare technology being introduced by private hospitals, and are therefore under pressure for retention of skilled healthcare employees.

Migration and Employee Turnover in Healthcare

Employee turnover continues to be an important challenge facing health-care systems globally and India, specifically. India is experiencing acute crisis of medical professionals due to increased turnover of professionals in the healthcare sector. Turnover leads to the loss of human capital as medical professionals leave, and the lost productivity associated with new medical professionals oriented (O'Brien-Pallas et al. 2008). Considerable researches describe the factors that push employees to voluntarily leave organizations (e.g., job dissatisfaction), factors that pull employees away from organizations (e.g., alternative job opportunities) and the processes by which individuals make turnover decisions. Staying in or leaving an organization is an integral part of an employee's behavioural decision set and a continuous challenge of human resource managers and scholars.

It is often assumed that there are always HR activities that are better than others and that affect employee commitment and motivation. The high costs associated with excessive voluntary turnover rates of medical professionals are frequently cited as a key management issue for healthcare administrators. As healthcare systems in many nations are experiencing similar issues, the need for empirical studies that examine the relationship between organizational factors, human resource practices in terms of their implications for the outcomes (e.g. quality of care, organizational commitment and turnover intentions) in Indian healthcare organizations are increasingly needed. Migration of health workers appears to be driven by a number of pull factors such as the opportunities for professional training and better employment opportunities in the host country besides better salaries and perks. Push factors such as less attractive pay and working conditions, high unemployment rate political instability and insecurity in the home country also play a key role (Stilwell 2004; Padilla 2006). Newspaper reports often highlight the scarcity of nurses even in cities of rich middle-east nations such as Dubai.

According to the Report of the High Level Committee on Indian Diaspora, there are about 2,000 Indian doctors in Oman (GOI 2001). Indian physicians account for 9.6% of foreign trained professionals in Canada (1998), 18.3% for the UK (2001) and 19.5% for the US in 2001 (Forcier 2004). Health professionals are the most precious healthcare resources, not money, beds or buildings. Shortage causes longer waits for surgery, can lead to delays in emergency care and deny patients a choice in who treats them. Shortages also cause stress among pressurized health workers and forces the health services to employ more temporary staff. Significant migratory flows of physicians from India towards Australia, Canada, and the US. There are an estimated 60,000 doctors of Indian origin working in the UK and around 35,000 in the US. Besides, India has bilateral agreements with six Middle Eastern countries and some others for recruiting private and government doctors on short-term assignments (Chanda 2002). About 3,000 Indian doctors migrated to the US during 1988–90 (Kanjanapan 1995). The rates of emigration have not increased but emigrating professionals are now finding newer destinations. For instance, the flow of Indian physicians to Australia has increased considerably from 81 in 1997–98 to 212 in 2002–03. In the hospitals, nurses are among the most important providers of patient care. As per unofficial records, over 60,000 nurses are working in the Middle Eastern countries.

An early study on migration of physicians into the US was conducted by Thomas (1972). He argued that reasons for migration include professional isolation, heavy workload and lack of better career prospects encouraging migration of health professionals. He further argued that migration of physicians from the less developed countries to the developed countries was not only due to ‘Pull Factors’ from affluent countries. In fact there were ‘Push Factors’ in the donor countries (Thomas 1972). The study posited that push factors made it far more attractive for the physician to seek opportunities elsewhere than within his/her own country. For instance, nurses in most developing countries report low levels of job satisfaction due to heavy workloads, long work hours, staff shortage, dissatisfaction with wages (compared to alternative career options) and a general move towards a more ‘business’ mindset (Aiken 2002; Davis 2003). The direction of migration flows may also change over time. In the 1960s, many physicians working in developing countries originated from developed countries, but in the 1990s developing countries were estimated to supply about 56% of all the migrating physicians (UNCTAD 1998). Historical, administrative and legislative frameworks, training institutions, professional associations and regulation have influenced practices in former colonies and affected the migration of physicians for training and employment to the UK, and from North African and Middle Eastern countries to France.

Carmeli and Weisber (2006) found no significant relationship between turnover intention and job performance. The ‘survivors’ exhibited a higher level of performance relative to those who have left the organization. High rates of turnover weaken the structure of healthcare systems and impede the proper implementation of healthcare processes and procedures, thus impact healthcare systems’ ability to provide effective, efficient, safe and responsive care leading to negative care outcomes. Turnover directly impacts an institution’s ability of patient care; thus negatively affects the quality of services provided. High rates of turnover among medical professionals are likely to lead to shortage of healthcare staff and loss of human capital of experienced and skilful medical professionals, which jeopardize the quality of care patients receive (Contino 2002). Sharma and Agarwal (2010) reported that among the professionals at the physician and paramedical levels in Indian public hospitals, perceived organizational support (POS) negatively predicted turnover intentions of paramedical professionals while intra-professional support negatively predicted turnover intentions of professionals at the physician levels. It was concluded that the perception of peer and organizational support are important dimension of the perceived work environment in hospitals for reducing turnover intentions among medical and paramedical professionals.

Challenges for Indian Healthcare

The complex and dynamic relationship between India's adaption to the new global environment and Indian population heath, health systems and healthcare-related industries is one deserving of social science scrutiny. In the 1990s, civil society organizations actively campaigned against the healthcare reforms of the structural adjustment policy and produced considerable writings on the negative impact of this process on health and health services. A few landmark studies at that time charted the patterns of utilization of health services for acute and long-term treatment (Dilip 2005; UNDP 2010, 2011) and the costs incurred and its implications for equity (Krishnan 1999; Banerji 1993; Rao 2005).

Indian healthcare has seen standards rising over the past decade. Strategic foreign investment and collaboration opportunities have already arrived in the sector. Indian health professionals are exploring whether to offer a variety of health services to its customers hailing largely from India and from the neighbouring countries like Pakistan, Nepal and Bhutan. Customers from developed countries are also heading to India for their growing health needs. The combination of high quality services and low cost facilities is also attracting a stream of international patients as cost of advanced surgery in India is 10–15 times lower than anywhere in the world.

Medical tourism India or health tourism India is an emerging concept whereby people from all over the world visit India for their medical and relaxation needs. Furthermore, 100% FDI is permitted for health and medical services under the automatic route. Rising demand from the growing middle-class in India's large cities is fuelling growth in private sector healthcare. Large national and state government programmes will spur growth along the primary (and secondary) care sector and public health domain. In addition, there is substantial demand for high-quality and specialty healthcare services in tier-II and tier-III cities. All these factors have created a huge demand for quality healthcare services in the country.

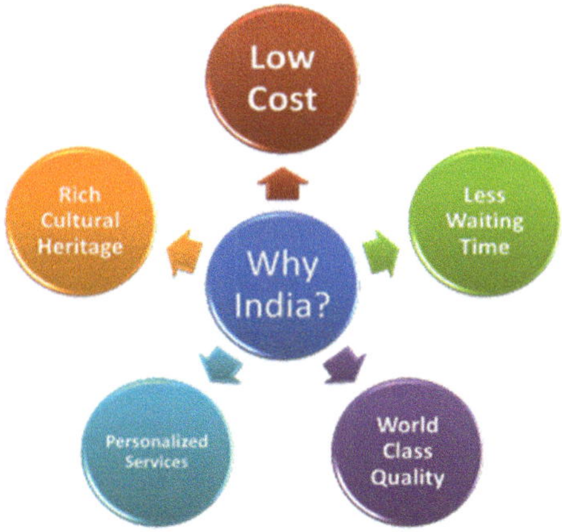
Low
Cost
Less
Waiting
Time
World
Class
Quality
Personalized
Services
Rich
Cultural
Heritage
Why
India?

The focal attraction for the medical tourists is the price factor or medical costs. Medical tourists believe that in India, the cost of surgery or other treatments is one tenth of what it is in European countries or in developed nations. Medical technology has improved drastically in private sector Indian hospitals and their standards have increased too, being at par with American and European countries. Among all the various treatments that are done in India, the commonest are heart surgery, Lasik eye surgery, cosmetic surgery, neurosurgery and dental care. India has some of the best hospitals and treatment centres in the world with the best facilities. Infrastructure, technology advancement, outstanding doctors and medical staffs, world-class hospitals, all these have made India the prime location or the top choice for medical tourists seeking overseas healthcare.

The emergence of medical tourism and swift development in technologies, has led to making the health sector as one of the fastest growing sectors in India. Several corporate and business organizations have forayed into the healthcare sector, resulting in the healthcare delivery system becoming more organized, systematic and efficient. This has subsequently led to a massive demand for qualified, well trained and dedicated healthcare management professionals.

Indian healthcare organizations require human resource management (HRM) practices that are unique and different from global HRM trends. The Indian culture is one that is deeply rooted in its societal and collectivistic values which respect for elders, joint family system, dignity for labour and shared responsibility as key components of the success of the Indian firm today. But HR practitioners in India depend largely on the models adopted by developed countries like USA and UK for emulating practices concerning the mode of hiring and managing healthcare professionals. However, the growing body of empirical research has found that HR practices are not always a source of sustained competitive advantage unless they are aligned with cultural and other contextual factors arising from the global operating environment since HRM practices are rooted deeply in the country's historical, cultural, social and political ethos. Therefore, a thorough understanding of the cultural and other contextual elements where HRM practices are being implemented is required in order to maximize the outcomes, as transfer of HRM practices occurs mostly from developed countries to developing ones (Aycan 2005). So the import or transfer of these practices from developed to the developing countries may produce unexpected results (Tanure and Duarte 2005).

Concluding Comments

Despite the fact that development of human resources practices plays an integral role within healthcare management, the importance of the HRM in healthcare, particularly the public sector, has been overlooked. Human Resource Management is strongly related to the success or failure of health system performance. It has been increasingly recognized that getting HR policy and management 'right' has to be at the core of any sustainable solution to health system performance. 'Performance' in the health sector can be fully assessed only with indicators that are sector-specific. These can focus on measures of clinical activity or workload (e.g. staff per occupied bed, or patient acuity measures), on measures of output (e.g. number of patients treated) or, less frequently, on measures of outcome (e.g. mortality rates; rate of post-surgery complications).

There is a need for assessing the HRD (Human Resource Development) climate in order to understand the preparedness of the hospital for initiating HRD practices. By and large, the HRD philosophy of a hospital is understood by ensuring the top management's commitment through HRD policy and the involvement of the line management. Aravind (2009) conducted a study on human resource development environment in a tertiary care teaching hospital. Ninety employees from a selected 1,000 bedded tertiary care teaching hospital were chosen using stratified proportionate random sample technique. Personnel engaged in healthcare delivery, were classified into three categories: clinical (34), administrative (20) and supportive staff (36). The study on human resource development environment pertained to teamwork, training, counselling and superior-subordinate relationship (SSR). Findings showed that teamwork, training and SSR had a moderate existence among the three categories of staff. However, availability of counselling facilities was poor for the clinical staff, but moderately good among administrative and supportive staff.

Internationally, the goal of contemporary workforce development thus, is to develop systems, processes and people that enhance client outcomes and operate in client rather than profession-centric ways. This requires systems-wide, interdisciplinary and outcomes-oriented frameworks (Cooper et al. 2004; Plesk and Greenhalgh 2001). This is more true in the context of healthcare organizations which are based on the talent, dedication and hard work of their employees. At the same time, it is also true that there is a huge diversity found in this type of organization which necessitates the formulation of sector-specific policies and programmes for the development of different calibre of knowledge and skills that can collaborate at the workplace, work in teams and achieve the goal of delivering quality of patient care. However, without an overarching conceptual framework to guide the formulation and implementation of such policies, the potential threat for working in professional isolation on matters related to health workforce planning remains. We need sector-specific outcome measures, such as quality of patient care, so as to devise a cross-functional/professional model, which encompasses human resource management, organizational development, clinical service planning and delivery of quality healthcare across different cultural settings.

References

Adrian, P. (1995). *The essence of service marketing*. New Delhi: Prentice-Hall of India.

Agarwal, M., Khanna, A., & Sharma, A. (2012). Organizational factors, fulfillment of the psychological contract and quality of patient-care in public hospitals. *Journal of Management Sciences, 3,* 66–83.

Agarwal, M., & Sharma, A. (2010). Relationship of workplace factors and job involvement of healthcare employees with quality of patient care in teaching and non-teaching hospitals. *Psychological Studies, 55,* 374–385.

Agarwal, M., & Sharma, A. (2011). Effects of hospital workplace factors on the psychological well-being and job satisfaction of healthcare employees. *Journal of Health Management, 13,* 439–461.

Agius, R. M., Blenkin, H., Deary, I. J., Zealley, H. E., & Wood, R. A. (1996). Survey of perceived stress and work demands of consultant doctors. *Occupational and Environmental Medicine, 53,* 217–224.

Aiken, L. H. (2002). Hospital nurse staffing and patient mortality, nurse burnout and job dissatisfaction. *JAMA, 288,* 1987–1993.

Alexopoulos, E. C., Burdorf, A., & Kalokerinou, A. (2003). Risk factors for musculoskeletal disorders among nursing personnel in Greek hospitals. *International Archives of Occupational and Environmental Health, 76,* 289–294.

Appleton, K., House, A., & Dowell, A. (1998). A survey of job satisfaction, sources of stress and psychological symptoms among general practitioners in Leeds. *British Journal of General Practitioners, 48,* 1059–1063.

Aravind, V. (2009). Study on human resource development environment in Atertiary care teaching hospitals. *Journal of the Academy of Hospital Administration, 21,* 21–27.

Aycan, Z. (2005). The interplay between cultural and institutional/structural contingencies in human resource management practice. *International Journal of Human Resource Management, 16,* 1083–1119.

Banerji, D. (1993). Simplistic approach to health policy analysis: World Bank team on Indian health sector. *Economic & Political Weekly, 28,* 1207–1210.

Bhandari, P., Bagga, R., & Nandan, D. (2010). Levels of job satisfaction among healthcare providers in CGHS dispensaries. *Journal of Health Management, 12,* 403–422.

Bhat, R., Venna, B. B., & Reuben, E. (2001). *An empirical analysis of district hospitals and grant-in-aid hospitals in Gujarat state of India*. Ahmedabad: Indian Institute of Management Ahmedabad.

Bisht, R., Pitchforth, E., & Murray, S. F. (2012). Understanding India, globalisation and healthcare systems: A mapping of research in the social sciences. *Globalization and Health, 8,* 32.

Caplan, R. D., Cobb, S., French, J. R. P., Van Harrison, R., & Pinneau, S. R. (1975). *Job demands and worker health: Main effects and occupational differences*. National Institute of Occupational Safety and Health Research Report, CT.

Carman, J. M. (1990). Consumer perceptions of service quality: An assessment of the SERVQUAL dimensions. *Journal of Retailing, 66,* 35–55.

Carmeli, A., & Weisberg, J. (2006). Exploring turnover intentions among three professional groups of employees. *Human Resource Development International, 9,* 191–206.

Chanda, R. (2002). Trade in health services. *Bulletin of the World Health Organization, 80,* 158–163.

Chaudhary, A. (1990). *A study of relationship between job satisfaction and role stress of bank officers.* Unpublished M.A. Dissertation, Department of Psychology, University of Rajasthan, Jaipur.

Chaudhury, S., & Bannerjee, A. (2004). Correlates of job satisfaction in medical officers'. *MJAFI, 60,* 329–332.

Contino, D. (2002). How to slash costly turnover. *Nursing Management, 33,* 10–13.

Cooper, H., Braye, S., & Geyer, R. (2004). Complexity and interprofessional education. *Learning in Health and Social Care, 3*(4), 179–189.

Cox, T., Tisserand, M., & Taris, T. (2005). Editorial: The conceptualization and measurement of burnout: Questions and directions. *Work & Stress, 19,* 187–191.

Cronin, J. J., Brandy, J. R. M. K., & Hult, G. T. M. (2000). Assessing the effects of quality, value, and customer satisfaction on consumer behavioral intentions in service environments. *Journal of Retailing, 76,* 193–218.

Cronin, J. J., & Taylor, S. A. (1992). Measuring service quality; a re-examination and extension. *The Journal of Marketing, 56,* 55–68.

Dasgupta, P. (2012). Effect of role ambiguity, conflict and overload in private hospitals' nurses' burnout and mediation through self efficacy. *Journal of Health Management, 14,* 513–534.

Davis, D. (2003). Nursing burnout and patient safety. *JAMA, 289*(5).

Dilip, T. (2005). Extent of inequity in access to healthcare services in India. In L. Gangolli, R. Duggal, & A. Shukla (Eds.), *Review of healthcare in India* (pp. 247–268). Mumbai: Centre for Enquiry into Health and Allied Themes.

Eriksen, W., Bruusgaard, D., & Knardahl, S. (2003). Work factors as predictors of sickness absence: A three month prospective study of nurses' aides. *Occupational and Environmental Medicine, 60,* 271–278.

Escribá-Agüir, V., Pérez-Hoyos, S., & Bolumar, F. (1993). Effects of work organization on the mental health of nursing staff. *Journal of Nursing Management, 1,* 3–8.

Firth-Conzens, J., & Greenhalgh, J. (1997). Doctors' perceptions of the links between stress and lowered clinical care. *Social Science and Medicine, 44,* 1017–1022.

Fisher, C., Harris, L., Kirk, S., Leopold, J., & Leverment, Y. (2004). The dynamics of modernisation and job satisfaction in the British National Health Service. *Review of Public Personnel Administration, 24,* 304–318.

Forcier, M. B. (2004). Impact, regulation and health policy implications of physician migration in OECD Countries. *Human Resources for Health*, 2.

Garvin, D. (1984). What does product quality really mean? *Sloan Management Review, 26,* 25–43.

Garvin, D. (1988). *Managing quality—The strategic and competitive edge.* New York: Free Press.

Government of India. (2001). *Report of the high level commission on the Indian.*

Grembowski, D. (2005). Managed care, physician job satisfaction, and the quality of primary care. *Journal of General Internal Medicine, 20,* 271–277.

Grol, R., Mokkink, H., van Eijk, J., Beek, M., Mesker, P., & Mesker-Niesten, J. (1985). Work satisfaction of general practitioners and the quality of patient care. *Family Practice, 2,* 128–135.

Gronroos, C. (1984). A service quality model and its marketing implications. *European Journal of Marketing, 18,* 36–44.

Haas, J. S., Cook, E. F., Puopolo, A. L., Burstin, H. R., Cleary, P. D., & Brennan, T. A. (2000). Is the professional satisfaction of general internists associated with patient satisfaction? *Journal of General Internal Medicine, 15,* 122–128.

Hillhouse, J. J., & Adler, C. M. (1997). Investigating stress effect patterns in hospital staff nurses: Results of a cluster analysis, *45,* 1781–1788.

Kanjanapan, W. (1995). The immigration of Asian professionals to the United States: 1988-1990. *International Migration Review, 29,* 7–32.

Kerr, E. A., Mittman, B. S., Hays, R. D., Zemencuk, J. K., Pitts, J., & Brook, R. (2000). Associations between primary care physician satisfaction and self-reported aspects of utilization management. *Health Services Research, 35,* 333–349.

Kersley, B., Alpin, C., Forth, J., Bryson, A., Bewley, H., Dix, G., et al. (2006). *Inside the workplace: Findings from the 2004 workplace employment relations survey.* London: Routledge.

Koeck, C. M. (1997). Doing better: A global medical interest. In V. A. Kazandjian (Ed.), *The effectiveness of CQI in healthcare: Stories from a global perspective*. Milwaukee, WI: ASQC Quality Press.

Krishnan, T. N. (1999). *Access to health and the burden of Treatment: An international comparison. In disinvesting in health: The world bank's prescription for health.* New Delhi: Sage.

Leggat, S. G., Bartram, T., Casimir, G., & Stanton, P. (2010). Nurse perceptions of the quality of patient care: Confirming the importance of empowerment and job satisfaction. *Healthcare Management Review*, 35.

Leiter, M. P., Harvie, P., & Frizzell, C. (1998). The correspondence of patient satisfaction and nurse burnout. *Social Science and Medicine, 47,* 1611–1617.

Mahal, A., Singh, J., Afridi, F., Lamba, V., Gumber, A., & Selvaraju, V. (2002). *Who benefits from public health spending in India: Results of a benefit incidence analysis for India.* New Delhi: NCAER.

Mehta, S. (2011). Service quality as predicator of patient satisfaction: A study of the healthcare sector. *Journal of Health Management, 13*(2), 211–229.

Murray, A., Montgomery, J. E., Chang, H., Rogers, W. H., Inui, T., & Safran, D. G. (2001). Doctor discontent. A comparison of physician satisfaction in different delivery system settings, 1986 and 1997. *Journal of General Internal Medicine, 16*, 451–459.

O'Brien-Pallas, L., Tomblin Murphy, G., & Shamian, J. (2008). *Final report: Understanding the costs and outcomes of nurses' turnover in Canadian hospitals.* Toronto: Nursing Health Services Research Unit, University of Toronto.

Padilla, P. (2006). Nurse migration and nursing shortage. *Imprint, 53,* 18–24.

Parasuraman, A., Valarie, A. Z., & Leonard, L. B. (1985). A conceptual model of service quality and its implications for future research. *Journal of Marketing, 49,* 41–50.

Pareek, U. (1983). Organisational role stress. In L. D. Goodstein & J. W. Pfeiffer (Eds.), *The 1983 annual for facilitators, trainers, and consultants* (pp. 115–118). San Diego, CA: University Associates.

Parikh, P., Taukariand, A., & Bhattacharya, T. (2004). Occupational stress and coping among nurses. *Journal of Health Management, 6,* 115–127.

Peccei, R. (2004). *Human resource management and the search for the happy workplace.* Rotterdam: Erasmus Research Institute of Management.

Pestonjee, D. M., & Mishra, P. K. (1999). Role stress and job satisfaction among doctors. *Journal of Health Management, 1,* 117–131.

Piko, B. (1999). Work-related stress among nurses: A challenge for healthcare institutions. *The Journal of the Royal Society for the Promotion of Health, 119,* 156–162.

Plsek, P. E., & Greenhalgh, T. (2001). The challenge of complexity in healthcare. *British Medical Journal,* 323, 625–628.

Rafnsdottir, G. L., Gunnarsdottir, H. K., & Tomasson, K. (2004). Work organization, well-being and health in geriatric care. *Work: A Journal of Prevention Assessment & Rehabilitation, 22,* 49–55.

Rameshan, P., & Singh, S. (2005). Quality of health delivery system: A case of customer orientation of primary health centres. *Journal of Health Management, 7,* 189–206.

Ramirez, A. J., Graham, J., Richards, M. A., Cull, A., & Gregory, W. M. (1996). Mental health of hospital consultants: The effects of stress and satisfaction at work. *Lancet, 347,* 724–728.

Ram-Persaud, C. (2007). India's middle class failure. *Prospect Magazine,* 138. http://www.prospectmagazine.co.uk/article_details.php?id=9776webcite.

Rao, S. (2005). *Financing and delivery of health services in India*. New Delhi: Ministry of Health and Family Welfare, Government of India.
Reddy, K. S. (2013). Health beyond healthcare. *Hindustan Times* (p. 9). Retrieved November 29.
Revicki, D. A., Whitley, T. W., & Gallery, M. E. (1993). Organizational characteristics, perceived work stress, and depression in emergency medicine residents. *Behavioral Medicine, 19*(2), 74–81.
Saha, D., Sinha, R., & Bhavsar, K. (2011). Understanding job stress among healthcare staff. *Online Journal of Health Allied Sciences, 10*, 6.
Shah, N., & Dhar, U. (2007). Constituent factors of HRD in healthcare: A comparative study of hospitals in India and the USA. *Journal of Health Management, 9,* 317–342.
Shamian, J., Kerr, M., Lachinger, H. K. S., Thomson, D. (2002). A hospital-level analysis of the work environment and workforce health indicator for registered nurses in Ontario's acute care hospitals. *Canadian Journal of Nursing, 33,* 35–50.
Shanafelt, T. D., Bradley, K. A., Wipf, J. E., & Back, A. L. (2002). Burnout and self-reported patient care in an internal medicine residency program. *Annual International Medicine, 136,* 358–367.
Sharma, A., & Agarwal, M. (2010). Hospitals' work environment, mental health status and turnover intentions among medical professionals. *Indo Indian Journal of Social Science Research, 5*(1), 33–44.
Sharma, E. (2005). Role stress among doctors. *Journal of Health Management, 7,* 151.
Sharma, K., & Zodpey, S. (2011). Demand and supply analysis of human resource capacity for hospital management in India. *Journal of Health Management, 13,* 155.
Sibbald, B., & Bojke, C. (2004). *General practitioner job satisfaction in England.* Manchester: National Primary Care Research and Development Centre.
Simoens, S., Scott, A., & Sibbald, B. (2002). Job satisfaction, work related stress and intentions to quit of Scottish GPS. *Scott Medical Journal, 47,* 80–86.
Stilwell, B. (2004). Migration of healthcare workers from developing countries: Strategic approaches to its management. *Bulletin of the World Health Organization, 82,* 595–600.
Stoddard, J. J., Hargraves, J. L., Reed, M., & Vratil, A. (2001). Managed care, professional autonomy, and income: Effects on physician career satisfaction. *Journal of General Internal Medicine, 16,* 675–684.
Sudhaker, C., & Gomes, L. A. (2010). Job stress, coping strategies and the job quality index of selected nurses working in selected multispeciality hospitals-towards human resource development. *Journal of the Academy of Hospital Administration, 22,* 10–14.
Tankha, G. (2006). A comparative study of role stress in government and private hospital nurses. *Journal of Health Management, 8,* 11–18.
Tanure, B., & Duarte, R. G. (2005). Leveraging competitiveness upon national cultural traits; the management of people in Brazilian companies. *International Journal of Human Resource Management, 16,* 2201–2217.
Tarnow-Mordi, W. O., Hau, C., Warden, A., & Shearer, A. J. (2000). Hospital mortality in relation to staff workload: A 4-year study in an adult intensive-care unit. *Lancet, 356*, 185–189.
Teas, R. K. (1993). Expectations, performance evaluation, and consumers' perceptions of quality. *Journal of Marketing, 57*, 18–34.
Thomas, D. (1972). The migration of physicians to the United States. *New England Journal of Medicine, 286,* 870–876.
Tómasson, K., Gunnarsdóttir, H. K., Rafnsdóttir, G. L., & Helgadóttir, B. (2004). Correlates of probable alcohol abuse among women working in nursing homes. *Journal of Public Health, 32,* 47–52.
Trinkoff, A., & Storr, C. (1998). Substance use among nurses: Differences between specialties. *American Journal of Public Health, 88,* 581–585.
Uncu, Y., Bayram, N., & Bilgel, N. (2007). Job related affective well-being among primary healthcare physicians. *European Journal of Public Health, 17,* 514–519.
UNCTAD Secretariat. (1998). International trade in health services: Difficulties and opportunities for developing countries In S. Zarrilli & C. Kinnon (Eds.), *International trade in health services: A development perspective.*

UNDP. (2010). *Human development report 2010 the real wealth of nations. Pathways to human development*. New York: UNDP.

UNDP. (2011). *Human development report 2011 sustainability and equity: A better future for all*. New York: UNDP.

Vroom, V. H. (1964). *Work and motivation*. New York: Wiley.

Wahlstedt, K., & Edling, C. (1994). Psychosocial factors and their relations to psychosomatic complaints amongst postal workers. *European Journal of Public Health*, 460–64.

Wall, T. D., Bolden, R. I., Borilla, C. S., Carter, A. J., Golya, D. A., Hardy, G. E., et al. (1997). Minor psychiatric disorder in NHS trust staff: Occupational and gender differences. *British Journal of Psychiatry, 171*, 519–523.

Warr, P. (2002). The study of well-being, behaviour and attitudes. In P. Warr (Ed.), *Psychology at work* (pp. 1–25). London: Penguin Books.

Warr, P., Cook, J., & Wall, T. (1979). Scales for the measurement of some work attitudes and aspects of psychological well being. *Journal of Occupational Psychology, 52*, 129–48.

West, E. (2001). Management matters: The link between hospital organization and quality of patient care. *Quality in Healthcare, 10*, 40–48.

WHO. (2000). *Health systems: Improving performance: The World Development Report 2000*. Geneva: WHO.

Chapter 23
Well-Being and Mental Health in the Aftermath of Disasters: A Social Constructionist Approach

Kumar Ravi Priya

Well-Being and Mental Health: A Critical Overview

Besides the absence of disease or disorders, the World Health Organization (WHO) posits well-being as an important element of health: 'Health is a state of complete physical, mental and social well-being and not merely the absence of disease or infirmity' WHO (2013, ¶ 2). As apparent from this definition of health, mental health may be considered as an aspect of well-being. As per WHO (2013), 'Mental health is defined as a state of well-being in which every individual realizes his or her own potential, can cope with the normal stresses of life, can work productively and fruitfully, and is able to make a contribution to her or his community' (¶ 1). However, a close look at the existing literature on well-being and mental health explicates the following limitations in the use of these concepts (Hird 2003; Misra 2010; Sinha 1990):

1. There is no consensus on the definition of well-being.
2. Well-being is studied as a separate concept from mental health with studies on mental health largely focusing on the prevalence of mental disorders.
3. Well-being is taken to be an intra-psychic entity experienced uniformly across human population as an indicator or adjustment to or control over environment.
4. Well-being is taken to be an acultural and apolitical concept and how it may be threatened or reformulated within the political or cultural context is not taken to be important.

Clearly, out of the four limitations listed above, the last one is the most debilitating for disaster survivors as their distress is shaped by the dynamic socio-political context of the post-disaster settings. The multidisciplinary approa-

K. R. Priya (✉)
Department of Humanities and Social Sciences, Indian Institute of Technology Kanpur, Kanpur 208016, Uttar Pradesh, India
e-mail: krp@iitk.ac.in

G. Misra (ed.), *Psychosocial Interventions for Health and Well-Being*,
https://doi.org/10.1007/978-81-322-3782-2_23

ches to disaster mental health, rather than taking well-being as a static intra-psychic phenomenon, tend to focus on how well-being or the coherence of selfhood may be threatened and reformulated within the socio-political and cultural context during the post-disaster period. This chapter focuses on the use of social constructionist paradigm that facilitates the use of a multidisciplinary approach, through the concepts of suffering and healing to understand the survivors' experiences of threat to or reformulation of well-being. To do this, the concepts of suffering and healing are elaborated with the help of examples from diverse post-disaster settings in the world. However, let us first take a look at the critique of mainstream psychological or psychiatric approaches to well-being or mental health in the aftermath of disasters.

Deconstructing Psychiatric Approach to Disaster Mental Health

In the domain of mental health, the positivist influences have been critiqued prominently in terms of 'category fallacy' (Kleinman 1987) of the categories of psychiatric disorders imported from Western psychiatry to the cultures marked by more socio-centric worldview of human nature (Lewis-Fernandez and Kleinman 1994). Several researchers of psychological impact of disaster trauma such as Bracken et al. (1995), Marsella and Christopher (2004), Priya (2013a, b), Summerfield (1999) and Weiss et al. (2003) delineated a paradox in the use of posttraumatic stress disorder (PTSD) to understand the impact of traumatic events in non-Western cultures. As they pointed out, PTSD is taken to be a universal intra-psychic phenomenon caused by trauma blocking the cognitive and emotional processing of the event but as Summerfield (1999) posited,

> Many ethnomedical systems have taxonomies which range across the physical, supernatural and moral realms, and do not conceive of illness as situated in body or mind alone.... Western trauma theory, which likens the brain to a machine and sees PTSD as the result of incomplete emotional and cognitive processing within that machine, cannot make sense in such settings. (Bracken et al. 1995, p. 1455)

Such a paradox that prevails in the uncritical use of PTSD could lead to a category fallacy as Summerfield maintains, 'Though the trauma literature suggests that PTSD has a worldwide prevalence, it is a mistake to assume that because phenomena can be regularly identified in different social settings, they mean the same thing in those settings. This is what Kleinman (1987) called a category fallacy'. (1999, p. 1454)

With the help of their research conducted in the non-Western world, Bracken et al. (1995), Priya (2012a) and Summerfield (1999) have illustrated that despite the prevalence of PTSD symptoms among the survivors of disasters, these were not what they themselves were concerned about or attending to. For example, in his study of war displaced rural peasants in Nicaragua, Summerfield and Toser (1991) found PTSD symptoms to be common among the survivors but they could not be taken to be psychological casualties as per their perception. They rather expressed how they were caring for their relationships amidst poverty and continued threat of future attacks. In another study in the same country, Summerfield and Hume (1993) noted that the war-injured ex-soldiers also showed PTSD features but they were not experiencing any dysfunction and their concerns were to explore the possibility for work and training. Bracken et al. (1995) searched for PTSD symptoms among the rape victims of civil war-related violence in Uganda and found these to be present but rather than these symptoms, the victims' concern was the fear rejection by the society (where women's fertility is given importance) owing to their perceived infertility that resulted from the sexual assault that they underwent. Similarly, in my studies among disaster survivors in India, I noticed the presence of PTSD symptoms in a widow's (whose husband had died in an earthquake in Kachchh, Gujarat) account but she was deeply distressed by the fact that as per the Hindu religious customs related to widowhood, she might not be allowed to participate in the marriage ceremony of her granddaughters (Priya 2007). Also, among the child survivors of communal riots, Priya (2012b) found PTSD symptoms being present but what dominated some children's concern was the ruining of friendship with the children of other religion who they used to play with.

Besides misinterpreting the experiences, an uncritical use of diagnostic categories such as PTSD[1] may also run the risk of ignoring the varied experiences of distress across cultures (Pedersen 2002). Since the advent of interpretive turn in social sciences, there has been a growing realization about the promise of social constructionist paradigm in psychological understanding of the socio-culturally and historically contextualized human experiences (Gergen 1985, 2009; Marsella 1998; Misra and Gergen 1993; Sampson 1993). Thus, this paradigm has the potential to facilitate the understanding of survivors' distress and recovery towards well-being within the post-disaster socio-historical context.

Suffering and Healing: Reconstructing Threat to and Reformulation of Survivors' Well-Being

Taxonomies of illness or distress in the ethnomedical systems of diverse cultures reflect and are intricately associated with shared notions of selfhood or personhood in the respective cultures (Bracken et al. 1995; Cassell 2004; Lewis-Fernandez and Kleinman 1994; Priya 2015). For example, Kleinman (1988b) illustrated how a demoralized North American woman accepted her problems as dysphoria that she perceived to be caused by her lack of self-efficacy (and control), an important aspect of the culturally valued model of selfhood in her culture. However, a Chinese

[1]See Quosh and Gergen (2008) and Young (1995) for a fuller version of the critique of exclusive focus of psychology and psychiatry on PTSD.

person experiences his distress or demoralization as 'loss of face' for his inability to engage in 'reciprocal affective relationship guided by moral norms', something that forms the basis of his socio-centric self (Lewis-Fernandez and Kleinman 1994, p. 69).

Conceptualizing Suffering and Healing

It becomes clear from above that an understanding of distress, well-being or mental health is hinged on the notions of selfhood of the distressed person within the socio-cultural context. The concepts of suffering and healing may play an important role in understanding the threat to and reformulation of survivors' well-being during the post-disaster period. According to Cassell (2004, 2013) and Kleinman (1988a, b), suffering may be understood as an experience of intense distress when the intactness or coherence of selfhood is threatened. As Cassell (2004) points out, that the coherence of selfhood or personhood is shaped with the cultural and the relational context,

> People can suffer from what they have lost of themselves in relation to the world of objects, events, and relationships. Such suffering occurs because our intactness as persons, our coherence and integrity, come not only from intactness of the body but also from the wholeness of the web of relationships with self and others. (p. 38)

These authors also point out that healing is the process of reformulation of selfhood where the person develops an enabling meaning in life through the cultural beliefs or symbols or the 'culturally authorized interpretations' (Kleinman 1988b, p. 134) of the events or aspects of social world associated with distress.

Although suffering and healing are conceptually related to selfhood or personhood, literature shows that there are reasons to understand these as closely related to well-being when considered from a cultural psychological perspective. It has been indicated that well-being may be taken to be the coherence of experience (Hird 2003). Sinha (1990) considered psycho-social well-being to be strongly associated with one's existential condition. Misra (2010) and Lewis-Fernandez and Kleinman (1994) conceptualized well-being to be able to maintain one's coherence of selfhood that for the societies with socio-centric worldview, is rooted in harmony within relationships. Thus, suffering, that is considered to be intense distress arising out of threat to coherence or intactness of selfhood, may also be considered to be a threat to one's well-being. Similarly, healing may be understood as the process of recovery towards well-being.

Before we begin to take a look at the various aspects of suffering and healing processes with some illustrative examples, it is pertinent to note that the literature points to various themes of suffering that the disaster survivors may undergo. Researchers following multidisciplinary approaches to disaster mental health have noted several aspects of suffering (Abramowitz 2005; Bracken et al. 1995; Han 2004; Priya 2010, 2012b, 2013a, 2015; Summerfield 1999):

- Demoralization or intense distress associated with one's failure to abide by cultural values,
- Intense distress associated with a denial of experiential space, and
- Intense distress associated with disaggregation of relationships caused by political violence and atrocious events.

It should be noted that these aspects of post-disaster suffering may also be understood as socio-morally generated distress or suffering since these denote how the coherence of survivors' selfhood is threatened due to the moral expectations from oneself and the socio-political forces.

Suffering as Demoralization

If culture may be understood as 'as value commitments and moral orientations more akin to faith that are embodied in, and experienced by, individuals as what is at stake in specific, local setting (Lewis-Fernandez and Kleinman 1994 definition of culture p. 68)', then the survivors' suffering may arise from their inability to adhere to the socio-moral demands in the local moral worlds. Such an experience of intense distress has been termed as demoralization (Kleinman 1988a) and is consistent with Cassell's (2004) definition of suffering where it is assumed that the coherence of selfhood or personhood is shaped within the cultural context. For example, in their study conducted in the battle-torn Uganda in 1980s, Bracken et al. (1995) observed that survivors reported that their suffering arose primarily from the disruption of social or moral order due to war and atrocities:

> A 28 year old woman who witnessed her husband being killed by the army was unable to bury his body as she was forced to flee the area immediately with her children, for fear that she herself, would be killed. When she was able to return 6 months later his body could not be traced. When she was seen by members of our team some 5 years later she was still haunted by nightmares and feelings of shame because she had not been able to bury her husband according to traditional rites. It was this aspect of her loss that she spoke most about when interviewed and which seemed to cause her most distress. (p. 1077)

Abramowitz (2005), in his study of the survivors of violent conflicts between the military and rebel groups in Guinea Languette (geo-political region of Guinea bound on its southern flanks by Liberia and Sierra Leone in Africa), observed the agonized survivors narrating how their source of distress was the collective violation of the shared cultural values of nurturing the community rather than one's own self:

> The poor have become rich and the rich have become poor. There is no respect in my community. No more values or morals exist in my community. Many of us have the experience of feeling less important in our communities. Women are involved in doing things that aren't good; for example, prostitution. Nobody has time for anyone any longer, no regard, and no respect. People have lost everything, and they are not happy. There are people who cry in their minds…you have to be with them before you know. There are no good relationships between people. (p. 2112)

Similarly, in his study of the survivors of an earthquake that hit Kachchh district of Gujarat, India, Priya (2005) noted a participant, Amba Bhai (a 46 year old tailor who lost his 78-year-old mother in the earthquake) expressing his distress associated with his brother's non-adherence to the cultural values of caring for the family members,

> My brother didn't come out to be responsible enough. According to the social norms, mother, father and unmarried sisters stay with youngest brother. But, only after 15 days, my father and sister had to come to my house as my brother didn't like to keep them well. In such a situation, I get some solace by remembering God. (p. 111)

Suffering as the Denial of an Experiential Space

Another aspect of the post-disaster suffering is the denial of voice or an experiential space to the survivors when the sociopolitical conditions or the cultural norms do not allow for having a meaning in life in accordance with one's self of selfhood. For example, Bracken et al. (1995) in a study in the socio-centric culture of Uganda mentioned above noted how a woman survivor's suffering was associated with her unfulfilled longing for living with her children besides the denial of her acceptance as a rape victim by her husband:

> A 34-year-old woman with five children had been rejected by her husband because of the fact that she had been raped by two soldiers five years prior to her interview with us. He had turned her off the smallholding which she had cultivated. As the rest of her own family had perished or been dispersed in the war, she had to survive on what she could find in the bush until ultimately she found her way to the home of some distant relatives who took her in. Unable to explain what had happened to her because of the shame she felt regarding her circumstances and the fear of further rejection if her plight was known, she relinquished any rights she had to the land and to her children and remained in the position of a servant in her relatives' home. Five years later she was still suffering terrible grief over the loss of her children and had had no other relationship during that period. (1079)

In the Indian post-disaster setting of Marathwada earthquake, Acharya (2000) noted that surgical operation to regain fertility was forced on women who had lost their son in the earthquake. Despite the proposal of the surgical operation being unnerving, their choice of not opting for it was denied by the patriarchal norms:

> Almost all women, though scared, opted for the operation with a fatalistic attitude. '…We have lost everything in the earthquake… if we have to die we will…' 'I was scared but there are no choices…' (p. 561)

Importantly, the women were also distressed fearing the condition that if the surgical operation didn't come out to be successful, it could result in stigma or an end of the marriage:

> The absence of any sign of pregnancy was a new source of distress for them. One woman stated, 'As the date of menses approaches, I wait and hope to miss my periods, for it would mean that I have conceived. But, when I get them, I feel helpless once again.' Another

> woman stated, 'When I came out of the debris it was my second birth, I died once again after the operation, as in spite of it, I am not able to conceive… the expectations have been raised in vain… my life is meaningless now… my husband is remarrying since I have not conceived in the last one year. (p. 562)

Suffering as Disaggregation of Relationships

The multidisciplinary research on disaster mental health also delineates survivors' suffering due to a damage to the relational networks (caused by the social hierarchy or socio-political conditions emerging in the post-disaster period; Priya 2005) that shape their coherence of selfhood. This aspect of suffering has also been termed as disaggregation of relationships by Lewis-Fernandez and Kleinman (1994). Let us take up some illustrative examples of this.

In my study of the survivors of Kachchh earthquake in India, a participant, Krishna Bhai, a 38-year-old poor farmer earning his livelihood through *sukhi kheti* (farmland completely dependent on rainwater) who lost his 12-year-old daughter in the earthquake, shared his frustration of being looked down upon by some of the villagers (Priya 2005):

> You must have noticed so many people playing cards near the *chowk* (referring to the main T-point the village where there is a PCO shop). They have lots of money because their family members are in Mumbai. But they do not have anything to do. They have the *vari* [farmland with a facility of electric pump set for irrigation]. I do not have sufficient money to buy the pump set for irrigation. I just have *sukhi kheti*. They do not have time to even look at us or talk to us in a dignified manner. Everything has changed after the earthquake. (p. 150)

Han (2004), in her ethnographic study of trauma among the inhabitants of Satiago, Chile resulting from historical changes in the country's political and economic scenario from being a socialist to a capitalist state elaborates on the disaggregation of relationships within a family. The socialist mother, Leticia, strongly identified with her ideology and activism during the earlier political regime but her children rejected her ideological discourse and her pain caused by the political change. Han explains,

> She then asked me, 'Do you see a *familia integrada aquí*(an integrated, close family)?' I responded, 'Here? Here, in this house?' 'Yes,' she replied. I hesitated, hoping to forestall judgement, not knowing quite what to say. She replied impatiently, '*Obvio* (obvious), no, look everyone here is *en su lado* (off on his own). I work for *lo social* (the social) and here, in my own house, everyone is alone.' Her feelings of guilt were palpable, as was a certain subjective crisis in which the compulsory obligation of motherhood and family relationships threw into doubt her discursive practices, and even more, shook her conception and experience of the everyday. (p. 176)

Leticia also attributed the difficult family relationships to her own decisions in the past. She was caught in a situation where it was difficult to manage political activism that she was committed to and her role as a mother to her children as she had to flee her home and her country to escape the brunt of being taken as 'terrorist',

> I feel *un conflicto por adentro* (an internal conflict). Perhaps if I had not left the country, if I had been a mother to the children, then maybe they would not fight with me. And maybe they would be more committed to remembering. Of course I feel guilt, but they also mistreatme. Just today, Julieta mistreated me, Darwin mistreated me, and Lorenzo mistreated me. Julieta thinks only of her family [her husband Jorge and their children]. They don't share. And look at Lorenzo, he's 22 years old and he acts like he is 15. (p. 176)

Healing: Process of Attaining Well-Being

Amidst threats to the coherence to selfhood or well-being of a survivor, there are cultural resources such as beliefs and values that may give hope to the survivors as Das and Kleinman (2002) noted, 'there usually is no complete defeat, no ultimate breakdown and dissolution' following a traumatic event. These cultural beliefs and symbols also facilitate the process of healing, that is, developing an enabling meaning in life (Cassell 2013; Kleinman 1988a, b).

Priya (2014) illustrated how the survivors' cultural belief in *karma* (internalized duties towards oneself, family, community and other beings of nature) facilitated the process of developing an enabling meaning in life through a sense of transcendental self, *shanti* (peace of mind) and inspiration to contribute to the growth of humanity and other beings of nature.

The belief in karma provided the survivors a re-affirmation in their faith and enabled them to focus on current duties towards family, community and humanity, and transcend the distress that they attributed to their negligence of such duties in the past. Krishna Bhai, 38 years of age, who lost his 12-year-old daughter in the earthquake, shared with us,

> We are experiencing *dukh* due to our indulgence in *paap* in the past or in *purv janm* (previous birth). In this life also, in the past, we committed paap (sin or non-adherence to karma). For example, when Kargil war[2] took place, people of Kachchh didn't give any financial support but, now in the troubled time of Kachchh, people from outside have come to provide all kinds of support. I have decided that I am going to build a structure where animals like cow and birds can have some cereals to eat. Let us do something for others. What shall we take with us after we die? (p. 356)

In Maya Ben's (a 48-year-old woman who lost her husband in the earthquake) account one may observe how the culturally valued belief in karma was influential in generating shanti or peace of mind,

---

[2]'Kargil war' is the name given to an Indian Armed Forces' mission in the state to Jammu and Kashmir to counter the infiltrators who had crossed the Line of Control from Pakistan. These infiltrators waged a mini-war with the Indian Armed Forces in 1999.

> My only son who lives in Mumbai, calls me there feeling that I would be lonely here. But, I do not like to leave this place. I have brought back one of my granddaughters from Mumbai and I look after her. Living at this place, I would be able to do some *punya* like, *sewa* or service to animals, birds, cow and poor people. Living here doing this gives me shanti.

Paras Bhai, a 42-year-old daily-wage labourer, received Rs. 80,000 as compensation money from the government for the death of her 13-year-old daughter in the earthquake. He added Rs. 20,000 to this amount and used this sum to rebuild the bus stop of the village that was devastated in the earthquake. He shared that he did feel sad whenever he came across the bus stop but at the same time, also felt motivated to carry out his karma with compassion towards all beings of nature,

> The death of my beloved daughter showed to me that our lives and those of our loved ones won't last forever. Therefore, whatever time we have in this world, we must try to do whatever we can for the society and humanity. Building the bust stop for the village was a small step in this direction (p. 358).

Psycho-Social Interventions After Disasters

What this chapter has attempted to highlight is that PTSD or mental disorders may constitute only an aspect of post-disaster suffering and the other socio-morally generated distress may be largely ignored by the psychiatric or medical model of health and illness. Before highlighting how a psycho-social intervention for the survivors going through socio-moral distress or suffering may be facilitated through the cultural healing process, let us develop some insight into the contemporary ways to address the psychiatric disorders such as PTSD faced by the disaster survivors.

Treatment for PTSD Within Cultural Context

Notwithstanding the widely held critique of the cross-cultural validity of PTSD, Kienzler (Kinezler 2008), in her reviews of psychological impact of disasters, pointed out that PTSD as a predominant psychiatric outcome could be prevalent across cultures particularly if the traumatic experience for the person is intense. The recent reviews of prevalence studies in the aftermath of natural, technological and human-made (involving wars, political conflicts, terrorist attacks etc.) have reported the prevalence rate of PTSD between 2.3 and 44.6% (Neria et al. 2007; Yasan et al. 2009).

In their review article, Cukor et al. (2009) have summarized the developments in treatment programmes for PTSD. They have noted that various treatment approaches based on cognitive-behavioural therapy (CBT) such as exposure therapy, cognitive processing therapy (CPT), eye movement desensitization and reprocessing (EMDR) have been some of the most effective treatments of PTSD. However, the promises of behavioural treatments (targeting behavioural change through learning new response patterns), imagery-based treatments (bringing about change through changes in the ways of information processing), therapies focussed on distress tolerance, and internet and computer-based treatments have also been highlighted by these researchers. They have also reported the attempts at addressing relational issues associated with PTSD through social and family-based treatments and interpersonal psychotherapy besides pointing out that the evidence for the efficacy of psychiatric drug treatment have not been clearly established. While improvement in the success-failure ratio of the therapeutic outcomes remains a major area of concern in research on psychotherapy for PTSD, in a recent meta-analytic research, Benish et al. (2008) have reported a path-breaking finding that despite the evidence of the efficacy of various therapies ranging from CBT, psychodynamic therapy, EMDR, exposure therapy to trauma desensitization compared to the control groups, it was not the type of therapy that predicted their success.

If not the type of therapy or some specific elements within a therapy that predicted efficaciousness of therapies, then what led to the desired change in the clients' experiences? The authors have indicated possibility of some factors common within these therapies that potentially led to the success. A paradigm shift in the understanding of factors predicting positive results of therapies for various psychiatric disorders faced by the clients has been brought about by a seminal volume titled, *The Heart and Soul of Change: Delivering What Works in Therapy,* published by the American Psychological Association (Hubble et al. 2010). Various chapters of this have detailed that factors, including *self-generated change by the clients*, and *goal consensus and collaboration within therapeutic relationship,* which may be common in different types of psychotherapies predict the successful outcomes of these therapies. Generally, these two factors also assume importance as these incorporate the crucial input in terms of the cultural context and cultural meanings of health and illness. Anderson et al. (2010, p. 156) posits, 'Working within the cultural context of the healing setting requires therapists to be empathically attuned to the client's cultural experiences, beliefs, and values.' In a similar vein, Marsella and Christopher (2004) recommend that the personnel who would provide psycho-social help or therapy in the post-disaster settings should be trained in cultural competency that is focused on

> understanding the nature and meaning of culture and on cultural variations in various aspects of mental disorders and services. Eventually, a core of knowledge can be developed for specific cultural groups and for the understanding of general cultural variations in disaster responses. (p. 534)

Post-disaster Healing: Towards Cultural Humility and Cultural Safety

Returning to the concern of psycho-social rehabilitation (or healing) for the forms of suffering other than PTSD or other psychiatric disorders, it is important to recall that post-disaster settings may generally induce socio-morally generated suffering due to a failure to abide by culturally valued norms (demoralization), a denial of experiential space by socio-political or cultural forces, and the disaggregation of relationships caused by political violence or atrocious events. Kirmayer's (2012) observation that conceptualizing culture merely as cultural beliefs, ethnic identities or traits of people belonging to a community might not help to plan or improve effective mental health services also holds true for addressing post-disaster suffering induced by the cultural or socio-political context. He recognizes, for mental health in general and psycho-social rehabilitation of or healing of suffering too, that the definition of 'culture' needs to incorporate 'unique social context of knowledge and power at the levels of individuals, families, communities and larger social systems' that pivotally shapes human suffering (p. 251). Healing of the socio-morally generated suffering, thus, entails not only the details of the cultural context on the part of the potential helpers but also a realization of a 'limited access to insider culture knowledge and the need to respect and be open to clients' own culturally-based understandings' (*cultural humility*) of the 'responsibility to work to make the clinical encounter safe by acknowledging and addressing structural violence and inequality', also termed as *cultural safety* (p. 251).

Finally, the focus on healing process also entails understanding experiences within cultural and socio-political context utilizing ethnographic or qualitative methods. As far as the impact of mental health services goes, Kirmayer (2012, p. 254) accentuates the need for 'both experience-near narrative methods and assessment of social ecosystems' along with the social justice the survivors expect from the social structure or the state.

Concluding Comments: A Note on Research Methodology

The chapter attempted to provide some insights into how the social constructionist approach may be useful in understanding disaster mental health through the concepts of suffering and healing that locate the experiences of threat to and reformulation of coherence of selfhood or well-being in the socio-political and cultural contexts. Since the social constructionist paradigm involves a shift in methodology toward the qualitative approaches, it is important to finally note their potential contribution to the field of disaster mental health research.

It is encouraging for the researchers, who take up multidisciplinary approach to disaster mental health, that ethnography (Abramowitz 2005; Priya 2010, 2012b, 2015; Young 1995), semi-structured interview (Abramowitz 2005; Mehta et al.

2005; Pedersen et al. 2008), case-study (Bracken et al. 1995), and other qualitative methodologies such as the draw-and-tell conversation technique and Word Association Test (Priya 2012b) or documentary analysis (Viswambharan and Priya 2015) have proved to be meaningful methodologies to study survivors' experiences.

Qualitative methodology is an essential ingredient of the social constructionist study of traumatized self in the post-disaster socio-political context as Marsella (1998) pointed out, 'increased use of qualitative research orientations and methods will enhance psychology's knowledge of context, meaning, and power asymmetries' (p. 1287). On the authenticity or rigour of such research endeavours, he posited, 'A compelling feature of the qualitative approach is the increased accuracy it brings to research because it acknowledges the subjective' (p. 1287). The open acknowledgement within qualitative research of 'the interpretive influence of the researcher in arriving at conclusions' (p. 1287) or reflexivity is taken to be a criterion of scientific rigour (Charmaz 2006; Denzin and Lincoln 2011). In Priya (2010, 2014), for example, I have illustrated how my belief in existentialism as philosophy of life helped me empathize with the survivors of Kachchh earthquake. I took up a social constructionist epistemological stand that shaped the process of data collection and I also explicated how the research process was shaped by bio-psycho-social model as the meta-theoretical framework for analysis of data.

References

Abramowitz, S. A. (2005). The poor have become rich, and the rich have become poor: Collective trauma in the Guinean Languette. *Social Science and Medicine, 61,* 2106–2118.

Acharya, N. (2000). Double victims of Latur earthquake. *The Indian Journal of Social Work, 61,* 558–564.

Anderson, T., Lunnen, K. M., & Ogles, B. M. (2010). Putting models and techniques in context. In B. L. Duncan, S. D. Miller, B. E. Wampold, & M. A. Hubble (Eds.), *The heart and soul of change: Delivering what works in therapy* (2nd ed., pp. 143–166). Washington, DC: American Psychological Association.

Banish, S. G., Imel, Z. E., & Wampold, B. E. (2008). The relative efficacy of bona fide psychotherapies for treating post-traumatic stress disorder: A meta-analysis of direct comparisons. *Clinical Psychology Review, 28,* 746–758.

Bracken, P. J., Giller, J. E., & Summerfield, D. (1995). Psychological responses to war and atrocity: The limitations of current concepts. *Social Science and Medicine, 40,* 1073–1082.

Cassell, E. J. (2004). *The nature of suffering and the goals of medicine* (2nd ed.). New York: Oxford.

Cassell, E. J. (2013). *The nature of healing: The modern practice of medicine*. New York: Oxford University Press.

Charmaz, K. (2006). *Constructing grounded theory: A practical guide through qualitative analysis*. Thousand Oaks, CA: Sage.

Cukor, J., Spitalnick, J., Difede, J., Rizzo, A., & Rothbaum, B. O. (2009). Emerging treatments of PTSD. *Clinical Psychology Review, 29,* 715–726.

Das, V., & Kleinman, A. (2002). Introduction. In V. Das, A. Kleinman, M. Lock, M. Ramphele, & P. Reynolds (Eds.), *Remaking a world: Violence, social suffering and recovery* (pp. 1–30). Oxford: New Delhi.

Denzin, N. K., & Lincoln, Y. S. (2011). *The Sage handbook of qualitative research* (4th ed.). Sage: USA.

Gergen, K. J. (1985). The social constructionist movement in modern psychology. *American Psychologist, 40,* 266–275.

Gergen, K. J. (2009). *An invitation to social construction* (2nd ed.). London: Sage.

Han, C. (2004). The work of indebtedness: The traumatic present of late capitalist Chile. *Culture, Medicine and Psychiatry, 28*(2), 169–187.

Hird, S. (2003). Individual wellbeing: A report for the Scottish executive and Scottish neighbourhood statistics. Retrieved from www.scotpho.org.uk/downloads/IndividualWellbeingAug03.doc.

Hubble, M. A., Duncan, B. L., Miller, S. D., & Wampold, B. E. (2010). Introduction. In B. L. Duncan, S. D. Miller, B. E. Wampold, & M. A. Hubble (Eds.), *The heart and soul of change: Delivering what works in therapy* (2nd ed., pp. 23–46). Washington, DC: American Psychological Association.

Kinezler, H. (2008). Debating war-trauma and post-traumatic stress disorder (PTSD) in an interdisciplinary arena. *Social Science and Medicine, 67,* 218–227.

Kirmayer, L. J. (2012). Cultural competence and evidence-based practice in mental health: Epistemic communities and the politics of pluralism. *Social Science and Medicine, 75,* 249–256.

Kleinman, A. (1987). Anthropology and psychiatry: The role of culture in cross-cultural research on illness. *British Journal of Psychiatry, 151,* 447–454.

Kleinman, A. (1988a). *The illness narratives: Suffering, healing and human condition.* New York: Basic Books.

Kleinman, A. (1988b). *Rethinking psychiatry: From cultural category to personal experience.* New York: The Free Press.

Lewis-Fernandez, R., & Kleinman, A. (1994). Culture, personality and psychopathology. *Journal of Abnormal Psychology, 103,* 67–71.

Marsella, A. J. (1998). Toward a "global-community psychology": Meeting the needs of a changing world. *American Psychologist, 53,* 1282–1291.

Marsella, A. J., & Christopher, M. A. (2004). Ethnocultural considerations in disasters: An overview of research, issues, and directions. *Psychiatric Clinics of North America, 24*(4), 521–539.

Mehta, K., Vankar, G., & Patel, V. (2005). Validity of the construct of post-traumatic stress disorder in a low-income country: Interview study of women in Gujarat, India. *British Journal of Psychiatry, 187,* 585–586.

Misra, G. (2010). The cultural construction of self and emotion: Implications for well-being. In Ralf Schwarzer & Peter A. Frensch (Eds.), *Personality, human development, and culture: International perspectives on psychological science* (Vol. 2, pp. 95–112). New York: Psychology Press.

Misra, G., & Gergen, K. J. (1993). On the place of culture in psychological science. *International Journal of Psychology, 28,* 225–243.

Neria, Y., Nandi, A., & Galea, S. (2007). Post-traumatic stress disorder following disasters: A systematic review.*Psychological Medicine,* 1–14. https://doi.org/10.1017/S0033291707001353

Pedersen, D. (2002). Political violence, ethnic conflict, and contemporary wars: Broad implications for health and social well-being. *Social Science and Medicine, 55,* 175–190.

Pedersen, D., Tremblay, J., Errazuriz, C., & Gamarra, J. (2008). The sequelae of political violence: Assessing trauma, suffering and dislocation in the Peruvian highlands. *Social Science and Medicine, 67,* 205–217.

Priya, K. R. (2005). Suffering and healing: A psycho-social study of the survivors of Bhuj earthquake. (Unpublished doctoral dissertation). University of Delhi, Delhi, India.

Priya, K. R. (2007). Healing as facilitated by socio-centric health beliefs: An ethnographic account of the survivors in post-earthquake rural Kachchh. *Eastern Anthropologist, 60*(2), 217–232.

Priya, K. R. (2010). Research relationship as a facilitator of remoralization and self-growth: Postearthquake suffering and healing. *Qualitative Health Research, 20,* 479–495.

Priya, K. R. (2012a). Social constructionist approach to suffering and healing: Juxtaposing Cassell, Gergen and Kleinman. *Psychological Studies, 57,* 211–223.

Priya, K. R. (2012b). Trauma reactions, suffering and healing among riot-affected internally displaced children of Gujarat: A qualitative inquiry. *Qualitative Research in Psychology, 9,* 189–209.

Priya, K. R. (2013a). Suffering and healing. In D. Kenneth Keith (Ed.), *Encyclopedia of cross-cultural psychology*. Malden, MA: Wiley-Blackwell. https://doi.org/10.1002/9781118339893.

Priya, K. R. (2013b). Disaster mental health. In D. Kenneth Keith (Ed.), *Encyclopedia of cross-cultural psychology*. Malden, MA: Wiley-Blackwell. https://doi.org/10.1002/9781118339893.

Priya, K. R. (2013c). Broadening of consciousness: A healing process among the survivors of Kachchh earthquake. *Cornelissen RMM Misra G Varma S Foundations and applications of Indian psychology* (pp. 351–362). New Delhi: Dorling Kindersley.

Priya, K. R. (2015). On the social constructionist approach to traumatized selves in post-disaster settings: State-induced violence in Nandigram, India. Culture, Medicine and Psychiatry. https://doi.org/10.1007/s11013-014-9423-6.

Quosh, C., & Gergen, K. J. (2008). Constructing trauma and its treatment: Knowledge, power and resistance. In K. J. Gergen, T. Sugiman, W. Wagner, & Y. Yamada (Eds.), *Meaning in action: Constructions, narratives, and representations* (pp. 97–111). New York: Springer.

Sampson, E. E. (1993). Identity politics: Challenges to psychology's understanding. *American Psychologist, 48,* 1219–1230.

Sinha, D. (1990). Concept of psycho-social well-being: Western and Indian perspectives. *NIMHANS Journal, 8,* 1–11.

Summerfield, D. (1999). A critique of seven assumptions behind psychological trauma programmes in war-affected areas. *Social Science and Medicine, 48,* 1449–1462.

Summerfield, D., & Hume, F. (1993). War and posttraumatic stress disorder: The question of social context. *Journal of Nervous and Mental Disease, 181,* 522.

Summerfield, D., & Toser, L. (1991). 'Low intensity' war and mental trauma in Nicaragua: A study in a rural community. *Medicine and War, 7,* 84–99.

Viswambharan, A. P., & Priya, K. R. (2015). Documentary analysis as a qualitative methodology to explore disaster mental health: Insights from analyzing a documentary on communal riots. *Qualitative Research*. https://doi.org/10.1177/1468794114567494.

Weiss, M. G., Saraceno, B., Saxena, S., & van Ommeren, M. (2003). Mental health in the aftermath of disasters: Consensus and controversy. *Journal of Nervous and Mental Disease, 191,* 611–615.

WHO (2013). Mental health: A state of wellbeing. Retrieved from http://www.who.int/features/factfiles/mental_health/en/.

Yasan, A., Saka, G., Ozkan, M., & Ertem, M. (2009). Trauma type, gender, and risk of PTSD in a region within an area of conflict. *Journal of Traumatic Stress, 22*(6), 663–666.

Young, Allan. (1995). *The harmony of illusions: Inventing post-traumatic stress disorder*. Princeton, New Jersey: Princeton University Press.

FSC
www.fsc.org
MIX
Papier | Fördert
gute Waldnutzung
FSC® C083411

Kolibri 360 GmbH
Ferdinand-Jühlke-Straße 7
99095 Erfurt, Deutschland
produktsicherheit@kolibri360.de